Conditions in
OCCUPATIONAL THERAPY

Effect on Occupational Performance

SECOND EDITION

Conditions in
OCCUPATIONAL THERAPY

Effect on Occupational Performance

Editors

RUTH A. HANSEN, PhD, FAOTA

Professor, Occupational Therapy Program
Head, Department of Associated Health Professions
Eastern Michigan University
Ypsilanti, Michigan

BEN ATCHISON, PhD, OTR, FAOTA

Associate Professsor and Graduate Coordinator
Department of Occupational Therapy
Western Michigan University
Kalamazoo, Michigan

LIPPINCOTT WILLIAMS & WILKINS
A **Wolters Kluwer** Company
Philadelphia · Baltimore · New York · London
Buenos Aires · Hong Kong · Sydney · Tokyo

Editor: Margaret M. Biblis
Managing Editor: Linda S. Napora
Marketing Manager: Debby Hartman
Production Editor: Karen M. Ruppert

351 West Camden Street
Baltimore, Maryland 21201-2436 USA

Printed in the United States of America

First Edition, 1989

Library of Congress Cataloging-in-Publication Data

Conditions in occupational therapy : effect on occupational performance / editors, Ruth A. Hansen, Ben Atchison.—2nd ed.
    p. cm
  Includes bibliographical references and index.
  ISBN 0-683-30417-8
    1. Occupational therapy. 2. Occupational therapy—Case studies. I. Hansen, Ruth Ann.
  II. Atchison, Ben.

RM735..C66 1999
615.8'515—dc21
                                                         99-049311

To purchase additional copies of this book, call our customer service department at (800) 638-0672 or fax orders to (800) 447-8438. For other book services, including large quantity sales, ask for the Special Sales department.

Canadian customers should call (800) 665-1148, or fax (800) 665-0103. For all other calls originating outside of the United States, please call (410) 528-4223 or fax us at (410) 528-8550.

Visit Lippincott Williams & Wilkins on the Internet: http://www.wwilkins.com or contact our customer service department at custserv@wwilkins.com. Williams & Wilkins customer service representatives are available from 8:30 am to 6:00 pm, EST, Monday through Friday, for telephone access.

PREFACE

Before the first edition of *Conditions in Occupational Therapy: Effect on Occupational Performance* was published, those of us who teach occupational therapy spent considerable time translating information from medical and pathophysiology texts for our conditions courses. Likewise, students struggled to interpret information about diseases and impairments from an occupational therapy perspective. Our purpose in this text is to facilitate both the teaching and the learning of conditions from the occupational therapy point of view. Faculty and students who used the first edition found the text to be useful; we accomplished our goal.

The second edition is organized into chapters that describe the more frequently occurring conditions that cause difficulties in daily-living tasks. All chapters have the same basic structure—etiology, prognosis, and progression of the condition; routine diagnostic tests; and medical management. This information is then synthesized from an occupational performance perspective by answering the question, "How might this condition impinge upon the occupational performance components (sensorimotor, psychosocial, and cognitive) and the occupational performance areas (work, play/leisure, and activities of daily living)?"

To answer this question, the text presents a systematic examination of the potential changes in each performance component and a discussion of the effect on a particular individual's occupational performance through case studies; each chapter has at least one case study. The cases enable the reader to use the information in the chapter to reflect on the ramifications of a specific condition for a specific individual.

This approach helps the reader to learn a thinking process that can be used to determine which occupational therapy services the client might need.

Each chapter provides the author's interpretation of the effects of the condition on occupational performance. This analysis is not absolute. Therapists may disagree about the importance of various disabilities and the secondary changes that might occur.

Conditions in Occupational Therapy: Effect on Occupational Performance—Second Edition provides the general descriptions regarding occupational dysfunction and specific cases as material for discussion and deliberation. In this way, the occupational therapy point of view is developed.

Acknowledgments. We acknowledge and thank our contributing authors. We greatly appreciate their cooperation, openness, and commitment to the process of revising this text. We are grateful to Kristen Rongaus who assisted us in the transcribing and keying of new content for this second edition.

Ben Atchison
Ruth A. Hansen

CONTRIBUTORS

Ben Atchison, PhD, OTR, FAOTA
Associate Professor and Graduate Coordinator
Department of Occupational Therapy
Western Michigan University
Kalamazoo, Michigan

Cynthia D. Batts Shanku, OTR
HCR Manor Care
Grosse Pointe Woods, Michigan

Susan Nassar Bierman, OTR
Occupational therapy Department
McLaren Rehabilitation Center
Flint, Michigan

Gerry E. Conti, OTR
Instructor
Department of Occupational Therapy
Eastern Michigan University
Ypsilanti, Michigan

Nancy Cox, OTR
Clinical Specialist
Occupational Therapy Division
Physical Medicine & Rehabilitation Department
University of Michigan Medical Center
Ann Arbor, Michigan

Virginia Allen Dickie, PhD, OTR, FAOTA
Associate Professor and Program Director
Occupational Therapy Program
Eastern Michigan University
Ypsilanti, Michigan

Diane K. Dirette, PhD., OTR
Assistant Professor
Department of Occupational Therapy
Western Michigan University
Kalamazoo, Michigan

Catherine Heck Edwards, OTR, CCM
Occupational Health Program Manager
Ingham Regional Medical Center
Lansing, Michigan

Joanne P. Estes, MS, OTR/L
Chairperson
Department of Occupational Therapy
Xavier University
Cincinnati, Ohio

Joyce Fraker, MS, OTR
Occupational Therapist
Department of Psychiatry
Ann Arbor VA Medical Center
Ann Arbor, Michigan

Ruth A. Hansen, PhD, FAOTA
Professor, Occupational Therapy Program
Head, Department of Associated Health Professions
Eastern Michigan University
Ypsilanti, Michigan

Jacqueline McKillop, OTR/L
Occupational Therapist
Health South Lewistown Outpatient Center
Lewistown, Pennsylvania

Laura Vincent Miller, MS, OTR
Private Practice
Livonia, Michigan

Janie B. Scott, MA, OTR/L, FAOTA
Private Practice
Columbia, Maryland

Yvonne Russell Teske, PhD, OTR, FAOTA
Associate Professor
Occupational Therapy Program
Shenandoah University
Winchester, Virginia

Mary Steichen Yamamoto, MS, OTR
Private Practice
Ann Arbor, Michigan

Linda York, BS, OTR/L
Instructor
Occupational Therapy Assistant Program
Lourdes College
Sylvania, Ohio

CONTENTS

Preface   v
Contributors   vii

CHAPTER **1**
THINKING LIKE AN OT   1
Ruth A. Hansen and Ben Atchison

CHAPTER **2**
CEREBRAL PALSY   8
Mary Steichen Yamamoto

CHAPTER **3**
PROGRESSIVE DEVELOPMENTAL DISORDERS   22
Janie B. Scott

CHAPTER **4**
MENTAL RETARDATION   42
Linda York

CHAPTER **5**
SCHIZOPHRENIA   54
Yvonne Russell Teske

CHAPTER **6**
MOOD DISORDERS   75
Virginia Allen Dicke

CHAPTER **7**
DEMENTIA   98
Joyce Fraker and Jacqueline McKillop

CHAPTER **8**
CEREBROVASCULAR ACCIDENT   121
Susan Nasser Bierman and Ben Atchison

CHAPTER **9**
CORONARY ARTERY DISEASE   147
Ben Atchison

CHAPTER **10**
TRAUMATIC BRAIN INJURY   165
Gerry E. Conti

CHAPTER **11**
SPINAL CORD INJURY   176
Laura Vincent Miller

CHAPTER **12**
BURNS   205
Nancy Cox

CHAPTER **13**
PROGRESSIVE NEUROLOGICAL DISORDERS   218
Diane K. Dirette

CHAPTER **14**
RHEUMATOID ARTHRITIS   230
Cynthia D. Batts Shanku

CHAPTER **15**
ORTHOPAEDICS   268
Joanne P. Estes

CHAPTER **16**
CHRONIC PAIN   279
Catherine Heck Edwards

CHAPTER **17**
DIABETES   298
Joanne P. Estes

GLOSSARY   311

APPENDIX **I**
*UNIFORM TERMINOLOGY FOR OCCUPATIONAL
THERAPY: THIRD EDITION*   341

APPENDIX **II**
MEDICATIONS   349

INDEX   357

CHAPTER 1

THINKING LIKE AN OT

Ruth A. Hansen and Ben Atchison

It is more important to know what kind of person has the disease than what kind of disease the person has.
—*Sir William Osler*
(*Address at Johns Hopkins University, February 1905*)

Melissa is an occupational therapy student beginning her first level II field work experience. During the first week, she spent most of her time in orientation sessions and observing as her supervising therapist treated patients. Now the time has come for patients to be assigned to her and to take responsibility for initiating treatment. When she receives her first referral, she reads the diagnosis and begins to decide what to do next.

How does a student learn to correlate general information about a diagnosis with the needs of a particular person and identify the problems that require occupational therapy intervention? How does a staff therapist set priorities for problems and decide which require immediate attention? How much problem identification can be done before the therapist actually sees the patient? How does a supervisor know when a student or therapist is doing a "good job" of screening referrals and anticipating the dysfunction that the patient might be experiencing? These are precursors to the actual intervention process and are essential to effective and efficient clinical reasoning, as described by Benamy (1).

The clinical reasoning procedure used by each health care professional is somewhat different. The information that is the main focus of intervention for a speech therapist will differ from that of a psychologist and a nurse. What makes occupational therapy unique among health care professions is that practitioners gather and use information to help people be self-sufficient in their daily activities. Such data gathering and analysis provide the therapist with the foundation for a treatment plan through a prioritized list of anticipated problems or dysfunctions for an individual.

To comprehend the unique aspects of occupational therapy requires an understanding of the core values of the profession as well as the language that is used to communicate information clearly and precisely.

CORE VALUES

The core values of occupational therapy are set forth in the document "Core Values and Attitudes of Occupational Therapy Practice" (2). Seven have been identified: altruism, dignity, equality, freedom, justice, truth, and prudence.

> *Altruism* is the unselfish concern for the welfare of others. This concept is reflected in actions and attitudes of commitment, caring, dedication, responsiveness, and understanding.
> *Dignity* emphasizes the importance of valuing the inherent worth and uniqueness of each

1

person. This value is demonstrated by an attitude of empathy and respect for self and others.

Equality requires that all individuals be perceived as having the same fundamental human rights and opportunities. This value is demonstrated by an attitude of fairness and impartiality.

Freedom allows the individual to exercise choice and to demonstrate independence, initiative, and self-direction.

Justice places value on the upholding of such moral and legal principles as fairness, equity, truthfulness, and objectivity.

Truth requires that we be faithful to facts and reality. Truthfulness or veracity is demonstrated by being accountable, honest, forthright, accurate, and authentic in our attitudes and actions.

Prudence is the ability to govern and discipline oneself through the use of reason. To be prudent is to value judiciousness, discretion, vigilance, moderation, care, and circumspection in the management of one's affairs, to temper extremes, make judgments, and respond on the basis of intelligent reflection and rational thought (2).

These values are the foundation of the belief system that occupational therapists use as a moral guide when making clinical decisions.

LANGUAGE

Although many language systems and mechanisms are available, we will discuss language from two perspectives. First is a philosophical discussion of using person-first language, second is the use of the *American Occupational Therapy Association's Uniform Terminology*, third edition (3).

Person-First Language

In many cases the literature and the media, both popular and professional, describe a person with a given condition as the condition—the arthritic, the C.P. kid, the schizophrenic, the alcoholic, the burn victim, the mentally retarded. All of these terms label people as members of a large group rather than as a unique individual. The use of person-first language requires that the person be identified first and the disease used as a secondary descriptor. For example, a woman, who is a physicist, is active in her church and has arthritis; the fourth grade boy, who is a good speller, loves baseball and has cerebral palsy. The condition does not and should not be the primary identity of any person.

Consider the following: a father is introducing his son to his coworkers. Which of the following is the best introduction:

> "Hey, everyone, this is my retarded son, John."
> "Hey, everyone, this is my son, John, who is retarded and loves soccer and video games."
> "Hey, everyone, this is my son, John. He loves soccer and video games."

Of course, the third is the best choice. Yet it is common when describing a person who has a disability to emphasize the disability first. The consequence is a labeling process. "Although such shorthand language is commonplace in clinics and medical records, it negates the individuality of the person. Each of us is a person, with a variety of traits that can be used to describe aspects of our personality, behavior, and function. To use a disease or condition as the adjective preceding the identifying noun negates the multiple dimensions that make the person a unique individual" (reprinted with permission, 4).

Uniform Terminology, Third Edition

The American Occupational Therapy Association has developed a set of terminology that is intended to describe the domain of concern in the practice of occupational therapy (see Appendix I). The terminology is organized into three domains—performance areas, performance components, and performance contexts. Performance areas are broad categories of human activity that are typically part of daily life. They are activities of daily living, work and productive activities, and play or leisure activities. Performance components are fundamental human abilities that—to varying degrees and in differing combinations—are required for successful engagement in performance areas. These components are sensorimotor, cognitive, psychosocial, and psychological. Performance contexts are situations or factors that influence an individual's engagement in desired or required performance areas. Performance contexts consist of temporal aspects and environmental factors (3). Consider the changes in response to task demand that can occur in each of the performance components and performance areas when the setting, the time of day, and the people in the setting shift. An example of this is the school-age child who, according to a parent, seems to do much better in school-related tasks when practicing at home than in the classroom. Every parent has experienced the child who talks incessantly with mother and father at home but appears speechless when introduced in public. Another example is the person who demonstrates a higher blood pressure reading in the doctor's office than what would be measured in a more comfortable, familiar environment. Every occupational therapy student has experienced the frustration of doing poorly on an examination when they "knew it all so well when studying!"

Each of the three domains has a relationship and influence on the others. The outcome is, of course, the ability to function and engage in occupations. Although at a given time you may focus on performance areas or components, the ultimate concern is whether the individual is able to perform necessary and desired tasks in daily life. For example, a therapist may evaluate a person's attention span, but not in isolation. Attention span is evaluated within the realm of the performance components and performance context of the person—the attention span required to work on an assembly line, to drive a car, to learn a card game, or to conduct a business meeting.

The process of clinical reasoning that is used in this book is based on the *Uniform Terminol-*ogy. Once you know the diagnosis and age of the person, you can use this terminology to examine systematically the deficits that occur in the components, as well as how these particular deficits can and do alter the person's ability to complete tasks in relevant areas of occupational performance. In other instances, you will focus primarily on the performance areas and the contextual factors for the individual, without paying much attention to the underlying deficits in performance areas. Definitions of all terms are provided in the Glossary at the back of the book.

ORGANIZATION AND FRAMEWORK OF THIS TEXT

Whereas the primary purpose of this book is to describe the potential impact of a condition on occupational performance, the descriptions should not be considered prescriptive or exhaustive. It is necessary to understand common facts of these conditions, including etiology, basic pathogenesis, commonly observed signs and symptoms, and precautions. However, it is equally important to recognize that the effects of a condition on occupational well-being will also be dependent on contextual factors such as age, developmental stage, health status, and the physical, social, and cultural environment (5). Rather than viewing an individual as a diagnostic entity or as the sum of biological cells, the condition must be personalized.

The general organization of each chapter is the same. First is a detailed description of the etiology, information about incidence and prevalence, signs and symptoms, course and prognosis, and other information that is usually found in a medical or pathophysiology text. This book is unique because the authors have used these details to generate a description of the various aspects of occupational performance that might be affected. At the end of each chapter is a discussion of at least one case study. Cases provide specific details about how the condition might impinge on the daily functioning of a person. The use of an occupational performance grid (Table 1.1) to

TABLE 1.1 Occupational Performance Profile

I. PERFORMANCE AREAS	II. PERFORMANCE COMPONENTS	III. PERFORMANCE CONTEXTS

A. Activities of Daily Living
  1. Grooming
  2. Oral Hygiene
  3. Bathing/Showering
  4. Toilet Hygiene
  5. Personal Device Care
  6. Dressing
  7. Feeding and Eating
  8. Medication Routine
  9. Health Maintenance
  10. Socialization
  11. Functional Communication
  12. Functional Mobility
  13. Community Mobility
  14. Emergency Response
  15. Sexual Expression
B. Work and Productive Activities
  1. Home Management
    a. Clothing Care
    b. Cleaning
    c. Meal Preparation/
      Cleanup
    d. Shopping
    e. Money Management
    f. Household Maintenance
    g. Safety Procedures
  2. Care of Others
  3. Educational Activities
  4. Vocational Activities
    a. Vocational Exploration
    b. Job Acquisition
    c. Work or Job
      Performance
    d. Retirement Planning
    e. Volunteer Participation
C. Play or Leisure Activities
  1. Play or Leisure Exploration
  2. Play or Leisure Performance
	A. Sensorimotor Component
	  1. Sensory
	    a. Sensory Awareness
	    b. Sensory Processing
	      (1) Tactile
	      (2) Proprioceptive
	      (3) Vestibular
	      (4) Visual
	      (5) Auditory
	      (6) Gustatory
	      (7) Olfactory
	    c. Perceptual Processing
	      (1) Stereognosis
	      (2) Kinesthesia
	      (3) Pain Response
	      (4) Body Scheme
	      (5) Right–Left Discrimination
	      (6) Form Constancy
	      (7) Position in Space
	      (8) Visual–Closure
	      (9) Figure Ground
	      (10) Depth Perception
	      (11) Spatial Relations
	      (12) Topographical Orientation
	  2. Neuromusculoskeletal
	    a. Reflex
	    b. Range of Motion
	    c. Muscle Tone
	    d. Strength
	    e. Endurance
	    f. Postural Control
	    g. Postural Alignment
	    h. Soft Tissue Integrity
	  3. Motor
	    a. Gross Coordination
	    b. Crossing the Midline
	    c. Laterality
	    d. Bilateral Integration
	    e. Motor Control
	    f. Praxis
	    g. Fine Coordination/Dexterity
	    h. Visual–Motor Control
	    i. Oral–Motor Control
		A. Temporal Aspects
		  1. Chronological
		  2. Developmental
		  3. Lifecycle
		  4. Disability Status
		B. Environment
		  1. Physical
		  2. Social
		  3. Cultural

(continued)

TABLE 1.1 Occupational Performance Profile (Continued)

I. PERFORMANCE AREAS	II. PERFORMANCE COMPONENTS	III. PERFORMANCE CONTEXTS

	B. Cognitive Integration and Cognitive Components
	   1. Level of Arousal
	   2. Orientation
	   3. Recognition
	   4. Attention Span
	   5. Initiation of Activity
	   6. Termination of Activity
	   7. Memory
	   8. Sequencing
	   9. Categorization
	  10. Concept Formation
	  11. Spatial Operations
	  12. Problem Solving
	  13. Learning
	  14. Generalization
	C. Psychosocial Skills and Psychological Components
	   1. Psychological
	     a. Values
	     b. Interests
	     c. Self-Concept
	   2. Social
	     a. Role Performance
	     b. Social Conduct
	     c. Interpersonal Skills
	     d. Self-Expression
	   3. Self-Management
	     a. Coping Skills
	     b. Time Management
	   4. Self-Control	

graphically review performance component data and their interaction with performance areas is suggested as a way of detailing the potential impact of the conditions described in this text and any other condition for which an occupational therapist might provide treatment. Each chapter outlines the impact of the condition on occupational performance components and areas. This outline is offered as a vehicle for further discussion, recognizing that the impact of the condition will vary among people.

Occupational therapists have a unique and valuable view of an individual as an occupational being. All of us attach meaning to our lives and the lives of others through the activities and occupations that are part of our daily existence. Occupation, then, means more than just work. It is a much broader concept that refers to human involvement in activities that will result in productive and purposeful outcomes. It also includes leisure, rest, and self-care activities that some may not consider productive and purposeful.

For example, the occupations of a 3-month-old infant include those that could be categorized under the general headings of play or activities of daily living. Activities such as play exploration and performance, feeding, socialization, and functional communication are critical at this age.

The complexity of occupation changes dramatically as the infant progresses toward preschool and school age. It is interesting to observe the rapid addition of new occupational roles and expectations as the child enters school. Many aspects of occupational development are emerging. For example, a 7-year-old child engaging in classroom activities is involved in a type of work. Being on time, turning in assignments that are completed properly, good grooming, and getting along with others are all behaviors that will be important as the child approaches adulthood.

Adults are expected to assume, independently pursue, and maintain all relevant occupations. In general, adults spend the greater portion of their waking hours engaged in some type of work activity. This work may be a job or vocation that is done for pay, organized volunteer activities, or home management. The percentage of time spent in each area is largely determined by the role the individual assumes. In addition, adults spend a portion of their time exploring and performing leisure activities. Activities of daily living, particularly socialization, sexual expression, grooming, and eating are all important for adults.

The basic tenets regarding occupational performance are that these tasks are critical and must be performed by the person or by others to survive. By engaging in various occupations the person develops, learns adaptive mechanisms, and meets individual needs. It is important to understand the influence of culture on adaptation. Cultural influences, such as institutions, rules, values, architectural design, art, history, and language, affect the ways and the extent to which a person uses adaptive mechanisms.

Conversely, illness, trauma, or injury can cause varying degrees of occupational dysfunction. The individual receiving occupational therapy is most often experiencing permanent, long-term changes in the ability to engage in everyday activities. The continuum between health and illness is dynamic. The individual's state of health or illness can be judged by the ability to engage in activities that meet both immediate and long-range needs, and to assume desired roles. Illness or disability is considered in relation to its effects on occupational activities and, therefore, the degree of occupational dysfunction that is experienced.

These precepts are the foundation for the reasoning process described in this book. The combination of these assumptions or beliefs and the occupational performance structure are the frame of reference that provide a unique occupational therapy perspective.

Of course, this book cannot cover every condition that an occupational therapist will encounter in practice. We selected the conditions based on AOTA survey data gathered in the late 1980s and on feedback we received from individuals who read and used the first edition of this textbook. We selected conditions representing the broad range of occupational therapy practice—mental health, physical rehabilitation, geriatrics, and pediatrics.

As an instructional tool, this book provides an opportunity to examine each condition closely. The reader is urged to use the information as a springboard for further study of the conditions included here and the many other conditions that occupational therapists encounter in practice. The analysis of the impact on occupational performance for a particular condition is dynamic, and the identification of the most important areas of dysfunction and, therefore, treatment will vary from practitioner to practitioner. In addition, factors such as secondary health problems, age, gender, family background, and culture contribute greatly to the development of a unique occupational performance profile for each individual served.

The occupational performance approach to the identification of dysfunction described in this book can be used to examine the effects of any condition on a person's daily life. This process will enable the therapist to identify and set a priority for problems in occupational performance, which, in turn, will serve as the foundation for creating an effective plan of intervention.

POINTS FOR REVIEW

1. Give an example of how an occupational therapist could demonstrate each of the seven core values of the profession in his or her daily practice.

2. Find an example in the media in which person-first language was not used to describe a person with a condition. Discuss the impact of this practice.

3. Discuss the reasons for the development and the use of uniform terminology for occupational therapy.

4. Define the term "occupation" and give examples of its meaning for individuals through the lifespan.

5. Describe how culture influences the way a person develops, learns adaptive mechanisms, and meets individual needs.

6. Describe an activity that you could use to observe each of the occupational performance components.

7. Discuss the impact of context on your personal occupational performance.

REFERENCES

1. Benamy BC. Developing Clinical Reasoning Skills. San Antonio, TX: Therapy Skill Builders, 1996.
2. Kanny E. Core values and attitudes of occupational therapy practice. Am J Occup Ther 1993;47: 1085–1086.
3. American Occupational Therapy Association. Uniform Terminology for Occupational Therapy, 3rd ed. Am J Occup Ther 1994;48:1047–1054.
4. Hansen RA. Ethical implications. In: Hinojosa J, Kramer P, eds. Evaluation: Obtaining and Interpreting Data. Bethesda, MD: AOTA, 1998:203.
5. Dunn W, Brown C, McGuigan A. Ecology of human performance: A framework for considering the effect of context. Am J Occup Ther 1994;48(7):595–607.

CHAPTER 2

CEREBRAL PALSY

Mary Steichen Yamamoto

CRITICAL TERMS

Areflexia	Deep tendon reflexes	Hypertonicity (spasticity)
Ataxia	Deformity	Kyphosis
Athetoid	Diplegia	Primitive reflexes
Contracture	Dysarthria	Stretch reflex
Cytomegalovirus (CMV)		

Sigmund Freud in his monograph entitled "Infantile Cerebral Paralysis" points out that a well-known painting entitled "The Lame" by Spanish painter Jusepe Ribera (1588–1656), which depicts a child with infantile hemiplegia, proves that cerebral paralysis existed long before medical investigators began paying attention to it in the mid-1800s (1). Freud's work as a neurologist is not generally well known and at the time that his monograph was published in Vienna in 1897, he was already deep into his work in the area of psychotherapy. However, he was recognized at the time as the prominent authority on the paralyses of children. Today, cerebral paralysis is known as cerebral palsy.

INTRODUCTION

Cerebral palsy is not one specific condition but rather a grouping of clinical syndromes that affect movement, muscle tone, and coordination as a result of an injury or lesion of the immature brain. It is not considered a disease. Cerebral palsy is classified as a static encephalopathy and is sometimes diagnostically referred to as such. Encephalopathy is a term used to describe a generalized disorder of cerebral function, which may be acute or chronic, and progressive or static (2). A child is considered to have cerebral palsy if all of the following characteristics apply:

1. The injury or insult occurs when the brain is still developing. It can occur anytime during the prenatal, perinatal, or postnatal periods. There is some disagreement about the upper age limit for a diagnosis of cerebral palsy during the postnatal period, but it generally ranges from 2 to 5 years of age (3, 4).

2. It is nonprogressive. Once the damage has occurred, there is no further worsening of the child's condition or further damage to the central nervous system. However, the characteristics of the disabilities affecting an individual often change over time.

3. It always involves a disorder in sensorimotor development that is manifested by abnormal postural tone and characteristic patterns of movement. The severity of the impairment ranges from mild to severe.
4. The sensorimotor disorder originates specifically in the brain. The muscles themselves and the nerves connecting them with the spinal cord are normal. Although some cardiac or orthopaedic problems can result in similar postural and movement abnormalities, they are not classified as cerebral palsy.
5. It is a lifelong disability. Unlike some premature babies who demonstrate temporary posture and movement abnormalities during the first year of life, for children with cerebral palsy, these abnormalities persist (5).

ETIOLOGY

Historically, birth asphyxia was considered the major cause of cerebral palsy. When British surgeon William Little first identified cerebral palsy in 1860, he suggested that a major cause was a lack of oxygen during the birth process. In 1897 Sigmund Freud disagreed, suggesting that the disorder might sometimes have roots earlier in life. Freud wrote, "Difficult birth, in certain cases is merely a symptom of deeper effects that influence the development of the fetus" (1). Although Freud made these observations in the late 1800s, it was not until the 1980s that research supported his views (6, 7). Many researchers now believe that prenatal problems may actually cause the obstetric difficulties during the birth of some babies with cerebral palsy (8). A study published by the National Institutes of Health reported that in 75% of reported cases of cerebral palsy, there were no symptoms of asphyxia during labor and delivery (9).

Recent research has focused on maternal infection as a critical risk factor for cerebral palsy, both during prenatal development and at the time of delivery. The infection does not necessarily produce signs of illness in the mother, which can make it difficult to detect. In a study conducted in the mid-1990s, it was determined that mothers with infections at the time of birth had a higher risk of having a child with cerebral palsy. The risk was threefold for infants who were full term and 2.3-fold for infants who were premature or weighed less than 3.3 lb. Another study identified maternal fever during labor and placental infection as highly associated with a diagnosis of cerebral palsy. Seizures and poor oxygenation were also more common among infants born to the mothers with infections (10). There is also evidence that maternal infection in the vagina or uterine cavity before the midpoint of pregnancy increases the risk for both premature labor and fetal brain damage (11). A recent study found that periventricular leukomalacia (PVL), which is a major cause of cerebral palsy in premature infants, is associated with intrauterine infection, particularly during the 27th to 30th weeks of fetal development (12).

A more thorough list of risk factors is found in Table 2.1. Prenatal and perinatal factors are responsible for two-thirds or more of the cases in both premature and full-term infants (4). However, premature infants are at greater risk of perinatal complications because of the physiological immaturity of their organ systems and brain and are at much greater risk for cerebral palsy (4, 8). During the postpartum period, sick neonates are at greater risk for developing complications, especially in the circulatory and pulmonary systems. These complications can lead to brain hypoxia and result in cerebral palsy. Intraventricular–periventricular bleeding and hypoxic infarcts that occur during this period also place the premature infant at increased risk (4).

In the perinatal and infancy period, common causes of cerebral palsy include cerebral vascular accidents, infections such as meningitis or encephalitis, poisoning, trauma such as near-drownings and strangulations, and illnesses such as endocrine disorders (4, 8, 13, 14). Closed head injury that occurs during this period is now classified as traumatic brain injury, even though the

Table 2.1 Cerebral Palsy: Contributing Risk Factors and Causes

Preconception (parental background)
Biological aging (parent or parents older than 35)
Biological immaturity (very young parent or parents)
Environmental toxins
Genetic background and genetic disorders
Malnutrition
Metabolic disorders
Radiation damage

First Trimester of Pregnancy
Endocrine: thyroid function, progesterone
  insufficiency
Nutrition: malnutrition, vitamin deficiencies,
  amino acid intolerance
Toxins: alcohol, drugs, poisons, smoking
Maternal disease: thyrotoxicosis, genetic disorders

Second Trimester of Pregnancy
Infection: cytomegalovirus, rubella, toxoplasma, HIV,
  syphilis, chicken pox, subclinical uterine infections

Placental pathology: vascular occlusion, fetal
  malnutrition, chronic hypoxia, growth factor
  deficiencies

Third Trimester of Pregnancy
Prematurity and low birth weight
Blood factors: Rh incompatibility, jaundice
Cytokines: neurological tissue destruction
Inflammation
Hypoxia: placental insufficiency, perinatal hypoxia
Infection: listeria, meningitis, streptococcus group B,
  septicemia, chorioamnionitis

Perinatal Period and Infancy
Endocrine: hypoglycemia, hypothyroidism
Hypoxia: perinatal hypoxia, respiratory distress
  syndrome
Infection: meningitis, encephalitis
Multiple births: death of a twin or triplet
Stroke: hemorrhagic or embolic stroke
Trauma: abuse, accidents

Adapted from UCP Research and Educational Foundation. Factsheet: Cerebral Palsy: Contributing Factors and Causes.
September, 1995.

resulting impairments are very similar to cerebral palsy (4). The cause remains unknown in 20 to 30% of cases with an early onset of symptoms (4).

INCIDENCE AND PREVALENCE

Estimates of the incidence of cerebral palsy in the United States range from 1.5 to 4 per 1000 live births (2, 4, 15). In 1991, the Centers for Disease Control and Prevention (CDC) conducted a study in which they monitored children ages 3 to 10. The overall rate of cerebral palsy was 2.4 per 1000 children in metropolitan Atlanta. The rate was higher among African-American children (3.1/1000) than among European-American children (2.0/1000) (13). The incidence of cerebral palsy is known to be higher in areas where there is inadequate obstetric and newborn care. It is also higher among very low–birth-weight babies, especially those who sustain injury to the brain's white matter (periventricular hemorrhage or leukomalacia) (15). The United Cerebral Palsy Association estimated in 1997 that 500,000 chil-

dren and adults in the United States show one or more symptoms of cerebral palsy. They estimate that each year, 5000 babies are diagnosed with cerebral palsy. In addition, each year some 1200 to 1500 preschool-age children are diagnosed with cerebral palsy (16).

There has been considerable advancement in obstetric and neonatal care during the past two to three decades. Many hoped these advancements would reduce the incidence of cerebral palsy. Unfortunately, the rate has increased slightly. This is probably a result of increased survival rates of very low–birth-weight and premature infants. Another factor may be the use of fertility treatments by older women that have resulted in an increase in the number of multiple births. Multiple births tend to result in infants who are smaller and premature and are at greater risk for health problems. On the average, they are half the weight of other babies at birth and arrive 7 weeks earlier (17). There is a 400% increase in the probability of cerebral palsy in twin births than in a single birth (17).

SIGNS AND SYMPTOMS

The early signs and symptoms common to all types of cerebral palsy are muscle tone, reflex, and postural abnormalities, delayed motor development, and atypical motor performance (4).

Tone Abnormalities

The tone abnormalities seen include hypertonicity, hypotonicity, and fluctuating tone. Fluctuating tone shifts in varying degrees from hypotonic to hypertonic. Most infants with cerebral palsy initially demonstrate hypotonia. Later the infant may develop hypertonicity, fluctuating tone, or continue to demonstrate hypotonia depending on the type of cerebral palsy.

Reflex Abnormalities

With hypertonicity, reflex abnormalities such as hyperreflexia, clonus, overflow, enhanced stretch reflex, and other signs of upper motor neuron lesions are present (4). Retained primitive infantile reflexes and a delay in the acquisition of righting and equilibrium reactions occur in conjunction with all types of abnormal tone. When hypotonia is present, there may be areflexia, or an absence of primitive reflexes. These reflexes should be present during the first several months of life.

Postural Abnormalities

The presence of primitive reflexes and abnormal tone causes the child to have abnormal positions at rest and to demonstrate stereotypical and uncontrollable postural changes during movement. For instance, a child with hypertonicity in the lower extremities often lies supine with the hips internally rotated and adducted and the ankles plantar flexed. This posture is caused by a combination of high tone in the affected muscles and the presence of the crossed extension reflex. A child with hypotonicity typically lies with the hips abducted, flexed, and externally rotated because of low muscle tone, weakness in the affected muscles, and the influence of gravity.

Delayed Motor Development

Cerebral palsy is always accompanied by a delay in the attainment of motor milestones. One of the signs that often alerts the pediatrician to the problem is a delay in the child's ability to sit independently.

Atypical Motor Performance

The way in which a child moves when performing skilled motor acts is also affected. Depending on the type of cerebral palsy, the child may demonstrate a variety of motor abnormalities such as asymmetrical hand use, unusual crawling method or gait, uncoordinated reach, or difficulty sucking, chewing, and swallowing.

TYPES OF CEREBRAL PALSY

Types of cerebral palsy are classified neurophysiologically or anatomically (18). There are three major neurophysiological types:

1. *Spastic,* which is characterized by hypertonicity and is caused by damage to the motor cortex or to the pyramidal or corticospinal tract (15, 18). This type is the most common and accounts for approximately 60 to 70% of the cases of cerebral palsy (15).
2. *Athetoid or dyskinetic,* which is characterized by involuntary and uncontrolled movements and caused by basal ganglia or extrapyramidal damage or, in some cases, both pyramidal and extrapyramidal damage (15, 18). This type accounts for approximately 20% of the cases of cerebral palsy (15).
3. *Ataxia,* which is characterized by unsteadiness and difficulties with balance, particularly when ambulating, and results from damage to the cerebellum. It is much less common than the other two types, occurring in only about 1 to 10% of the cases of cerebral palsy (15, 19).

There are additional types such as *hypotonic,* in which muscle tone remains hypotonic throughout life. These types are rare. The three major types may occur in combination. Approximately 30% of individuals with cerebral palsy have a combination of spasticity with dyskinesia or ataxia (19).

Spastic

Spastic cerebral palsy is characterized by hypertonicity, retained primitive reflexes in affected areas of the body, and slow, restricted movement. Contractures and deformities are common. It is categorized anatomically by the area of the body that is affected. Spastic hemiplegia, spastic diplegia, and spastic quadriplegia are the most common types.

Spastic Hemiplegia

Spastic hemiplegia involves one entire side of the body, including the head, neck, and trunk. Usually the upper extremity is most affected. Early signs include asymmetrical hand use during the first year or dragging one side of the body when crawling or walking. The initial hypotonic stage is short-lived, with spasticity developing gradually (4, 19). Most children begin walking after 18 months of age, with nearly all children walking by their third birthday (4). When walking, the child typically hyperextends the knee and the ankle in equinovarus or equinovalgus position on the involved side. The child often lacks righting and equilibrium reactions on the involved side and will avoid weightbearing on this side. The shoulder is held in adduction, internal rotation; the elbow is flexed; the forearm is pronated; the wrist is flexed and ulnar deviated; and the hand is often fisted. Spasticity increases during physical activities and emotional excitement. Arm and hand use is limited on the involved side, depending on the severity. The child may use more primitive patterns of grasping and lacks precise and coordinated movement.

In more severe cases, the child may totally neglect the involved side or use it only as an assist during bilateral activities. This is the only type of cerebral palsy where cortical sensory deficit is found and should be suspected when the child neglects the affected arm (20). Parietal lobe damage occurs in about 50% of cases and results in impaired sensation, including astereognosis, loss or lack of kinesthesia, diminished two-point discrimination, decreased graphesthesia, and topagnosia (4).

Spastic Diplegia

Spastic diplegia involves both lower extremities, with mild incoordination, tremors, or less severe spasticity in the upper extremities. It is most often attributed to premature birth and low birth weight and is, therefore, on the rise as more infants born prematurely survive as a result of medical advances. The ability to sit independently can be delayed up to 3 years of age or older because of inadequate hip flexion and extensor and adductor hypertonicity in the legs (21). Frequently the child will rely on the arms for support. The young child will move forward on the floor by pulling along with flexed arms while the legs are stiffly extended. Getting up to a creeping position is difficult because of spasticity in the lower extremities. Similarly, standing posture and gait are affected to varying degrees, depending on severity. Because of a lack of lower extremity equilibrium reactions, excessive trunk and upper extremity compensatory movements are used when walking. Lumbar lordosis, hip flexion and internal rotation (scissoring), plantar flexion of the ankles, and difficulty shifting weight when walking are common. Many of these problems result in contractures and deformities, including dorsal spine kyphosis, lumbar spine lordosis, hip subluxation or dislocation, flexor deformities of hips and knees, and equinovarus or equinovalgus deformity of the feet (21).

Approximately 85% of children with diplegia will walk independently. Another 10 to 15% will be able to walk in the community with the assistance of crutches or a walker (21). Independent walking occurs typically between 3 and 5 years of age in spastic diplegia (22).

Spastic Quadriplegia

With spastic quadriplegia, the entire body is involved. The arms typically demonstrate spasticity in the flexor muscles, with spasticity in the extensor muscles in the lower extremities. Because of the influence of the positive tonic labyrinthine reflex (TLR), shoulder retraction and neck hyperextension are common, particularly in the supine position. This results in difficulty with transitional movements such as rolling or coming up to sitting. In the prone position there is increased flexor tone, also a result of TLR influence, causing difficulty with head raising and weightbearing on the arms. Independent sitting and standing are difficult for the child because of hypertonicity, the presence of primitive reflex involvement, and a lack of righting and equilibrium reactions. Only a small percentage of children with quadriplegia are able to walk independently, and less than 10% ever walk in the community after adolescence (23, 24). Oral musculature is usually affected, with resulting dysarthria, eating difficulties, and drooling. Individuals are susceptible to contractures and deformities, particularly hip dislocation and scoliosis, and must be closely monitored.

Athetosis

Athetosis is the most common type of dyskinesia or dystonia characterized by slow, writhing movements of the face and extremities. These movements often don't begin until 12 months to 3 years of age (20, 25). Head and trunk control is often affected as is the oral musculature, resulting in drooling, dysarthria, and eating difficulties. Whereas spasticity is characterized by hypertonicity in the affected muscle groups and restricted movement, athetosis is characterized by fluctuating tone and excessive movement. Contractures are rare, but hypermobility may be present. More than two-thirds of those with this type of cerebral palsy have IQs above 90, although their movements and speech disorders often erroneously give the impression of mental retardation (MR) (18).

In the mixed type of cerebral palsy, two different patterns occur together as a result of the diffuse brain damage. The most frequent mixed type is spastic–athetoid. Persons with this type have signs of athetosis, and fluctuating postural tone fluctuates from hypertonicity to hypotonia.

ASSOCIATED DISORDERS

There are a number of disorders associated with cerebral palsy, in addition to the motor impairment that can significantly affect functional abilities.

Mental Retardation

Estimates of the incidence of MR with cerebral palsy range from 40 to 70% (3, 15). It occurs most often and most severely in spastic quadriplegia and mixed types (19). It is seen less often in spastic diplegia and hemiplegia; when it does occur, it is usually less severe (3, 15, 19).

Seizure Disorder

Reports of the incidence of seizures in people with cerebral palsy range from 25 to 60% (3, 15, 19). The incidence varies across the diagnostic categories. It is most common in spastic hemiplegia and quadriplegia, and rare with spastic diplegia and dyskinesia (3, 15, 19). All clinical types of seizures are reported, with grand mal being the most common (15).

Visual and Hearing Impairments

Visual and hearing impairments occur at a higher rate with cerebral palsy than in the general population. Strabismus is the most common visual defect, occurring in 20 to 60% of children with cerebral palsy, with the highest rates in spastic diplegia and quadriplegia (3, 25). Other visual and ocular abnormalities include nystagmus, homonymous hemianopsia associated with spastic hemiplegia, and difficulties with visual fixation and tracking (3, 14). Some children with athetosis have paralysis of upward gaze, which is a clinical manifestation of kernicterus. Hearing impairments include sensorineural hearing loss, present in approximately 12% of individuals with cerebral palsy. There is a four times greater prevalence in athetosis than in spasticity (3). Conductive hearing losses, caused by persistent fluid in the ears and middle ear infections, occur when there is severe motor involvement in children who spend a lot of time lying down (15).

COURSE AND PROGNOSIS

The course of cerebral palsy varies depending on type, severity, and the presence of associated problems. With mild motor involvement, the child will continue to make motor gains and compensate for motor difficulties. With more severe forms, little progress may be made in attaining developmental milestones and performing functional tasks. As the child grows older, secondary problems such as contractures and deformities will become more common, especially with spasticity. The lifespan for most persons with cerebral palsy is within the average range (15).

DIAGNOSIS

No definitive test will diagnose cerebral palsy. Several factors must be considered. Physical evidence includes a history of delayed achievement of motor milestones. Delayed motor development can occur with MR and other developmental disabilities. The quality of movement is the factor that helps provide a differential diagnosis. The findings of atypical or stereotypical movement patterns and the presence of infantile reflexes and abnormal muscle tone point toward a diagnosis of cerebral palsy. However, other causes must be ruled out, such as progressive neurological disorders, mucopolysaccharidosis, muscular dystrophy, and a spinal cord tumor. Many of these disorders

can be ruled out by laboratory tests, although some must be differentiated by clinical or pathological criteria. A baseline EEG, CT scan, or MRI can be used to help determine the location and extent of structural lesions and can be helpful when the diagnosis is unclear.

Cerebral palsy often is not evident during the first few months of life and is rarely diagnosed that early. Most cases, however, are detected by 12 months and nearly all by 18 months (15). In some cases early postural and tonal abnormalities in premature infants can resemble cerebral palsy, but the signs are transient with normal subsequent development.

MEDICAL/SURGICAL MANAGEMENT

Because of the complexity and diversity of difficulties affecting the individual with cerebral palsy, medical management requires a team approach using the skills of many professionals. Depending on the type of cerebral palsy and the presence of associated problems, team members typically include an occupational therapist, physical therapist, speech pathologist, educational psychologist, nurse, and social worker. The emphasis of intervention is usually on helping the child gain as much motor control as possible; positioning the child to minimize the effects of abnormal muscle tone; instructing the parents and caregivers on handling techniques and ways to accomplish various activities of daily living; recommending adaptive equipment and assistive technology to increase the child's ability to perform desired activities; providing methods to improve feeding and speech if difficulties are present; and helping parents manage behavioral concerns and family stresses.

The primary physician treats the usual childhood disorders and helps with prevention of many health problems. Physicians with various medical specialties may receive a referral. The usual specialists include a neurologist to assess neurological status and help control seizures if present, an orthopaedist to prescribe orthotic devices and any necessary surgeries, and an ophthalmologist to assess and treat any visual difficulties.

Medical management includes both surgical and nonsurgical approaches, with most of the focus on nonsurgical management. Pharmacological agents such as dantrolene (Dantrium) and baclofen are used to reduce spasticity (3, 15) with limited clinical success. A drawback in the use of both these medications is their tranquilizing effect. More recently, a technique in which a pump is implanted under the skin of the abdomen to administer baclofen has been used to reduce undesirable side effects. However, clinical effectiveness in cerebral palsy has not yet been established, and it cannot be used for children under age 12 (26). Sometimes a local anesthetic, phenol, or alcohol solution is injected into the muscles in the region of the myoneural junction, resulting in a temporary decrease in tone, which can last several months (3, 22). Antiseizure medications are also prescribed.

Orthotics and splinting are used to improve function and prevent contractures and deformities. Resting or night splints are used to maintain range of motion. Soft splints, dynamic splints, and those allowing movement of the fingers and thumb are used during waking hours and functional activities to reduce tone and promote more typical patterns of movement.

Orthoses prescribed include ankle–foot orthosis (AFO) for children with hemiplegia to reduce spastic equinus positioning with supination or, occasionally, pronation of the foot. Children with bilateral spasticity who are ambulatory generally do not require or benefit from extensive bracing. However, AFOs are often used to improve abnormal alignment of the feet when the child pulls to stand and begins walking (3). Supramalleolar orthoses (SMO) are used when plantar flexor spasticity is mild and mediolateral malalignment is the main concern (3).

Inhibitory and progressive casting has gained acceptance as an alternative to bracing in recent years (27, 28). A molded footplate is constructed that inhibits the primitive reflexes, thus reducing spasticity. The footplate is surrounded by a snug bivalve below the knee cast. Inhibitory and progressive casting also is used with the upper extremities.

Surgical approaches are used to improve the function and appearance of affected areas of the body and to prevent or correct deformities. Tendon lengthening to increase range of motion and tendon transfers to decrease spastic muscle imbalances are done. These procedures, commonly used on the lower extremities, are performed more selectively in the upper extremities. Selective posterior rhizotomy is a neurosurgical technique that is used to reduce spasticity and improve function in carefully selected individuals (29–31). The procedure involves dividing the lumbosacral posterior nerve root into four to seven rootlets. Each rootlet is stimulated electrically. The dorsal rootlets causing spasticity are cut, leaving the normal rootlets intact. This approach is highly successful for individuals who meet the selection criteria (29–31). The most likely candidates are children with either severe quadriplegia, severe spasticity, or diplegia, or those with mild quadriplegia.

Other surgical procedures include hip reconstruction for hip dislocation and spinal fusion to correct severe scoliosis. These surgeries are most often performed on children with severe quadriplegia. Although there are proponents of surgical intervention, some parents and physicians question whether the results are significant enough to warrant subjecting individuals to the risks of a surgery (27).

IMPACT ON OCCUPATIONAL PERFORMANCE

Virtually all areas of occupational performance and each of the performance components can be affected by cerebral palsy (Table 2.2). The extent to which the occupational performance areas are affected will depend in part on the severity of the disability and on the presence of associated disorders. In all individuals with cerebral palsy, the

TABLE 2.2 Occupational Performance Profile

I. PERFORMANCE AREAS	II. PERFORMANCE COMPONENTS	III. PERFORMANCE CONTEXTS

I. PERFORMANCE AREAS

A. Activities of Daily Living
  1. Grooming
  2. Oral Hygiene
  3. Bathing/Showering
  4. Toilet Hygiene
  5. Personal Device Care
  6. Dressing
  7. Feeding and Eating
  8. Medication Routine
  9. Health Maintenance
  10. Socialization
  11. Functional Communication
  12. Functional Mobility
  13. Community Mobility
  14. Emergency Response
  15. Sexual Expression
B. Work and Productive Activities
  1. Home Management
    a. Clothing Care
    b. Cleaning
    c. Meal Preparation/Cleanup
    d. Shopping
    e. Money Management
    f. Household Maintenance
    g. Safety Procedures
  2. Care of Others
  3. Educational Activities
  4. Vocational Activities
    a. Vocational Exploration
    b. Job Acquisition
    c. Work or Job
      Performance
    d. Retirement Planning
    e. Volunteer Participation
C. Play or Leisure Activities
  1. Play or Leisure Exploration
  2. Play or Leisure Performance

II. PERFORMANCE COMPONENTS

A. Sensorimotor Component
  1. Sensory
    a. Sensory Awareness
    b. Sensory Processing
      (1) Tactile
      (2) Proprioceptive
      (3) Vestibular
      (4) Visual
      (5) Auditory
      (6) Gustatory
      (7) Olfactory
    c. Perceptual Processing
      (1) Stereognosis
      (2) Kinesthesia
      (3) Pain Response
      (4) Body Scheme
      (5) Right–Left Discrimination
      (6) Form Constancy
      (7) Position in Space
      (8) Visual–Closure
      (9) Figure Ground
      (10) Depth Perception
      (11) Spatial Relations
      (12) Topographical Orientation
  2. Neuromusculoskeletal
    a. Reflex
    b. Range of Motion
    c. Muscle Tone
    d. Strength
    e. Endurance
    f. Postural Control
    g. Postural Alignment
    h. Soft Tissue Integrity
  3. Motor
    a. Gross Coordination
    b. Crossing the Midline
    c. Laterality
    d. Bilateral Integration
    e. Motor Control
    f. Praxis
    g. Fine Coordination/Dexterity
    h. Visual–Motor Control
    i. Oral–Motor Control

III. PERFORMANCE CONTEXTS

A. Temporal Aspects
  1. Chronological
  2. Developmental
  3. Lifecycle
  4. Disability Status
B. Environment
  1. Physical
  2. Social
  3. Cultural

(continued)

TABLE 2.2 Occupational Performance Profile (Continued)

I. PERFORMANCE AREAS	II. PERFORMANCE COMPONENTS	III. PERFORMANCE CONTEXTS
	B. Cognitive Integration and Cognitive Components	
	1. Level of Arousal	
	2. Orientation	
	3. Recognition	
	4. Attention Span	
	5. Initiation of Activity	
	6. Termination of Activity	
	7. Memory	**All Performance Components and Performance Areas affected**
	8. Sequencing	
	9. Categorization	
	10. Concept Formation	
	11. Spatial Operations	
	12. Problem Solving	
	13. Learning	
	14. Generalization	
	C. Psychosocial Skills and Psychological Components	
	1. Psychological	
	a. Values	
	b. Interests	
	c. Self-Concept	
	2. Social	
	a. Role Performance	
	b. Social Conduct	
	c. Interpersonal Skills	
	d. Self-Expression	
	3. Self-Management	
	a. Coping Skills	
	b. Time Management	
	c. Self-Control	

sensorimotor components, in particular the neuromusculoskeletal and motor components, affect occupational performance. Sensory components also may be involved if there is an associated vision or hearing impairment, or if there are difficulties with sensory or perceptual processing. The involvement of cognitive components will be determined primarily by whether the individual also has MR. In some individuals with cerebral palsy, level of arousal and attention span also may be affected. Psychosocial skills and psychological components least often have an impact on occupational performance. However, the difficulties involved in coping with the disabling effects and chronic nature of cerebral palsy can result in psychological and social problems.

CASE STUDIES

CASE 1

L. N. is a 64-year-old woman with cerebral palsy, spastic quadriplegic type. She has lived alone in an apartment complex for the elderly and disabled for the past 15 years. Before then, she was in a nursing home. She supports herself on supplemental security income (SSI) and disability payments from the state. A personal-care attendant provided by the Department of Social Services comes in each morning and evening to help her with activities of daily living, such as meal preparation, bathing, and dressing. L. N. has never been employed, but has done volunteer work. She writes articles for a local newsletter on her computer and has worked in her church's Sunday school. She has no family support but has many friends. She enjoys learning and taking classes and is currently enrolled in classes at a local community college.

In considering the occupational performance profile for L. N., temporal aspects of performance context include the life cycle stage of retirement and the lifelong nature and severity of her disability. Environmental performance contexts include no available family support and wheelchair accessibility of her home, school, church, and community.

Affected occupational performance components include neuromuscular, skeletal, and motor components in the sensorimotor area. Spasticity, fluctuating tone, and primitive reflexes severely restrict L. N.'s purposeful movement. She has limited range of motion in her left upper extremity and both lower extremities. When reaching with the left arm, she cannot bring it to shoulder height or behind her back. She has a gross grasp in her right upper extremity and can grasp a joystick to operate her electric wheelchair. She cannot write or perform other activities requiring fine motor dexterity. Her left upper extremity is used as an assist for bilateral activities, with no grasping ability present. She can maintain an upright position in sitting, but her weight is shifted to the left (with resulting scoliosis). She can bring her head to an upright position, but neck flexion increases with activities requiring effort. Oral–motor muscles are affected, resulting in severe dysarthria, drooling, and difficulty eating. Endurance is a problem, and L. N. becomes easily fatigued.

The self-management component in the psychosocial and psychological area is also affecting occupational performance. L. N. is having difficulty with coping skills and self-control. She went through depressive episodes when her father and mother died several years ago. She was treated for depression by a psychiatrist who prescribed Haldol. These episodes continue, but are not as severe. L. N. becomes frustrated when unable to communicate her needs to others. At times, this leads to an emotional outburst.

All occupational performance areas are affected. In the work and productive activities category, L. N. is a student at a local community college. She uses a tape recorder to take notes and takes examinations verbally. In home management, L. N. is dependent in clothing care, cleaning her apartment, household maintenance, and meal preparation. She can use a hand-held portable vacuum cleaner for small cleanups. She has a cat that she cares for. She shops independently, but needs assistance getting money out of her wallet at the cash register.

In the leisure area, L. N. has varied interests. She is an avid reader and enjoys computer games. She socializes with friends frequently and enjoys going out into the community. She participates in church retreats and field trips through an independent living center.

All areas of activities of daily living are affected except socialization. L. N. is dependent in grooming, bathing/showering, toilet hygiene, and dressing. She brushes her teeth and can transfer on and off the toilet in her apartment with grab bars and the toilet seat at the proper height and position. She can feed herself with her fingers if the food is set up for her, but the process is slow and messy. She drinks from a straw. She takes her own medications if they are set out for her.

In functional communication, L. N. uses a computer for written communication. She uses a speaker phone for telephone communication and can use a tape machine if it is set up for her. If she falls or is in danger at home, she has an emergency alert system that she can activate. Her speech is difficult to understand. She has a Canon communicator but prefers not to use it.

In functional mobility, L. N. can transfer herself between her wheelchair and her bed. She needs assistance transferring to the shower seat she uses for bathing. She uses a motorized wheelchair for mobility. In the community, L. N. uses public transportation with no difficulty. She has some difficulty transferring herself to and from the toilet when using public restrooms, which sometimes results in incontinence.

CASE 2

A. K. is a 4-year-old girl with a diagnosis of cerebral palsy, hypotonic type. She was the product of a full-term pregnancy with no complications. A. K. was born by spontaneous vaginal delivery after an unremarkable 2-hour labor. Her birth weight was 7 lb. Apgar scores were 8 and 9 at 1-minute and 5-minute intervals, respectively. She breathed and cried immediately after birth. A. K. was born with a cephalohematoma, which disappeared 2 to 3 weeks after birth.

A. K.'s mother first became concerned about her development when she was not rolling from supine to prone until nearly 8 months of age. She did not crawl until 18 months and walked independently at 2 1/2 years of age. At 15 months, A. K. was evaluated by a neurologist. He diagnosed a mild cerebral palsy resulting from anomalous development occurring during the first trimester. An MRI was performed and the results were essentially normal. Physical examination included slightly hypotonic muscle tone, lack of protective reactions, inaccurate reaching, and a palmar grasp of objects. The parents sought a second opinion 1 year later that confirmed the initial diagnosis, with the type of cerebral palsy labeled hypotonic. A T-4 and urine metabolic screenings were conducted at that time with normal results. Genetic testing was also completed, which ruled out any genetic syndromes.

A. K. lives with her parents and two older brothers. She recently moved to Michigan from Florida where she received early intervention services. She is currently a student in a special education preschool classroom where she received occupational, physical, and speech therapy services.

A. K. loves music, books, and videos. Family activities she enjoys include going for walks and riding bikes with her mother, swimming, playing with her brothers, and going to their sporting events. A. K. has a good sense of humor and looks forward to going to school each day. Her favorite school activities include music movement group and computer activities using a touch window screen.

In considering the occupational performance profile for A. K., temporal aspects of performance contexts include her age, developmental level, and disability status. Because she has a disability that impacts her development, she has been enrolled in a preschool program for students with special needs to help her reach her maximum potential. Environmental contexts include a supportive family and parents. They have hopes that she will catch up developmentally with other children her age and that she will have every opportunity to reach her "full potential."

In the sensorimotor area, sensory integration, neuromuscular, and motor components are affected. The sensory integration component includes tactile defensiveness as evidenced by A. K. pulling away when touched on the upper extremities and hands. Neuromuscular components include hypermobility in the joints throughout her body. Muscle tone is mildly hypotonic. Remnants of the tonic labyrinthine reflex limit her ability to assume antigravity postures. She has decreased static and dynamic balance reactions. Motor components include decreased gross motor coordination, fine motor coordination and dexterity, decreased motor control, and poor visual motor integration. Oral–motor control affects the intelligibility of A. K.'s speech and difficulties with drooling.

In the cognitive component, she has a limited attention span. A. K. requires much repetition to acquire new concepts and behaviors, and she sometimes has difficulty sequencing tasks.

In the psychosocial skill and psychological components, A. K. has difficulty with social conduct. She usually expresses excitement by hugging herself, but is beginning to use her communication board or to verbally express her excitement.

Activities of daily living must be considered within the performance context of her age. At age 4, children are still dependent on their parents for assistance with many self-maintenance tasks and would not be expected to be independent. Given this, A. K.'s affected activities of daily living include grooming, oral hygiene, toilet hygiene, dressing, feeding and eating, and functional communication. A. K. is not yet assisting with toothbrushing. She needs prompting to remember the sequence for handwashing. She is working on toilet training and needs physical and verbal assistance when pulling her pants up. She requires full assistance with clothing fasteners. She feeds herself with a spoon, with some spilling, and is not yet using a fork. She uses a communication board and some sign language for functional communication.

A. K.'s work and productive activities are in the educational area. Sensorimotor components influencing educational performance include difficulty assuming a floor sitting position during circle time activities. Attention is limited for many classroom tasks. She can make single snips using regular scissors but needs adaptive scissors to cut using forward progression. She needs assistance positioning the scissors in her hand. A tripod grasp of writing utensils is emerging. She has difficulty manipulating puzzle pieces to complete a simple puzzle. Cognitive components include limited attention span for classroom activities and difficulty following two-step commands. In the social area, A. K. is working on expressing excitement in more socially acceptable ways.

In the play/leisure occupational performance area, A. K. is beginning to participate in parallel play. She is unable to climb on raised playground equipment such as slides or climbers without assistance. She has difficulty with ball skills such as throwing and catching.

POINTS FOR REVIEW

1. Who was the first person to be recognized as an authority on cerebral palsy?

2. What are the five characteristics that determine the presence of cerebral palsy?

3. What are the contemporary ideas about the cause of cerebral palsy, and what are some of the risk factors associated with cerebral palsy?

4. Discuss the reasons for the slight increase in the incidence of cerebral palsy?

5. What are the three major types of cerebral palsy? Which is most common?

6. Describe motor impairment of spasticity, dyskinesia, and ataxia.

7. How effective is the use of medications to reduce spasticity in persons with cerebral palsy, and what other medical approaches are used in treatment of cerebral palsy?

8. Describe surgical procedures used to treat orthopaedic problems of persons with cerebral palsy.

9. Discuss the impact of cerebral palsy on occupational performance. Which components are more involved?

REFERENCES

1. Freud S. Infantile Cerebral Paralysis. Coral Gables: University of Miami Press, 1968.

2. Behrman R, Kliegman R, Arvin A, eds. Nelson W, senior ed. Nelson's Textbook of Pediatrics. 15th ed. Philadelphia: WB Saunders, 1996.

3. Molnar G, ed. Pediatric Rehabilitation. 2nd ed. Baltimore: Williams & Wilkins, 1992.

4. UCP Research and Educational Foundation. Factsheet: Cerebral Palsy: Contributing Risk Factors and Causes. September, 1995.

5. Little W. On the influence of abnormal parturition, difficult labor, premature birth and physical condition of the child, especially in relation to deformities. Trans Obstet Soc 1862;3:293.

6. Freeman J, Nelson K. Intrapartum asphyxia and cerebral palsy. Pediatrics 1988;82:240–249.

7. Illingsworth R. A pediatrician asks—Why is it called a birth injury? Br J Med Obstet Gynecol 1985;92: 122–30.

8. Brody J. Research sheds new light on causes of cerebral palsy. In: The Ann Arbor News, December 28, 1989:D3.

9. Researchers find asphyxia not responsible for most CP. OT. Week, September 22, 1988:2.

10. Grether J, Nelson K. Maternal infection and cerebral palsy in infants of normal birth weight. JAMA 1997;278:3.

11. UCP Research and Education Foundation. Factsheet: Some Thoughts on the Prevention of Cerebral Palsy. January, 1997.

12. Zupan V, Gonzalez P, Lacaze-Masmonteil T, et al. Periventricular leukomalacia: risk factors revisited. Dev Med Child Neurol 1996;38:12.

13. Marmer L. ACDC tracks disability in kids aged 3 to 10. In: Advance for Occupational Therapists. King of Prussia, PA: Merion Publications, Inc., 1997.

14. Lefkofsky S. Introduction to Cerebral Palsy. Detroit: Wayne State University School of Medicine, 1973.

15. Blackman J. Medical Aspects of Developmental Disabilities in Children Birth to Three. 3rd ed. Iowa City: The University of Iowa, 1997.

16. UCP-Research and Educational Foundation. Fact Sheet: Cerebral Palsy—Facts and Figures. United Cerebral Palsy, 1997.

17. Multiple Births and Developmental Brain Damage. UCP Research and Educational Foundation. May, 1997.

18. Avery ME, First LR, eds. Pediatric Medicine. Baltimore: Williams & Wilkins, 1989:1298.

19. Berkow R, Fletcher A, eds. The Merck Manual of Diagnosis and Therapy. 16th ed. Rahway: Merck Sharp & Dohme Research Laboratories, 1992:2263.

20. Crother B, Paine R. The Natural History of Cerebral Palsy. Cambridge: Harvard Press, 1959.

21. Bobath K. A Neurological Basis for the Treatment of Cerebral Palsy. Philadelphia: JB Lippincott, 1980.

22. Koop S. Orthopedic aspects of static encephalopathies. In: Miller G, Ramer J, eds. Static Encephalopathies of Infancy and Childhood. New York: Raven Press, Ltd., 1992.

23. Bleck E. Locomotor prognosis in cerebral palsy. Dev Med Child Neurol 1975;17:18–25.

24. Russman B, Gage J. Cerebral palsy. Curr Probl Pediatr 1989;19:65–111.

25. Hiles D, Wallar P, McFarlane F. Current concepts in the management of strabismus in children with cerebral palsy. Ann Ophthalmol 1975;7:789.

26. United Cerebral Palsy Research and Educational Foundation. Factsheet: Baclofen and the Baclofen Pump. April, 1994.

27. Cusick B. Progressive Casting and Splinting for Lower Extremity Deformities in Children with Neuromuscular Dysfunction. Tucson: Therapy Skill Builders, 1990.

28. Hanson C, Jones L. Gait abnormalities and inhibitive casts in cerebral palsy: literature review. J Pediatr Med Assoc 1989;79:53–59.

29. Staudt L, Peacock W. Selective posterior rhizotomy for treatment of spastic cerebral palsy. In: Pediatric Physical Therapy. Baltimore: Williams & Wilkins, 1989.

30. Berman B, Vaughan C, Peacock C, et al. The effect of rhizotomy on movement in patients with cerebral palsy. Am J Occup Ther 1990;44:6.

31. Kinghorn J. Upper extremity functional changes following selective posterior rhizotomy in children with cerebral palsy. Am J Occup Ther 1992;46:6.

SUGGESTED READINGS

Fraser B, Hensinger R, Phelps J. Physical Management of Multiple Handicaps. A Professional's Guide. 2nd ed. Baltimore: Brookes Publishing, 1990. Valuable reference for those working with children and adults with severe physical or multiple impairments. *Contains chapters on physical management and treatment; seating systems; therapeutic positioning and adaptive equipment; and activities of daily living.*

Kurtz L, Dowrick P, Levy S, et al. Handbook of Developmental Disabilities: Resources for Interdisciplinary Care. Gaithersburg, MD: Aspen Publishers, 1996. Comprehensive reference book. *Includes interdisciplinary evaluation, management, and treatment issues. Helpful discussion on medical/surgical issues, most of which apply to individuals with cerebral palsy.*

Levitt S. Treatment of Cerebral Palsy and Motor Delay. 3rd ed. Oxford, England: Blackwell Science LTP, 1995. *Good discussion of treatment approaches, principles of treatment, and description of procedures.*

Morris S, Klein M. Pre-Feeding Skills. Tuscon: Therapy Skill Builders, 1987. *Excellent reference for oral–motor and feeding therapy for children. Very thorough and good overall approach to feeding issues.*

CHAPTER 3

PERVASIVE DEVELOPMENTAL DISORDERS

Janie B. Scott

CRITICAL TERMS

Asperger's disorder
Autistic disorder
Childhood disintegrative
  disorder
Echolalia

Gene
Macrocephaly
Pervasive developmental
  disorder-not otherwise
  specified

Psychotropic
Rett's disorder

INTRODUCTION

Pervasive developmental disorders (PDD) are organized by the *Diagnostic and Statistical Manual of Mental Disorders, Fourth Edition* (DSM-IV) under the broad category of "communication disorder, not otherwise specified" (1). The conditions included under this broad category are: autistic disorder, Rett's disorder, childhood disintegrative disorder, Asperger's disorder, and pervasive developmental disorder-not otherwise specified (PDD-NOS) (including atypical autism). This chapter contains a discussion of all these conditions.

Temple Grandin is recognized throughout the world for her expertise with animals and for designing machinery that allows more humane handling of animals. She also is the author of articles and books about her experiences as a person with autism. Grandin lectures internationally about the needs of animals and about autism.

During infancy, Grandin's tactile defensiveness was so intense that she would claw violently to protect herself from being touched. She discusses her auditory sensitivity, especially to particular frequencies of sound. She attempted to compensate for this by blocking out many sounds (including language). She had not begun to speak by the age of 3. Her mother placed her in a nursery school that was sensitive to the needs of speech-handicapped children. Grandin began to develop speech between the ages of 4 and 5. After nursery school, she received special education services that varied in frequency and intensity.

Grandin recalls her feelings of social isolation during her adolescence. She had difficulty relating to peers both in groups and individually. Grandin described puberty as a difficult time because of the heightened arousal produced by this period of life. She had a greater sense of fear, partially from the increased emotional intensity. Antidepressants helped her cope with this state of heightened arousal and anxiety. When Grandin became perimenopausal, the symptoms she experienced in puberty resurfaced. She found some relief by taking estrogen.

During adolescence, Grandin went to visit a family member's farm. There she watched cows proceeding through a chute. It was here that she got the idea for her "squeeze machine." She designed this machine, similar to the cattle chute, to provide herself with controlled tactile and proprioceptive sensory input.

Grandin's IQ is reported to be 137. She earned a degree in psychology and a Ph.D. in animal science. In her book, *Thinking in Pictures and Other Reports from My Life with Autism* (2, 3), Grandin stated that she understands the pain and anxiety experienced by animals and develops equipment that makes more humane handling possible. Grandin describes thinking and seeing things in pictures. When communicating with the outside world, she had to translate from her picture-oriented thinking into words.

The communication problems she has experienced contributed to her philosophy on marriage. When people with autism marry each other, or when an autistic person marries another person with a disability or eccentricity, both individuals are more in tune and responsive to their mate's special needs. Communication may be less demanding. Grandin remains unmarried and admits to difficulties in interpersonal relationships. Close relationships require a degree of spontaneity that is challenging for a person with autism or other PDD.

Grandin spoke of other business and interpersonal relationships. Her difficulties understanding subtle social cues and conventions have made succeeding in business and friendships more challenging. Her vulnerability compounds her difficulty in living successfully and actively in the community. She usually cannot detect when others are lying or trying to take advantage of her. Understanding complex interpersonal communications is not nearly as easy or natural as thinking in pictures or understanding the needs and feelings of animals. She says that if she were diagnosed today, her condition would be labeled as Asperger's syndrome.

ETIOLOGY

The first mention of any of the PDDs probably occurred in folklore and literature in tales of witches and others with special abilities and powers. Some cultures cared for their "special people," whereas other cultures shunned them.

At one time, autism was thought to be an infantile form of schizophrenia. Years of study have separated it from early-onset of schizophrenia or psychosis. Differences have been noted in the development of social, communication, and play behaviors of these children. Kanner, a psychiatrist at the Johns Hopkins Henry Phipps Psychiatric Clinic in Baltimore, officially identified autism in 1943. His contact with young children with psychiatric dysfunction led him to the identification of this disorder. The children's symptoms were poor communication, poor socialization, and bizarre and repetitive behaviors. Almost simultaneously, Asperger was studying children with identical symptoms. The term "autistic" comes from the Greek word "autos," meaning "self."

Many theorists attempted to explain the bizarre and asocial symptoms of young children with autism. Over the years, the diagnosis and treatment of autism have changed as the field of psychiatry has changed. When autism was first identified, psychoanalytic treatment was the preferred method of treatment. Children were separated from the alleged cause—the family. In psychoanalytic theory, the mother was considered the cause of the child's unusual behavior. In the 1970s and 1980s, more emphasis was placed on behavior modification. Theorists looked for causal factors within the social environment.

Genetic

Familial

The most prominent current theory is that a genetic defect or defects cause PDD. Some speculate that the defects may be caused by infection. The genetic/neurological link is strongly supported, in part because sensory and attention deficits are thought to be neurologically based as well. Studies that focused on the incidence of these symptoms among twins also suggested a genetic link.

The notion of genetic links has been discussed for many years. Specific genes have not been identified, nor are there any data on how the conditions are transmitted genetically. Researchers continue to study families in which one or more members have PDD. Some studies are initiated when a child is diagnosed with autism. The researchers focus on whether the parents demonstrate some of the same communication deficits and behavior patterns manifested by individuals with autism. Researchers know that there is a genetic base for PDD. Preliminary data from multigeneration studies have identified "autistic-like" symptoms among nondiagnosed family members. Some family members display mildly autistic or more deviant behaviors than would be expected in the general population.

Developmental

Other researchers believe that PDD is a developmental condition with prenatal origins. These conditions are usually evident by the time the child is 3 years old. So far, no specific structural deficits in the development of the brain have been identified as causal factors for the existence of PDDs.

Kallen, speaking for the medical committee of the Autism Society of America, Inc. (4), agrees with others that this is a neurodevelopmental disorder that occurs during early brain development. The committee's statements regarding incidence of the disorder in the population, among identical twins, and the connection between familial patterns and serotonin levels are consistent with others noted in this chapter (4). Other researchers suggest that early childhood autism may be caused by deficits in cell development within the first few months of conception.

Brain Morphology

The brains of individuals with autism are abnormal. However, it is important to remember that autism is not considered a neurological condition, nor is it a psychological condition.

Bauman (5) looked at the structure of the brains of people with PDD. The brains of those with autism showed widespread damage to the midbrain and the cerebellum. The brains of those diagnosed with autism and Asperger's syndrome had a similar pattern of lesions. The brains of people with Rett's syndrome were different; they had the greatest and most widespread brain abnormalities. The diffuse patterns may be reflective of damage that occurred during the earliest period of brain development. This leads to global dysfunction and, perhaps, brain atrophy in people with this syndrome.

The brain does not develop as a whole. Different areas of the brain mature and gain function gradually. The earlier that damage occurs in the development of the brain, the greater the impact on the individual's functioning. Rett's disorder exemplifies how devastating damage to the developing brain can be. The cause of Rett's disorder is genetic and involves global brain damage, which ultimately results in atrophy.

Macrocephaly also has been reported in studies of those with autism. People with macrocephaly may also be above average in height and weight. External measurements, cranial imaging techniques, measurement at necropsy, and magnetic resonance imaging (MRI) have all been used to determine brain size. The significance of microcephaly on cognitive functioning has been established previously. It is not clearly understood, however, whether macrocephaly has an effect on the brain's functioning. "Macrocephaly appears to be the single most consistent physical characteristic of children with autism. . . One or both parents of 62% of the individuals with macrocephaly were also determined to be macrocephalic" (6). Macrocephaly may be a feature used to determine subgroups among those diagnosed with autism. The usefulness of these findings is still uncertain and will require further research.

Magnetic resonance imaging was used to study brain volume in 35 autistic and 36 normal subjects. Brain sizes were enlarged in the temporal, parietal, and occipital lobes of the subjects with autism. Their frontal lobes did not show any changes in size. Among the subjects with autism, the brains of the males were significantly larger than those of the females (7).

Several researchers have noted tuberous sclerosis in the temporal lobes of people diagnosed with autism. Neuroanatomical abnormalities discovered on MRI suggest the potential importance in linking these abnormalities as causative factors. None of these researchers have definitively determined whether these abnormalities cause autism themselves, or if they exist in combination with other autism-producing factors (8).

Recent studies have looked at the anatomy and physiology of the brain to discover the cause of PDD. One study examined the MRIs and computed tomographic (CT) scans of brains of people with autism, mental retardation (MR), and psychiatric disorders. The researchers discovered the presence of the genetic disease tuberous sclerosis in more people with autism and MR than in those with psychiatric diagnoses. Eight of the nine individuals with autism studied had these lesions in their temporal lobes, but more and larger studies are needed (7).

Kallen identified specific brain regions responsible for social cognition, such as the medial temporal lobe structures, the amygdala, and the hippocampus (4). He also cited the work being done through the Human Genome Project (see Resources), that there are likely to be up to five genes that contribute to the dysfunction seen in people diagnosed with PDD. There are hypotheses regarding the number of defective genes necessary to produce the abnormalities seen in this diagnostic category.

Nutrition

More than 18 studies have explored the impact that vitamin B6 and the mineral magnesium have on people with PDD. Subjects who received these substances have experienced a reduction in their symptoms. In a letter in the September-October 1966 issue of the *Advocate* (9), Rimland wrote that immune system abnormalities have been recognized in people with PDD for more than 20 years, and he strongly supported the use of this treatment. Rimland and others encourage further research in this area (10). Others have questioned whether some symptoms can be attributed to allergies to food, scents, fabrics, and other substances.

Multiple Causes

Researchers admit that a prenatal or perinatal illness, metabolic illness, or traumatic brain injury may cause autism; however, the percentage of individuals with PDD that can be traced to these causes is relatively low. Some also are questioning whether the range of PDD symptoms may be caused by the overuse of antibiotics.

The current consensus is that there is no single cause of PDD. A combination of genetic and neurobiological abnormalities appears to produce the symptoms that generally are apparent at a fairly young age. Many times parents express concern to the pediatrician that "something isn't right" with their 1-year-old child. Infants may avoid eye contact or be unresponsive to sounds and people. They may interact with toys and objects in nontraditional ways, such as spinning the wheels on the car rather than pushing it. Typically the diagnosis is made by the time the child is 3 years old and is based on a review of developmental milestones and patterns.

INCIDENCE AND PREVALENCE

Sex Differences

More males than females are diagnosed with autism, at a 3:1 ratio. Almost all those diagnosed with Rett's disorder are girls. Girls with autism also are more likely to have lower IQs than boys.

Social Class or Level of Education

It is doubtful that social class or level of education affects the incidence of PDD. However, when parents and caregivers are educationally and eco-nomically privileged, their infants and young children may be diagnosed earlier.

Handedness

Sixty-five percent of people diagnosed are left-handed.

Seasonal Variations

Whether seasonal variances have an influence on the pregnant woman or newborn infant has not been established clearly. Trevarthen (11) suggested that infections like influenza, acquired more easily during certain seasons, may have an impact on the developing fetus. He also suggested that pregnant women and newborns may be more susceptible to stresses at certain times of the year. The questions of how much stress or infection might affect the infant and whether it is significant enough to produce PDD require further study.

Early Diagnosis

The changes in the DSM IV classification of PDD and greater emphasis on early identification and intervention have resulted in more individuals with these conditions being identified, mostly in early childhood. Furthermore, clearer definitions may make more people eligible under the PDD classification. Changes in definitions do not increase the incidence of PDD; however, improved guidelines may identify more people who fit the diagnostic criteria.

Genetic Influence

There is a 75% chance that after one child in a family has been diagnosed that other offspring will be diagnosed with PDD as well. According to Larkin (12), 70% of adults with autism are institutionalized in adulthood. In the future, the emphasis on early diagnosis and intervention is likely to reduce the number of people that require institutionalization in adulthood. Early and intensive intervention benefits at least 50% of children diagnosed with PDD. The reduction in the rate of institutionalization also is consistent with current trends toward community housing and community services for individuals with disabilities.

There are more reports that the primary feature that distinguishes this diagnostic category from others is the prevalence of diagnostic features in the parents. The cognitive and social deficits are observable in the parents of PDD offspring. Piven and associates (13) interviewed families who had two or more children with autism and families who had children with Down syndrome. The age range of the children was 4 to 28 years. Families with more than one autistic child were chosen because of the greater likelihood that the causes of autism were genetic. A standardized interview—the Autism Diagnostic Interview—was completed with the families. They also used the Autism Diagnostic Observation Schedule to gauge the intensity of each child's behavior. Additionally, physical examinations and family histories were completed. The parents of the autistic children showed more stereotyped behaviors and social deficits than did the parents of children with Down syndrome.

Bryson's 1996 study of autism (14) stated that the incidence of this condition appears greater than previously suspected because of the expansion of the definition and the recognition that people with higher functioning may be autistic. The current estimates of incidence range from 5 to 15/10,000.

SIGNS AND SYMPTOMS

Autism is thought to be more of a syndrome than a specific condition. "Autism usually affects very specific neurological pathways, leaving others unharmed or even strengthened" (15). The onset of PDD occurs by age 4 or 5, and there are wide variations in severity. The disorder usually affects behavior and communication, and severity often decreases with age. People with PDD have difficulty understanding the facial expressions of others and their affect is usually flat. Many people diagnosed with PDD have an obsessive need for sameness. The symptom that usually motivates parents to seek medical attention is delay in or impairment of the child's language development. Parents may be concerned earlier about other developmental delays; however, the lack of or impairment in verbal communication necessitates professional consultation.

The diagnosis and classification of PDD are difficult because intelligence and social behaviors vary in those with PDD. Presenting symptoms may include language delay or deficits, difficulties in social interactions and with relationships, unusual reactions to sensory stimuli, and a wide range of functional skills and abilities. Individuals with PDD may have excellent fine motor skills, but their level of distractibility prevents them from performing tasks for more than a short period. Others may remember dates and events but have difficulty initiating and terminating activities. Children and adults with PDD vary in their ability to perform activities of daily living and learn new skills such as reading and writing. They may have difficulty carrying out many occupations in their daily lives. Developing a specific assessment is difficult as the symptoms may be scattered across the performance areas and performance components. Also, the ability to perform tasks often is context-specific. The accuracy of all assessment tools is challenging because of the individual's difficulties with social and communication skills.

The Autism Society of America identified characteristics of autism. If the person has more than

50% of these characteristics, the diagnosis of autism is likely to apply (16). These characteristics are:

Difficulty in mixing with other children
Appears to be deaf
Resists learning
No fear of real life dangers
Resists change in routine
Indicates needs by gesture (leading adults by the hand, rather than pointing)
Inappropriate laughing or giggling
Resists cuddling
Marked physical overactivity
Avoids eye contact
Inappropriate attachment to objects
Spins objects
Sustained odd play
Standoffish manner

Freeman (17) published a list of four behavioral symptoms that characterize autism.

1. Disturbances (delays) in the rate of appearance of physical and social skills.
2. Abnormal responses to sensations. Any one of a combination of senses or responses is affected, such as, sight, hearing, touch, balance, reaction to pain, proprioceptive or kinesthetic.
3. Delays or disturbances in speech, language, and nonverbal communication.
4. Abnormal ways of relating to people, objects, and events in the environment.

Frith (18) referred to the work of Lorna Wing, who studied the IQ range of individuals with autism. She found a strong correlation between autism and mental retardation. Most of those individuals with low intelligence (<70) also had the most severe impairments in social communications. In her study, the girls were more seriously impaired than the boys. She found that boys consistently had higher levels of ability than girls.

According to child development, by 2 months of age the typical infant attends to the visual picture, expressions, and sounds from the mother and is able to respond visually with a smile and auditorily with coos. Playing with mother and others helps to establish understanding of communication and object manipulation, while establishing muscle strength and visual attention. In contrast, by the end of the first year, the child with autism has difficulty receiving and interpreting auditory and visual input, and the drive to explore and learn is diminished.

As the individual grows and acquires some skills, problems or deficit areas continue to exist. However, symptoms change with age and these skill deficits interfere with functional performance.

Persons with PDD have similarities in their style of communication. When allowed the choice, they prefer to be alone. They find communication awkward. The content of conversations is stilted, and there is a lack of reciprocity in oral communication. Speech echolalia, pronoun reversal, and a lack of inflection are typical. Approximately half the people with PDD do not speak. Many who can will speak in short phrases or sentences.

The nuances of social interactions are lost, leaving these individuals unable to understand innuendo, facial expressions, and jokes. They never develop some of the subtle interaction skills necessary in establishing close relationships.

Behaviorally, compulsions and obsessions can be so severe that skills for independence and self-sufficiency do not develop. Changes in schedule or environment are difficult and can be the catalyst for behavioral outbursts.

Toys are used to facilitate self-stimulation, not for interaction. The nonverbal individual's needs are communicated through pushing and pulling. Higher functioning people with PDD may use pictures, sign language, and computers to communicate.

People with PDD learn throughout their lives. Their rate of learning depends on their IQs and the intrusion of self-stimulating behaviors, or sensory stimulation. Splinter skills are developed by some individuals with PDD, who may be thought of as savants. Their cognitive or functional skills will excel in one or two specific areas, while other areas remain significantly impaired.

Expressive communication is greatly affected. People with Asperger's and PDD-NOS possess higher levels of verbal skills than others within the PDD classification. Even though they may possess verbal skills, it is not unusual for them to reverse or avoid using pronouns. For example, when Sam was asked if he liked the new nature magazine, he would avoid saying, "Yes, I like it." Instead, he might say either yes, no, or it was good (19).

COURSE AND PROGNOSIS

Autism is a rare condition and is usually diagnosed by the time the child is 3 years old. There is no specific treatment, and it is often accompanied by other conditions like MR and epilepsy. One of the greatest deficits is the individual's inability to socialize, communicate, and engage in a variety of activities. The life spans of people diagnosed with PDD are not shortened. They are usually diagnosed with a PDD before they begin preschool. Once diagnosed, intensive early interventions begin, focusing on the child's social and communication skills. If behavior management is needed, it will be instituted early in treatment.

Sensory histories are helpful in the diagnostic process. Individuals with autism may have normal sensory systems or may be hypersensitive. Tactile defensiveness and rigid, stereotyped behaviors (verbal or motor) are associated with PDD (20), along with an inability to generalize learning from one situation to another. Learning occurs more by association. A significant number of individuals with autism have hearing and visual impairments.

Fifty percent of those with autism never develop functional speech. Individuals with other types of PDD may acquire the ability to speak, then gradually lose that ability. For example, Mac was a typically developing baby until about 18 months of age. He had begun to say a few words, but his speech development ceased by age 5. At age 16, Mac's verbalizations are confined to guttural sounds in varying frequencies and no functional speech. Children with Rett's syndrome or childhood disintegrative disorder show the most significant and global deterioration (11).

DIAGNOSIS

Autism is a deficit in social and emotional functioning characterized by obsessive behaviors. The DSM-IV separates the condition according to social relatedness, communication skills, and imagination. This guide lists the following as diagnoses under the PDD category: autistic disorder, Asperger's disorder, childhood disintegrative disorder, Rett's disorder, and PDD-NOS.

The World Health Organization's (WHO) *International Classification of Diseases (ICD), volume 10* (ICD-10) includes a section on PDD that lists the conditions of childhood autism, atypical autism, Rett's syndrome, other childhood disintegrative disorder, Asperger's syndrome, other PDD, and PDD, Unspecified. The ICD-10 emphasizes that the symptoms/impairments must exist before the child's third year of life (11).

There is obvious agreement between the two organizations (the American Psychiatric Association and WHO) regarding the major criteria for diagnosing a child with a PDD. Because children with symptoms in this category can often be misdiagnosed, it is advisable that a team of professionals be involved in the evaluation process. Evaluations must assess all aspects of sensory, motor, cognitive, psychological, and social development. Special attention is focused on the level and quality of reciprocal communication; the level of social skills/interactions; the presence or absence of stereotyped interests, behaviors, and activities; and the degree of sensory integration that the child has achieved.

Some individuals advocate for the screening of all 18-month-old children, considering the severity of this classification of disability. Because of expanded understanding of development, screening at this age would allow early detection of autism and autism spectrum disorders. Intensive early intervention would be a saving (financially and emotionally) to families, as well as educational and support systems.

Pervasive developmental disorder is divided into five separate diagnoses, each similar to the other, but with varying degrees of severity. All the conditions included in this category are severe and pervasive. Advocacy organizations and the literature suggest that the growing number of people diagnosed with milder symptoms found in PDD-NOS, rather than autism, narrows the definition and understanding of these disorders. Families are often more "comfortable" with a diagnosis of PDD-NOS, instead of the more stigmatized autism. Diagnostic decisions ultimately have an impact on the family's access to services. There is a lack of agreement among service providers and specialists about the classification of individuals with IQS of 70 or higher who are considered to be "high functioning."

Asperger's Disorder

Asperger's disorder was first defined in 1944. Wing (21) described symptoms clinically in 1981. A diagnosis of Asperger's syndrome is generally used when the individual's IQ is above 70. The primary feature of this disorder is the verbosity of the individual's speech. These people may talk nonstop; however, their conversations are tangential. They perform best when they are in charge of the conversation, either asking a series of questions or giving information. They have great difficulty with reciprocal conversation. They have difficulty using pronouns correctly, their thoughts are expressed simply and in short phrases, and echolalia is present. People with this diagnosis have excellent rote memory for narrow and specific types of information such as maps, dates, and numbers.

Delayed motor development, "odd" postures, below-normal manipulation skills, and narrow interests also are prominent features of Asperger's disorder. The individual's movements are clumsy.

Their social skills are impaired, speech is concrete, and they become absorbed in a limited range of interests. Socially, these individuals lack a sense of humor. They speak with a monotone and do not have the ability to empathize. Individuals with Asperger's disorder cannot interpret nonverbal communication and are unaware of the nonverbal communication they project. They are more egocentric in their thinking. They display more social skills in early childhood and have fewer neurological abnormalities than the same age group with autism.

On measures of intelligence, people with Asperger's disorder score in the ranges of normal and above. Those diagnosed with autism often score below normal. Experts (11) believe that there is an intellectual continuum that includes autism, Asperger's syndrome, and the other PDDs. Those with Asperger's syndrome will have normal or above-normal intelligence. As with other PDDs, social communication is their most obvious limitation.

Autistic Disorder (Autism)

The diagnosis of autism is not easy to establish. There is no one specific test to determine if a child has autistic disorder. The diagnosis is made based on the evidence of impairments in communication, social skills, interests, and activities. An understanding of developmental history and milestones is critical to an accurate assessment.

The *Advocate,* a publication of the Autism Society of America, publishes a definition of autism as follows, "Autism is a severely incapacitating lifelong developmental disability that typically appears during the first three years of life." Autism and its behavioral symptoms occur in approximately 15 of every 10,000 births and is 4 times more common in boys than girls. It has been found throughout the world in families of all racial, ethnic, and social backgrounds. No known factors in the psychological environment of a child have been shown to cause autism.

Individuals with autism may have delays in their physical, social, and language development. Speech and language difficulties are not linked to cognitive deficits. People with autism often have an abnormal response to sensations. Any one or a combination of senses or responses are affected: sight, hearing, touch, balance, smell, taste, reaction to pain, and the way an individual holds his or her body.

Autism occurs by itself or in association with other disorders that affect the function of the brain, such as viral infections, metabolic disturbances, and epilepsy. It is important to distinguish autism from retardation or mental disorders, because diagnostic confusion may result in referral to inappropriate and ineffective treatment techniques. However, 70% of persons with autism have MR. The severe form of the syndrome may include extreme self-injurious, repetitive, highly unusual, and aggressive behaviors. Special education programs using behavioral methods have proved to be the most helpful treatment for persons with autism (22).

Freeman's work on autism helps parents understand whether their child may have autism. According to Freeman (17), autism is a spectrum disorder. It ranges from very severe involvement to mild symptoms.

Autism is a developmental diagnosis, that is, expression of the syndrome varies with age and the developmental level of the person affected. As with any other child, the individual with autism will change as he or she grows older.

Autism is a retrospective diagnosis. It cannot be made without taking a careful developmental history from parents and others involved in a child's or adult's life.

Autism can coexist with other conditions, appearing most commonly with MR. Just because a person has autism does not mean that there will be no other diagnosable conditions.

Childhood Disintegrative Disorder

Childhood disintegrative disorder is also known as Heller's syndrome and degenerative psychosis. The diagnosis is often made based on a history of early development. Children develop normally until age 3 or 4, when their functional speech gradually stops, and mood changes and degeneration of development occur. Self care, including toileting, and interests in social activities decrease. Seizures also may begin. Although this condition is rare, males are affected more often than females (11).

Pervasive Developmental Disorder-Not Otherwise Specified

Children diagnosed with PDD-NOS have behaviors similar to those found in children with autism; however, the severity and range of "autistic-like" behaviors are less severe. A diagnosis is often made by process of elimination, as fewer features are present than in other PDDs. Social skills are not as impaired as with others in this classification. There may be impairments in communication, stereotyped behaviors, and social skills. Intelligence is more likely to be within normal limits. Children identified as having PDD-NOS are likely to have better-developed verbal skills; however, verbal and nonverbal communication skills are impaired.

Rett's Disorder

This disorder has no known cause, no cure, and affects only females. As with so many of this group of disorders, development is initially normal. Changes occur after the first year when language development may stop and episodes of crying escalate. Physical growth continues, but skills in communication and activities of daily living (including feeding and dressing) do not progress. Growth of the head slows. If the child has learned to walk, the gait becomes wide, stiff, and awkward. She begins hand wringing, teeth grinding, facial grimacing, and self-injurious behaviors. Purposeful movement of the hands discontinues. There is little response to pain and scoliotic changes appear in the spine.

In addition to these physical and behavioral changes, an examination of the blood reveals an increased level of ammonia (11). How this finding affects the individual is unknown. Severe MR is common. The incidence of Rett's disorder is 1/10,000, second only to Down syndrome in its impact on girls and the severity of MR.

Development is normal until 6 months of age. At 9 months, there is an increase in distractibility, decreases in posture, and a decrease in coordination of the extremities. If the child has developed any verbal language, by 18 months of age, further development will cease. Behavioral changes intensify and the child will display stereotypical behaviors frequently associated with autism. Periods of agitation occur and there is significant involuntary movement at and around the mouth. The child will stop using objects and gestures of communication or speech. At age 2, the autistic-like behaviors stop

and there is less agitation. The child is responsive to affect, and she smiles and babbles. There is no hand use, no speech or learning, no understanding of language. By 2 to 4 years, brain growth stops and there is evidence of reduced blood to the brain (11).

MEDICAL/SURGICAL MANAGEMENT

There is no evidence that their lifecycle is shortened, primarily because PDD's impact is on cognitive-social-perceptual functioning, not on health. The most common medical intervention is medication, with those that alter or modify behaviors being most frequently prescribed. The gene that regulates serotonin is thought to be important in understanding the cause of autism. People with autism may produce less serotonin than others and often respond well to antidepressant drugs because they increase serotonin levels. This helps reduce some of the symptoms associated with autism, such as repetitive behaviors (23).

Symptoms that are apparent in this classification of disorders generally respond, to some degree, to medications. Symptoms will not disappear and no treatment can cure the individual of this disability. Medications that increase serotonin uptake reduce aggression and repetitive (obsessive and compulsive) thoughts and behaviors. People with PDD may have seizures and other medical conditions for which appropriate medications are administered, perhaps at reduced dosages. Nonmedication treatment of PDD is based on the philosophy that the conditions are caused by allergic reactions to food products. Others have suggested that frequent ear infections treated with antibiotics may in some way be linked with the causes of PDD.

Neuroleptics block the dopamine activity, but they do have undesirable side effects. Many currently available medications have side effects, from tardive dyskinesia and organ damage to blurred vision and dry mouth. Neuroleptic medications, such as haloperidol (Haldol) and thioridazine (Mellaril), produce more significant side effects than the group of atypical neuroleptics (clozapine [Clozaril]). The atypical neuroleptics have a lower risk of long-term, severe side effects and may be equally effective in treating the behavioral symptoms seen in PDD. Stimulants, such as methylphenidate (Ritalin), are used to treat hyperactivity and inattention. Some studies (see Bergman in Suggested Reading) agree that stimulants may exacerbate some of the intrusive symptoms, such as stereotypy. When any of these medications are used, it is important to monitor whether they reduce symptoms and create side effects.

Fluoxetine (Prozac), sertraline hydrochloride (Zoloft), and other serotonin reuptake inhibitors have become more popular in treating some of the compulsive symptoms seen in individuals with PDD. Cautious optimism exists until additional research is conducted regarding the side effects. Fenfluramine became popular as a diet medication, and its effectiveness looked promising in the treatment of PDD until reports surfaced that it increased the risk of serious cardiac problems in those who took it.

McDougle (24) looked at how dysregulation in serotonin function affects people with autism. His study provided additional validation to the work of others who are interested in serotonin's impact. Short-term reduction of available serotonin may result in the exacerbation of some of the behaviors commonly seen among those with autism. Further investigation is needed.

Gordon (25) conducted a double-blind study with clomipramine that showed this medication to be more effective than others in reducing compulsive and ritualistic behaviors and in significantly reducing hyperactivity commonly seen in persons with autistic disorder.

Hollander and Kwon (26) describe a family study that was under way in mid-May 1997. They also briefly describe the work examining how medications (such as fluoxetine) that increase the supply of serotonin help to decrease the severity of autistic symptoms. They further cite the cingulate gyrus as playing a role in the presence of the repetitive behaviors exhibited by persons with autism. Magnetic resonance imaging and positron-emission testing (PET) scans have provided additional detail about brain structure and activity. The authors also described studies in which oxytocin, infused in individuals with autism, positively affected their "social" symptoms. The preliminary findings in much of the research currently under way ultimately may give the medical community greater insight into the causes of PDD (26).

IMPACT ON OCCUPATIONAL PERFORMANCE

The occupational performance of a person with PDD changes through his or her life. This type of developmental disability has varying effects on the individual's occupational performance at different ages and stages. The challenges the person faces will change in both focus and intensity.

People with autism and other PDDs often have rigid needs for order and sameness within the environments where they work, rest, and play. When individuals with these disorders move through these environments, their supporter/caregivers need to be aware of the elements within the settings that may support or challenge the individual. The "person-activity-environment fit" is critical (Table 3.1). Close attention must be paid to the amount and arrangement of stimuli and all the factors that combine to make up the contextual framework.

TABLE 3.1 Occupational Performance Profile

I. PERFORMANCE AREAS	II. PERFORMANCE COMPONENTS	III. PERFORMANCE CONTEXTS
A. Activities of Daily Living*	A. Sensorimotor Component	A. **Temporal Aspects**
1. Grooming	1. Sensory	**1. Chronological**
2. Oral Hygiene	a. Sensory Awareness	**2. Developmental**
3. Bathing/Showering	b. **Sensory Processing**	**3. Lifecycle**
4. Toilet Hygiene	**(1) Tactile**	**4. Disability Status**
5. Personal Device Care	**(2) Proprioceptive**	B. **Environment**
6. Dressing	**(3) Vestibular**	**1. Physical**
7. Feeding and Eating	**(4) Visual**	**2. Social**
8. Medication Routine	**(5) Auditory**	**3. Cultural**
9. Health Maintenance	**(6) Gustatory**	
10. Socialization	**(7) Olfactory**	
11. Functional Communication	c. **Perceptual Processing**	
12. Functional Mobility	(1) Stereognosis	
13. Community Mobility	(2) Kinesthesia	
14. Emergency Response	(3) Pain Response	
15. Sexual Expression	(4) Body Scheme	
B. Work and Productive Activities	(5) Right–Left Discrimination	
1. Home Management	(6) Form Constancy	
a. Clothing Care	(7) Position in Space	
b. Cleaning	(8) Visual–Closure	
c. Meal Preparation/	(9) Figure Ground	
Cleanup	(10) Depth Perception	
d. Shopping	(11) Spatial Relations	
e. Money Management	(12) Topographical Orientation	
f. Household Maintenance	2. Neuromusculoskeletal	
g. Safety Procedures	a. Reflex	
2. Care of Others	b. Range of Motion	
3. Educational Activities	c. Muscle Tone	
4. Vocational Activities	d. Strength	
a. Vocational Exploration	e. Endurance	
b. Job Acquisition	f. Postural Control	
c. Work or Job	g. Postural Alignment	
Performance	h. Soft Tissue Integrity	
d. Retirement Planning	3. Motor	
e. Volunteer Participation	a. Gross Coordination	
C. Play or Leisure Activities	b. Crossing the Midline	
1. Play or Leisure Exploration	c. Laterality	
2. Play or Leisure Performance	d. Bilateral Integration	
	e. Motor Control	
	f. Praxis	
	g. Fine Coordination/Dexterity	
	h. Visual–Motor Control	
	i. Oral–Motor Control	

(continued)

TABLE 3.1 Occupational Performance Profile (Continued)

I. PERFORMANCE AREAS	II. PERFORMANCE COMPONENTS	III. PERFORMANCE CONTEXTS

	B. Cognitive Integration and Cognitive Components
	   1. Level of Arousal
	   2. Orientation
	   3. Recognition
	   4. Attention Span
	   5. Initiation of Activity
	   6. Termination of Activity
	   7. Memory
	   8. Sequencing
	   9. Categorization
	  10. Concept Formation
	  11. Spatial Operations
	  12. Problem Solving
	  13. Learning
	  14. Generalization
	C. Psychosocial Skills and Psychological Components
	   1. Psychological
	     a. Values
	     b. Interests
	     c. Self-Concept
	   2. Social
	     a. Role Performance
	     b. Social Conduct
	     c. Interpersonal Skills
	     d. Self-Expression
	   3. Self-Management
	     a. Coping Skills
	     b. Time Management
	     c. Self-Control	

*All may be affected.

Performance Components

Sensorimotor

The infant's occupation is to learn how to understand and interact with the world. A child with autism has difficulty processing sensory messages and, as a result, has a flattened or nonadaptive response. A lack of visual integration is common among people with PDD; they are reluctant to make eye contact. They gaze at their environment indirectly and have a short visual attention span. Thus, they miss visual cues that are important for normal development.

In addition, those with PDD may have inadequate modulation of tactile, vestibular, and proprioceptive sensations. This makes it difficult for them to develop refined motor skills. Their difficulty with auditory processing can hinder the development of communication.

Psychosocial

As infants, individuals with PDD are usually described as being unusually quiet. They do not appear to need the company of others. Their communication lacks reciprocity and is often dominated by questions on a particular topic. The topic is generally logical and concrete and void of descriptive embellishment. Because the person does not use or understand nonverbal communication, his or her interaction is stiff, flat, and lacks affect. Such people tend to be inflexible and are unable to engage in spontaneous conversation. Tomchek (27) studied the sensory processing of children with PDD and found a correlation between sensory deficits and social skill development.

Children with autism have difficulty in peer relationships. They do not engage in imaginative play like most children. This prevents them from being able to communicate through make-believe games. Stereotypic behaviors and rigid adherence to patterns of activity can cause these children to be further alienated from their peers.

Whereas people with PDD demonstrate a lack of concern about the opinions of others, it does not mean that they feel no attachment to others. Some will make efforts to please and even to seek approval from those close to them.

Cognitive

Mental retardation and PDD often occur simultaneously. Social and communication difficulties are compounded when individuals also have below-average intelligence. Nevertheless, many do form relationships and demonstrate appropriate affect.

Word recognition may be good but comprehension is usually poor. Because they lack intuitive thought, individuals with PDD have difficulty with mathematical computations based on story problems. In general, situations that require abstract thinking are difficult, if not impossible, for them.

CASE STUDIES

CASE 1

B. R. was born on April 17, 1978. There are three significant factors in his prenatal history. When his mother was pregnant, she contracted both measles and chicken pox. In addition, the school where she worked was closed four times during her pregnancy because standing water surrounded it. Ms. R. also fell during her fifth month of pregnancy.

As a baby, B. R. cried frequently and slept little. He was calmed when his mother held and rocked him. He was a good eater. Ms. R. was concerned because her son's responses were very different from those of his older brother.

B. R.'s survival was in danger during the first few years his life because of head banging and other self-injurious behaviors. At one time, it was estimated that he hit himself 1500 times a day. He needed to wear a football helmet to protect himself from greater injury. The family sought treatment and learned that B. R. had autism and MR. His IQ was estimated at 30. He was enrolled in several educational/treatment programs.

B. R. began to speak in single words at about age 3. Currently, his vocabulary consists primarily of nouns. He has difficulty pronouncing several consonant and vowel sounds. Although he has poor articulation, he sings and communicates some feelings with his vocal tones. B. R. walked at 13 to 14 months. He had very poor balance until age 4 and walked on his toes all of the time. Currently, he will occasionally revert to that pattern.

Changes in B. R.'s environment, schedule, or routine lead to aggressive behavior. He also engages in self-abusive behaviors when he wants attention. His behaviors include biting, hitting, head butting, scratching, and pinching. He has no sense of his personal safety and must be supervised at all times.

B. R.'s skills and needs were assessed at age 19. The following describes the results of that assessment:

I. Performance Areas
   A. Activities of Daily Living
      1. Grooming—B. R. needs supervision with many grooming activities such as brushing his hair and cutting his nails.
      2. Oral Hygiene—Care of teeth and other oral hygiene require supervision. Any dental work (teeth cleaning, having a cavity filled) requires a general anesthetic.
      3. Bathing/Showering—B. R. needs guidance and cuing when washing and drying his body; otherwise he will get distracted.
      4. Toilet Hygiene—B. R. does not consistently communicate his need to use the toilet. Even though he is on a bathroom schedule, accidents continue to occur.
      8. Medication Routine—B. R. takes his medication when it is given to him. However, he shows no understanding of the medication or the schedule for taking it.
      9. Health Maintenance—B. R. maintains a high level of fitness, because of his high energy level and his enjoyment of recreational activities. He eats balanced meals.

      10. Socialization—B. R.'s socialization needs to be supervised. His paucity of verbal skills reduces his opportunities for interactions. He prefers to be around familiar adults/caregivers.
      11. Functional Communication—B. R. uses a picture schedule at school and in his residence.
      13. Community Mobility—B. R. uses public transportation when traveling to and from his volunteer work site. He requires little, if any, cuing to pay his fare, locate a seat, or to get off at the correct stop. He does need supervision to keep him from darting into traffic and from being aggressive.
      14. Emergency Response—B. R.'s lack of comprehension and communication skills results in a dependency on caregivers. He is unable to use 911 to call for help.
      15. Sexual Expression—B. R. has difficulty managing his sexual urges and needs to be redirected to constructive activities.
   B. Work and Productive Activities
      B. R. engages in purposeful activities that are familiar to him. His performance is greatest when there are no deviations from his rigid schedule of activities. He is challenged by several of the performance areas here. B. R.'s difficulties result from the level of his retardation that influences his ability to learn, categorize, and generalize learned information from one situation to another.
      1. Home Management—B. R. is dependent in this area. He performs best at vacuuming and removing dishes from the dishwasher. Tasks involving handling fabric, string (laundry, folding towels) require the greatest supervision because of their inherent stimulatory appeal.

B. R.'s work and productive activities are affected by his difficulties with social conduct and self-management. His lack of communication skills is an obvious barrier in all life roles. His lack of self-control is a danger to himself and others. When placed in new situations or when feeling stressed, B. R. becomes more vulnerable. His coping skills are greatest when he is familiar with the situation and with his caregivers.

B. R.'s "performance contexts" are made safe by his one-to-one supervision 24 hours a day, 7 days a week. Without this support, this severely disabled young man would be barred from participation in age-appropriate social and cultural activities.

CASE 2

P. J. was born on January 28, 1980. His mother had a normal labor and delivery. His motor milestones were accomplished early; however, his language development was delayed. P. J. always had difficulty establishing eye contact. He responded to physical contact by stiffening his body and arching his back. From the ages of 13 to 20 months, he enjoyed twirling his body in circles with his arms extended out to his sides.

His recurrent ear infections resulted in his having tubes inserted in his ears by the age of 4. P. J.'s vocabulary contained approximately 75 words. He had the ability to hum and whisper. He received medical treatment for his allergies. When P. J. was five, he continued to have an aversion to cuddling and hugging.

Socially and behaviorally, P. J. needed additional supervision when he was outside, because he would run away. When engaged with others, supervision was required to prevent him from grabbing, pinching, slapping, or biting. His sensory integration was such that he needed to have his body rubbed, gently swung, or allowed to twirl after long bus rides. From early childhood, P. J. has not responded well to change. Changes occasionally lead to tantrums.

P. J.'s ritualistic mannerisms, limited eye contact, and poor social interactions led to his diagnosis of autism. His myopia and astigmatism are corrected with eyeglasses. He scored in the borderline range (74) on the Stanford Binet Intelligence Scale. P. J. has functional speech, although it is often unintelligible because of his problems with articulation and oral motor control. He has difficulty processing and constructing longer, more complicated sentences. His language age equivalency scores are between 6 and 7 years. His comprehension is 8 years, and his auditory memory is at the 5- to 6-year level. P. J.'s visual and auditory attentions are good; however, he is occasionally distracted by his inner thoughts.

P. J. is currently placed in a level six school because of his need for close (1:2) supervision. He has difficulty controlling his aggression toward others and maintaining an appropriate voice volume when agitated. When P. J. becomes frustrated, he needs assistance refraining from property destruc-

tion, refusing to perform tasks, slowing down his work productivity, or wandering or darting away.

P. J.'s disability has an impact on his occupational performance in several ways. He has a rigid need for sameness in his daily schedule and for the objects within his environment.

I. Performance Areas
  A. Activities of Daily Living

P. J. consistently performs a number of activities of daily living independently, such as washing his face, bathing, making his bed, washing his clothes, folding towels, brushing his teeth, preparing frozen foods, and mopping and vacuuming. He needs a structured schedule to help him accomplish his daily activities. He makes his own lunch every day.

   8. Medication Routine—P. J. is compliant taking his medication; however, he shows no understanding of the medication or its usage.
   9. Health Maintenance—P. J. eats a well-balanced diet; however, he does not maintain an active lifestyle. He needs encouragement to stay physically active to avoid excessive weight gain.
   10. Socialization—P. J. establishes fleeting eye contact. When speaking, he looks at the floor and speaks softly. He is able to discuss only a limited range of topics. P. J.'s conversations lack reciprocity and are generally simple responses to questions. He enjoys being around others; however, his social awkwardness limits his ability to establish social relationships with his peers. The majority of his social skills were learned through repetition. He does not generalize knowledge in social situations.
   14. Emergency Response—P. J.'s lack of comprehension and constricted communication skills result in his dependence on caregivers. He has the ability to dial 911 but would have difficulty describing an emergency situation.
   15. Sexual Expression—P. J. has moderate difficulty managing his sexual urges. An educational module was developed to help him learn about his sexuality and its expression.
  B. Work and Productive Activities

P. J. needs a structured daily schedule to ensure that he maintains a productive lifestyle. He is not successful in structuring his own time. He learned how to manage a number of activities in his home environment, such as mopping floors, placing dishes in the dishwasher and emptying it, and making his bed. He does not independently clean the bathroom sink; however, this may be more task avoidance than a limitation in cognitive integration.

3. Educational Activities—P. J.'s attention span is usually good. He is a visual learner. He needs to have his daily schedule written out to help him initiate and terminate each activity he needs to accomplish. He has an excellent memory and spatial operations for map reading and solving puzzles. P. J. knows how to read; however, his teacher assistant must review the material, because his comprehension is not as good as his reading ability. Practice and modeling are necessary to help him improve his ability to generalize.

4. Vocational Activities—P. J. currently works in a warehouse, stacking boxes. His supportive employment counselor has begun consideration of new job sites that will use his cognitive strengths more.

C. Play or Leisure Activities

P. J. enjoys putting puzzles together, building with Legos, playing computer games, dribbling the basketball, and taking walks. He needs to expand his repertoire of leisure interests. Although P. J. requires close monitoring by staff, opportunities should be sought that will allow him to engage in activities with peers who are not disabled. Increased physical activities will help P. J. increase his strength and endurance. Improved postural control would occur through participation in an exercise and activity program.

POINTS FOR REVIEW

1. What is the category used in DSM-IV to describe PDD?

2. Trace the history of the identification of what is known as autism.

3. Which theoretical perspective regarding the etiology of PDD is more widely accepted?

4. Describe the rationale for developmental, neurological pathogenesis, nutritional, and other causes of PDD. Discuss current research that you might have read that strengthens the argument for consideration of these etiologies.

5. Discuss various factors that may contribute to the incidence and prevalence of PDD.

6. Give examples of behaviors that you might observe that could be indicative of autism.

7. In the diagnostic process of autism, sensory histories are helpful. Why?

8. To what degree is communication behavior involved in individuals with autism?

9. Describe the signs and symptoms of the five diagnostic categories of PDD: Asperger's disorder; autism; childhood disintegrative disorder; PDD-NOS; and Rett's disorder.

10. List the medications most commonly prescribed for persons with PDD and their purpose.

11. If you were going to observe a person with PDD in an activity, which performance components would you expect to be affected? Give examples of behaviors that you would likely observe.

REFERENCES

1. Diagnostic and Statistical Manual of Mental Disorders. 4th ed. American Psychiatric Association, 1994:65
2. Grandin T. Thinking in Pictures and Other Reports from My Life with Autism. New York: Bantam Doubleday Dell Publishing Group, Inc., 1995.
3. Grogan D, Bane V. In touch, at last. People Weekly 1995;43:42.
4. Kallen RJ. The genetics of autism. Advocate 1996;28:19–21.
5. Bauman, ML. Neuroanatomic observations of the brain in pervasive developmental disorders. J Autism Dev Disord 1996;26:199–203.
6. Stevenson RE, Schroer RJ, Skinner C, et al. Autism and macrocephaly. Lancet 1997;349:1745.
7. Piven J, Arndt S, Bailey J, et al. Regional brain enlargement in autism: a magnetic resonance imaging study. J Am Acad Child Adolesc Psychiatry 1996;35:530.

8. Lainhart J E. Developmental abnormalities in autism. Lancet 1997;349:373–374.

9. Rimland B. Letter to the Advocate. Advocate 1996;28:4–5.

10. Henderson K , Brooks A, Raynesford A, et al. Trace mineral hair analysis in autistic children. J Am Osteopath Assoc December 1980;80:298.

11. Trevarthen C, Aitken K, Papoudi D, et al. Children with Autism Diagnosis and Interventions to Meet Their Needs. London: Jessica Kingsley Publishers Ltd, 1996.

12. Larkin M. Approaches to amelioration of autism in adulthood. Lancet 1997;349:186.

13. Piven J, Palmer P, Jacobi D, et al. Broader autism phenotype: evidence from a family history study of multiple-incidence autism families. Am J Psychiatry 1997;154:185.

14. Bryson, SE. Epidemiology of autism. J Autism Dev Dis 1996;26:165–167.

15. Hart CA. A Parent's Guide to Autism. New York: Simon and Schuster, 1993.

16. Board of Directors. Bethesda, MD: Advocate Autism Society of America, 1994.

17. Freeman BJ. Diagnosis of the syndrome of autism: questions parents ask. Bethesda MD: Autism Society of America 1994:21–31.

18. Frith U. Autism. Sci Am 1993;268:108.

19. Sullivan RC. Autism: Definitions past and present. Marica Datlow Smith, Issue editor. J Vocational Rehab January 1994;4:4–9.

20. Baranek G, Foster LG, Berkson G. Tactile defensiveness and stereotyped behaviors. Am J Occup Ther 1997;51:91–95.

21. Wing L, ed. Aspects of Autism: Biological Research. London: The Royal College of Psychiatrists, 1988.

22. Advocate, Autism Society of America Sept.-Oct. 1995. Bethesda, MD.

23. Holden C. A gene is linked to autism. Science 1997;276:905.

24. McDougle CJ. Effects of tryptophan depletion in drug-free adults with autistic disorder. JAMA 1997;277:1336F.

25. Gordon CT. A double-blind comparison of clomipramine, desipramine, and placebo in the treatment of autistic disorder. JAMA 1993: 270:2798.

26. Hollander E, Kwon J. The Seaver Autism Research Center of the Mount Sinai School of Medicine. Advocate 1997;29(3):12–13.

27. Tomchek SD. Sensory processing in children diagnosed with an autism spectrum disorder: an item analysis. Advocate 1997:21–22.

RESOURCES

American Speech-Language-Hearing Association
10801 Rockville Pike
Rockville, MD 20852
301-897-5700
800-638-8255

Autism Society of America
7910 Woodmont Avenue
Suite 650
Bethesda, MD 20814-3015
301-657-0881
301-657-0869 (fax)

**Autism & Sensory Impairments Network
for Individuals with Hearing
or Visual Impairment and Autism**
Dolores & Alan Bartel
7510 Oceanfront Avenue
Virginia Beach, VA 23451
757-428-9036

National Institute of Mental Health
5600 Fishers Lane, Room 7C02
Rockville, MD 20857-8030
301-443-4515
301-443-5158 (Fax on Demand)

**National Institute of Neurological Disorders and
Stroke Neurology Institute**
Bldg. 31, Rm. 8A16
31 Center Drive
MSC 2540
Bethesda, MD 20892-2540
301-496-5751
301-402-2186 (fax)
http://www.ninds/nih.gov

**National Information Center for Children
and Youth with Disabilities (NICHY)**
P.O. Box 1492
Washington, DC 20013-1492
800-999-5599

REHABDATA
National Rehabilitation Information Center
8455 Colesville Rd., Suite 935
Silver Spring, MD 20910-3319
800/346-2742
http://www.naric.com/naric

Upledger Institute
1121 Prosperity Farms Rd.
Palm Beach Gardens, FL 33410-4449
407-622-433

CHAPTER 4

MENTAL RETARDATION

Linda York

CRITICAL TERMS

Alzheimer's disease
Cortical atrophy
Craniostenosis
Cytomegalovirus
Down syndrome
Fragile X syndrome

Hydrocephaly
Hyperphenylalaninemia
Hypoxia
Mongoloid
Muscular dystrophy

Pica
Spina bifida
Tay-Sachs disease
Teratogenic
Toxemia

The following two cases are representative of the experience parents have had when their child has Down syndrome, a chromosomal defect causing mental retardation (MR).

In the mid-1950s, Mr. and Mrs. D. had their first child. Mrs. D., a homemaker in her late 30s, and Mr. D., a bank officer, had tried for many years to have a child. They had both given up when Mrs. D. became pregnant. Shortly after his birth, they were told by their doctor that their son was born a "mongoloid." He would be severely retarded and incapable of learning anything. The doctors suggested that they put E. D. in an institution immediately and felt it would be better if they had no further contact with him. Mr. and Mrs. D. were not willing to do that and wanted him home with them. They took E.D. home with no support from their doctors, family, or the community.

In the late 1980s, Mr. and Mrs. T., both in their 20s, were eagerly awaiting the birth of their second child. Mr. T., a construction worker, and his wife, a bookkeeper, had a 3-year-old son. Mrs. T. had what she described as an easy pregnancy and delivery, resulting in the birth of another son, T. T. Shortly after his birth, the doctors told them that they suspected their son had Down syndrome. Mr. and Mrs. T. were devastated. They had heard of Down syndrome but knew little about it. They were frightened and did not know what to expect or how this would affect their family. They were told that T. T. would have MR that could range from mild to severe. They wanted answers and predictions but were told that they would have to wait, as it was not possible to predict what T. T. would be capable of. Some children with Down syndrome were learning academics in regular classrooms whereas others remained dependent for many of their basic needs. They were also told that with early intervention, children with Down syndrome were achieving much more independence and higher levels of functioning than had previously been thought possible.

Before T. T. and his parents left the hospital, a referral was made to the local school district for early intervention services to begin within a few months. They were given pamphlets written for parents, describing Down syndrome, that helped to answer many of their questions. Their doctor asked if they would like to be contacted by a parent volunteer from a local group for parents of children with Down syndrome. Although it would take some time for them to come to terms with their son's diagnosis, they knew that there were programs and support available in their community to help their family.

Today E. D. lives in a group home about 30 miles from his parents, who are now elderly and can no longer care for him. He takes a bus by himself to visit them twice a week. Although he is very independent, the group home provides the structure and supervision he needs. E. D.'s mother recalls that there were no school programs for him when he was growing up. However, she proudly says that all who know E. D. are very fond of him and he has many special friends. She describes him as a sweet and loving son.

T. T. is now in a special preschool class. His parents feel that he is doing well and are proud of each new accomplishment. Mrs. T. recently gave birth to a baby girl, who was not born with Down syndrome. They are enjoying T. T. but still feel some anxiety about his future.

From these two cases, it is apparent how much attitudes toward and treatment of Down syndrome has changed in this country. This phenomenon applies not just to Down syndrome but to other forms of MR as well. (These case studies were contributed by Mary Steichen Yamamoto in the first edition.)

INTRODUCTION

"Mental retardation" is a functional condition rather than a medical one. It may occur in isolation or in conjunction with other neurological or developmental disabilities (1). For an individual to be considered mentally retarded, he or she must meet three different criteria. There must be the presence of "significantly subaverage intellectual functioning" (2), usually defined as an intelligence quotient (IQ) of approximately 70 or less, onset must occur before age 18, and there must be significant limitations in at least two areas of adaptive functioning. These adaptive skill areas include communication, self-care, home living, social/interpersonal skills, leisure, health and safety, self-direction, functional academics, use of community resources, and work (2, 3). It is therefore possible for someone to have significantly impaired intellectual function and not

be considered mentally retarded because there is not significant limitation in two or more adaptive skill areas (2).

ETIOLOGY

The causes of MR may be classified according to when they occurred in the developmental cycle (prenatally, perinatally, or postnatally) or by their origin (biomedical vs. environmental) (1, 4). There are hundreds of causes of MR (5).

Despite knowing the many factors that can cause MR, in a large proportion of cases the cause remains unknown. The ability to determine cause is highly correlated with the level of the retardation. The etiology of MR is much less likely to be known with individuals who are mildly retarded (IQs of 50 to 70) than with those who are severely retarded (IQs of <50) (1, 4, 6).

In a large United States population-based study describing probable causes of MR in school-aged children, the following results were obtained (4):

Prenatal conditions	12.4%
Genetic	7.1%
Teratogenic	2.9%
CNS birth defects	1.5%
Other birth defects	0.8%
Perinatal conditions	5.9%
Intrauterine/intrapartum	5.2%
Neonatal	0.7%
Postneonatal events	3.6%
No defined cause	78.0%

Prenatal factors that can cause MR include genetic aberrations, birth defects that are not genetic in origin, environmental influences, or a combination of factors (4). Up to 50% of the individuals diagnosed with MR may have more than one causal factor (3). With genetic aberrations, the problem is either with the genes, which are the basic unit of heredity, or the chromosomes, which carry the genes. Each nongerm cell (cells other than the ovum and spermatozoa) contains 23 pairs of chromosomes, including one pair of sex chromosomes that determine the sex of the person. Males have an X and a Y chromosome, and females have two X chromosomes.

In many cases of MR, the gene or chromosome that has caused the condition can be identified specifically. In fact, more than 350 inborn errors of metabolism that result from genetic changes have been identified. Many of these metabolic errors lead to MR (7). The two most common genetic causes of MR are Down syndrome and fragile X syndrome (8). Down syndrome is generally caused by an extra 21st chromosome, and fragile X syndrome is the result of a mutation at what is known as the fragile site on the X chromosome (9). In other cases, the specific genetic aberration has not been identified. Factors such as higher incidences of a condition in specific families or increased recurrence rates among siblings suggest that the defect is genetic (6).

Birth defects that are not considered genetic in origin also can contribute to or cause MR. These could include such things as malformation of parts of the central nervous system (CNS) (cortical atrophy, hydrocephaly, spina bifida, craniostenosis) (4), congenital cardiac anomalies (10), or metabolic disorders not associated with genetic defect (hypothyroidism) (11).

Environmental factors may also be involved in prenatal development of MR. They may include exposure to chemical agents, such as alcohol or nonprescription drugs ingested by the mother during the pregnancy, maternal conditions such as hyperphenylalaninemia (12), toxemia, hypertension, and diabetes, or congenital infections such as cytomegalovirus, rubella, and syphilis (4).

Genetic Causes

Genetic causes can be divided into two types: single gene disorders and chromosomal abnormalities. In single gene disorders, there is a problem with the quality of the genetic material; a specific gene is defective. In chromosomal abnormalities, the problem is with the quantity of material. There is either too much or too little genetic material in a specific chromosome (13).

Single Gene Disorders

Single gene disorders follow specific patterns of transmission: autosomal dominant, autosomal recessive, or sex-linked. Table 4.1 presents the transmission patterns and risk factors associated with each type.

The autosomal dominant type is caused by a single altered gene. Either parent may be a carrier or there may have been a spontaneous mutation of the gene. Dominant inheritance occurs when one parent passes on the defective gene. This occurs even if the other parent passes a healthy gene. Because the defective gene can be passed by either parent, there is a 50% risk of the child being affected in each pregnancy (8). An example of this type of inherited disorder is tuberous sclerosis.

Table 4.1 Single Gene Disorders			
TYPE	**AUTOSOMAL DOMINANT**	**AUTOSOMAL RECESSIVE**	**SEX LINKED**
Transmission Pattern	Either parent carries gene or spontaneous transmission	Both parents are carriers	Either parent can transmit gene: mother usually a carrier, father cannot be a carrier but can have the disorder
Risk Factors	50% risk of child being affected with each pregnancy	25% risk of child being affected with each pregnancy	If mother has affected gene, 25% risk of having affected son or carrier daughter; if father has affected gene, all his daughters will be carriers and his sons will be normal
Sex Distribution	Male and female children equally at risk	Male and female children equally at risk	Primarily male children at risk for having disorder, female children at risk for becoming carriers

In the autosomal recessive type, both parents are carriers but show no outward signs or symptoms of having the disorder. Inheritance occurs when both parents pass the defective gene to their offspring. Each pregnancy has a 25% risk of the child being affected (8). Examples of this type of disorder are phenylketonuria (PKU) and Tay-Sachs disease.

With X-linked disorders, the affected gene is on the sex chromosomes, specifically the X chromosome, and can occur in either parent. Because males have only one X chromosome, if the father has an affected gene, he will always have the disorder and cannot be a carrier. Because the female has two X chromosomes, she can either be a carrier of the disorder (if only one X chromosome is affected) or have the disease herself (if both X chromosomes are affected). A carrier mother has a 25% risk of having an affected son. If the father has the affected gene, all his daughters will be carriers, but his sons will not be affected (8). Examples of X-linked disorders are Duchenne muscular dystrophy, fragile X syndrome, Lesch-Nyhan syndrome, and Hunter's syndrome.

Chromosomal Aberrations

Chromosomal aberrations include missing or extra chromosomes, either in part, such as a short arm, or the total chromosome, as is found in the trisomal types. Either the autosomes or sex chromosomes can be affected, with the autosomal type resulting in more serious neuromotor impairments (14). The most common are trisomy 21, 18, and 13. The patterns of transmission are not as readily identified as those of specific gene defects.

Environmental Influences

Prenatal Factors

There are numerous environmental causes of MR in the prenatal period, including maternal infections such as rubella, cytomegalovirus, toxoplasmosis, and syphilis. Low birth weight that results from prematurity or intrauterine growth retardation can also be a contributing factor. Maternal factors associated with low birth weight include smoking, lack of prenatal care, infections, poor nutrition, toxemia, and placental insufficiency. Exposure to industrial chemicals or drugs, including certain over-the-counter prescriptions and illegal substances, also can affect birth weight, particularly during the first trimester of pregnancy.

Perinatal Factors

Two major causative factors of MR in the perinatal period are mechanical injuries at birth and perinatal hypoxia. Mechanical injuries are caused by difficulties of labor because of malposition, malpresentation, disproportion, or other labor complications that result in tears of the meninges, blood vessels, or other substances of the brain. Factors that cause perinatal hypoxia or anoxia include premature placental separation, massive hemorrhage from placenta previa, umbilical cord wrapped around the baby's neck, and meconium aspiration. Very premature infants also may have impaired respiration or an intracranial hemorrhage that can result in brain damage.

If a mother has an active case of herpes simplex II and is shedding the virus at the time of delivery, the baby can acquire the infection in the birth canal, which can cause severe developmental disability. This can be avoided by testing to determine whether the mother has an active case and, if so, delivering by cesarean section.

Postnatal Factors

Traumas or infections that result in injury or a lack of oxygen to the brain are a major cause of MR during the postnatal period. Traumas include near-drowning or strangulation, child abuse, and closed head injuries. Infections include encephalitis and meningitis. Mental retardation that results from meningitis caused by *Haemophilus influenzae* is now preventable, however, with the introduction of the HiB vaccine (15).

Another major postnatal factor is sociodemographic characteristics or environmental influences. When an analysis of the relationship of sociodemographic characteristics and MR was completed for a large population of children with MR, it was found that boys, children with two or more older siblings, African-American children, children whose mothers had not completed high school, and children of older mothers (with Down syndrome factored out) were more likely to experience MR (1).

INCIDENCE AND PREVALENCE

Mental retardation is the most frequently occurring developmental disability. Estimates of the prevalence of MR in this country range from 1 to 3%. A recent review of prevalence studies found that 2.5 to 3% is probably an accurate estimate of distribution in the general population (16). Boys are 1.5 times more likely to experience MR than girls (17), which may be related to the sex-linked genetic disorders that result in MR (1).

SIGNS AND SYMPTOMS

Mental retardation often occurs in tandem with, or as a secondary manifestation of, another diagnosis. One study's results found that two-thirds of the children with severe MR (IQ <50) had an additional neurological diagnosis; less than 20% of children with mild MR were found to have an additional neurological diagnosis. These diagnoses included conditions such as cerebral palsy, epilepsy, and hearing and visual impairments (1). With certain genetic conditions, such as Down syndrome, MR is one of the clinical signs of the condition.

Mental retardation is defined by the American Association on Mental Retardation (AAMR) as a condition that is present from childhood (age 18 or younger), with (IQ) level below 70–75 as measured on a standardized test, and significant limitations in two or more adaptive skills areas (3). As previously stated, adaptive skill areas include communication, self-care, home living, social/interpersonal skills, leisure, health and safety, self-direction, functional academics, use of community resources, and work. Adaptive skills should be assessed in all of the individual's performance contexts. Someone with limited intellectual function who does not have adaptive skill deficits is not considered mentally retarded (3).

There are currently two major systems of classification for MR. The American Psychiatric Association (APA) uses the older, more traditional system of classifying MR based on performance on standardized intelligence tests using somewhat arbitrary cutoffs to assign levels of function. It is essentially used for diagnostic purposes (2). In 1992, the AAMR introduced a system of classification based on adaptive skills levels and supports needed to function (3). The AAMR system, because it focuses on function and supports needed in adaptive skills across performance contexts, is more useful to the practice of occupational therapy.

In the traditional system, MR is classified according to the severity of the impairment in intellectual functioning. This is determined through standardized intelligence testing. To be considered mentally retarded, the person's performance on these tests must be two standard deviation units or more below the mean. The levels of MR as identified by IQ tests are mild, moderate, severe, and profound. Approximately 85% of individuals with MR are in the mild range, 10% are in the moderate range, 3.5% are in the severe range, and 1.5% are in the profound range of function (17, 18). Table 4.2 presents the classifications, IQ levels, and general level of functioning as an adult (2, 3, 9, 19). It is important to remember that not all individuals in a particular classification will function at exactly that level.

The classification system developed by the AAMR involves a three-step process. The first step is to have a qualified person administer standardized intelligence and adaptive skills assessments that are appropriate for the individual's age, communication abilities, and cultural experience. The second step is to describe the individual's strengths and weaknesses across the

dimensions of 1) intellectual and adaptive behavior skills, 2) psychological/emotional considerations, 3) physical/health/etiological considerations, and 4) environmental considerations. The third step is to have the interdisciplinary team determine needed supports across these four dimensions. Supports are classified based on level of intensity and include intermittent, limited, extensive, and pervasive. Intermittent support is provided on an "as-needed" basis. Limited support occurs over a limited time span. Extensive support is assistance provided on a daily basis in a life area. Pervasive support refers to the need for support in all life areas across all environments on a daily basis (3).

In addition to the performance deficits produced by MR and the associated conditions already mentioned, a high proportion of individuals with MR also have some form of mental illness. Estimates of prevalence of mental illness among people with MR range from 10 to 20% (19) to 40 to 70% (18). Some of the common types of mental illness seen in people with MR include personality disorders, affective disorders, psychotic disorders, avoidant disorder, paranoid personality disorder, severe behavior problems that may include self-injurious behavior (20) and dementia associated with Down syndrome (21). Several misconceptions about people with MR may complicate or prevent appropriate care for their mental illness, including the beliefs that people who are mentally retarded cannot also be mentally ill, do not experience normal feelings and emotions, and are not affected by changes in their environment. Substance abuse problems, especially with alcohol, may be overlooked and there is controversy about the benefit of using antipsychotic drugs with individuals who are mentally retarded (17). Because of limited communication skills and limitations in abstract thinking caused by the MR, the diagnosis of mental illness and mental health problems can be a very difficult process and is frequently inexact. Good communication with caregivers and significant others in the life of the individual with MR is essential.

TABLE 4.2 Levels of Retardation

CLASSIFICATION	IQ RANGE	WHEN IDENTIFIED	ADAPTIVE BEHAVIOR AS ADULT
Profound	Less than 20/25	Infancy	Independent functioning • Requires total supervision • Dependent upon others for personal care Communication • Very minimal language Occupation • Minimal participation
Severe	20/25–35/40	Early childhood	Independent functioning • Can contribute partially to self-care with total supervision Communication • Can engage in simple conversation • Recognizes signs and selected words Occupation • May prepare simple foods, can help with simple household tasks, e.g., bed making, vacuuming, setting and clearing table • Requires much supervision
Moderate	35/40–50/55	Early childhood	Independent functioning • Feeds, bathes, and dresses self; prepares simple foods for self and others; able to care for own hair (wash and comb) • May function semi-independently in supervised living situation Communication • Carries on simple conversation, uses complex sentences; recognizes words, reads sentences, ads, and signs with comprehension Occupation • May do simple routine household chores (dusting, garbage, dishwashing); prepares food requiring mixing • May function in supported employment or sheltered workshop setting • Can learn some functional living skills: shopping, using post office, laundry
Mild	50/55–70/75	Elementary school	Independent functioning • Exercises care for personal grooming, feeding, bathing and toileting; may need health or personal care reminders; may need guidance and assistance when under unusual social or economic stress Occupation • Prepares meals, performs everyday household tasks • Can hold semiskilled or simple skilled job

COURSE AND PROGNOSIS

Mental retardation is generally considered a lifelong condition, but the course and prognosis will vary depending upon the cause(s) of the retardation. (For information about specific causative conditions, consult reference 21 or 22.) Most cases of MR are nonprogressive, that is, once the initial insult to the brain occurs, there is no further damage. The emphasis is on managing the medical aspects of the condition and helping individuals to achieve their highest potential. However, certain genetic conditions (e.g., muscular dystrophy and Tay-Sachs disease) are progressive, with incremental loss of function and, in some cases, associated early death. The goal for these individuals is to help them achieve the highest level of independence and maintain it as long as possible. Those with Down syndrome experience degenerative changes in the brain, beginning at about age 40, that eventually result in progressive dementia similar to Alzheimer's disease (20). On a positive note, it is possible for individuals with mild MR to gain adaptive behavior skills through remedial programs to the extent that they no longer meet the diagnostic criteria for being mentally retarded, although their intellectual function has probably not changed significantly (2).

DIAGNOSIS

An evaluation must be performed to determine whether a person meets the criteria for being mentally retarded. Besides ascertaining that the onset of the condition occurred before age 18, there are two main aspects to this process. The first part involves administration of appropriate standardized intelligence tests by a qualified individual. "The choice of testing instruments and the interpretation of results should take into account factors that may limit test performance (e.g., the individual's sociocultural background, native language, and associated communicative, motor, and sensory handicaps)" (2).

The second aspect of the process is the evaluation of adaptive behavior as it relates to the targeted adaptive life skill areas. "Adaptive functioning refers to how effectively individuals cope with common life demands and how well they meet the standards of personal independence expected of someone in their particular age group, sociocultural background, and community setting" (2). The skills needed for adaptive behavior become more complex and varied as the person ages. For instance, eating and dressing independently are major skills for the young child, but the child does not need to be able to use a telephone or manage money. Evidence for deficits and strengths in adaptive function should be gained from one or more independent, reliable sources who are familiar with the individual's abilities in different performance contexts. This information should be used to complete a standardized scale designed to provide a composite "picture" of the individual's adaptive function. As with the selection of an intelligence test, care should be taken that the adaptive behavior scale chosen is appropriate for the individual's sociocultural background, education, associated handicaps, motivation, and cooperation level (2).

MEDICAL/SURGICAL MANAGEMENT

There is no drug treatment for the condition of MR; however, medications may be needed for some of the conditions that may occur in tandem. Concomitant mental health problems such as affective or psychotic disorders, and severe behavior problems would all benefit from appropriate medical intervention; seizure disorders would require drug therapy. Neuromuscular aberrations (spasticity, rigidity, etc.) seen in cerebral palsy may also be helped by medication. (Appendix II includes a comprehensive list of medications used to treat these concomitant disorders.)

IMPACT ON OCCUPATIONAL PERFORMANCE

Virtually all areas of occupational performance and many of the performance components can be affected by MR, depending on the cause and severity of the retardation. As stated previously, the diagnostic criteria for individuals with MR identify 10 adaptive behavior skill areas that may be affected in persons with MR, and at least 2 of these areas must be substantially limited to meet the criteria for being mentally retarded (2, 3). If these areas are compared with the occupational performance areas addressed in occupational therapy practice, we see that 9 of the 10 areas (communication, self-care, home living, social/interpersonal skills, leisure, health and safety, functional academics, use of community resources, and work) fall into the occupational performance areas of activities of daily living, work and productive activities, and play/leisure. One of the areas, self-direction, corresponds with the psychosocial performance components.

Although all of the occupational performance areas and components can be influenced by MR, those that are affected will depend on factors such as the presence of additional medical diagnoses and the severity of the retardation. Those individuals who have a physical impairment in addition to the MR will have involvement in the sensory integration, neuromuscular, and motor components. When MR occurs without additional diagnoses, the cognitive, psychological, social, and self-management performance components will be most affected. When both physical and mental impairment are present, dysfunction will be more pervasive. The following case studies illustrate how MR affects an individual's occupational performance in different stages of the lifecycle.

CASE STUDIES

CASE 1

K. K. is a 21-year-old young woman with Down syndrome. Despite the fact that she has reached the legal age of adulthood, she is still in the process of transitioning from the developmental stage of adolescence to young adulthood. She still receives special education services but is also working on developing work and job skills through traditional vocational services. Her "disability" is expected to be lifelong.

K. K.'s condition was identified at birth. She has received continuous support and direct services to facilitate development of her abilities since then. She has always lived at home with her parents and still does so. She has her own room and bathroom at home and generally has exclusive use of the family room for her leisure pursuits. Her parents are professionals who are actively involved in their professions and the community. They are very realistic about her abilities and extremely supportive, allowing her to make most of her life choices. K. K. has a younger sister who is now away at college. K. K. has always been exposed to and involved in many social and cultural opportunities in the community, both with her family and on her own. Her social circle includes friends with and without disabilities and she has several close friends as well as many social acquaintances.

K. K. has recently declared her life goals to be getting a job, getting an apartment of her own, and spending leisure time at the local community drop-in/recreational center for individuals with disabilities. Her mother feels that, with appropriate supports, all of these goals are attainable.

K. K. is independent in most areas of personal care. Due to limited fine motor coordination that seems to be complicated by visual perceptual deficits, she needs assistance with regulating the water temperature for her bath, fastening zippers and buttons, and tying her shoes. She also occasionally needs reminders to straighten her clothing and brush the back of her hair. She has a speech impediment that makes it difficult for individuals who are unfamiliar with her to initially understand her. K. K. has learned to adapt to this limitation and works very hard to make people understand what she is trying to communicate. When cued, she will slow down and work on enunciating her words. She is independent in functional mobility but because of problems with depth perception, she is very cautious when climbing steps and negotiating between different surface levels. She is able to travel independently in community areas she is familiar with and can ride the community "Dial-a-Ride" bus if the ride is arranged for her. Her mother feels that K. K. would be aware of danger in her home, such as a fire, and would get out of the house. She does not consistently answer the phone when it rings, although she is capable of doing so. For this reason, she is generally not allowed to be at home alone because her parents have no way of checking in with her if she does not answer the phone.

K. K. is able to perform many home management tasks and has recently become motivated to attempt more activities given her desire to have an apartment of her own. She generally dislikes "housework" but knows it is necessary in order to be a good roommate. She folds laundry and puts it away, and is learning to sort light and dark clothing and operate the washing machine. Her mother questions her ability to make judgments about what should or should not go into the dryer, however. She is able to sweep, vacuum, and dust but is not thorough and this may be a result of her lack of interest and/or her visual-perceptual impairment. She keeps her bathroom clean and makes her bed. She is currently dependent in meal preparation and this is the area that will probably require the most support for her to live in her own apartment. She cannot safely regulate stove and oven temperatures because of her fine motor problems.

At the current time, K. K. attends class in a self-contained special education classroom in the local high school for half a day, focusing on vocational and prevocational skills, and spends the other half-day at Goodwill Industries in a work adjustment trial placement. K. K. has told her mother that she no longer enjoys going to school and would rather go to Goodwill. In addition to school and vocational activities, K. K. volunteers at the local community theater and at her church office doing clerical tasks. She is very interested in obtaining employment and would prefer to work at a video store, a music store, at the mall, or Pizza Hut. She is very interested in clerical tasks and has been working at her father's medical practice putting monthly billings in envelopes to be mailed.

K. K. has many leisure interests and activities. She enjoys music and videos, likes to eat out, participates in Special Olympics, goes to a community center for structured activities, and socializes with her friends. She prefers not to do strenuous physical activities, probably because of the difficulty she has as a result of generalized hypotonia. She has participated in team sports at the center but does so mostly for the social interaction. K. K. is very aware of her limitations and takes herself out of situations that she knows will be difficult or where she might not succeed.

CASE 2

F. B. is a 60-year-old gentleman who is mentally retarded. He has a history of behavior problems, including pica and obsessive-compulsive type behaviors of picking at his skin and clothing and stuffing toilets. He was retired from a sheltered workshop approximately 18 months ago when the emphasis of the program shifted to work readiness for community placement. It was determined that he would not be a good candidate for community work because of his age and lack of necessary supports (i.e., transportation). He currently attends a day program for social/leisure activities. F. B. has no known family and has spent most of his life in public residential institutions or in adult foster care (AFC) homes. He currently has a court-appointed guardian who makes most significant life decisions for him, including those regarding medical care and living arrangements. His guardian supports and encourages F. B. to make his wishes known about how he would like to spend his leisure time and allowed him input into his last housing change. In addition to his intellectual limitations, F. B. also experiences fairly frequent medical problems related to his obsessive-compulsive behaviors (i.e., skin infections). Medical problems, which may be age related, are emphysema and frequent fractures of bones in his lower extremities. F. B. currently lives in an adult AFC with 11 other adults who are developmentally disabled. His home is only required by law to provide basic care and so does not offer training in or support for participation in many home management tasks. His social groups generally consist of other adults with developmental disabilities or paid paraprofessional staff, either at home or the day program. His cultural experiences have been very limited and because of his background, it would be fair to say that he has been encultured as a "mentally retarded person."

F. B. is independent in most self-care tasks but needs supervision when using the bathroom because of his history of stuffing the toilet. He needs assistance and supports for taking medication owing to his cognitive limitations. He also needs very close monitoring of health status because he has a very high pain tolerance. He tends to prefer solitary activities but has become more verbal, social, and outgoing since going to the day program. He generally seeks out staff to interact with, and this usually takes the form of teasing. He will share activities with day program peers if prompted and has shown protective behaviors toward clients who are more limited and vulnerable than he is. Although he is verbal, he has a speech impediment that makes it difficult for people who are unfamiliar with him to understand what he is saying. He is independently ambulatory; however, he has reduced endurance as a result of an old hip fracture and neuropathy of the right lower extremity caused by degenerative disease in the lumbar spine. He is dependent for all community mobility as a result of cognitive limitations and lack of experience and training. It is not clear whether he understands emergency situations, but he is cooperative with emergency drill procedures at the day program. It is likely that he would need ongoing supervision to maintain his personal safety.

Because of a lack of experience and opportunity, F. B. is dependent in all home management tasks. He has no responsibility for caring for others but seems to be very aware when one of his peers needs assistance or protection and alerts staff to these needs. He has been retired from the vocational arena for 18 months and now attends a day program that emphasizes social and leisure activities.

F. B. is generally not open to exploring new activities and has to be coaxed and teased by staff to try them. He generally prefers solitary activities and appears to enjoy assembly activities that result in a finished product like picture puzzles and building with Erector-Set components. He does not seem to be very interested in watching television or listening to music but does enjoying going on automobile rides with his guardian, especially when she drives her convertible with the top down.

Acknowledgments

The author would like to acknowledge and thank Mary Steichen Yamamoto for her work on developmental disabilities in the first edition of this text. A great deal of the information that she contributed about genetic and environmental causes of retardation was left intact and used in this chapter, as were the tables and the case studies concerning single gene disorders and levels of retardation.

POINTS FOR REVIEW

1. What three criteria are used to determine if a person is "mentally retarded"?

2. Describe the two types of genetic disorders that can cause MR and the patterns of transmission for each subtype.

3. Describe the three-step classification process that was developed by the AAMR to classify different levels of MR.

4. Discuss the factors that determine the impact of MR on an individual's occupational performance.

REFERENCES

1. Drews C, Yeargin-Allsopp M, Decoufle P, et al. Variation in the influence of selected sociodemographic risk factors for mental retardation. A J Public Health 1995;85:329–334.

2. American Association on Mental Retardation, American Psychiatric Association. Diagnostic and Statistical Manual of Mental Disorders. 4th ed. Washington, DC: 1994.

3. American Association on Mental Retardation. Mental retardation: Definition, classification, and systems of supports. 9th ed. Washington, DC: 1992.

4. Yeargin-Allsopp M, Murphy C, Cordero J, et al. Reported biomedical causes and associated medical conditions for mental retardation among 10-year-old children, metropolitan Atlanta, 1985 to 1987. Dev Med Child Neurol 1997;39:142–147.

5. Introduction to Mental Retardation. Arlington, TX: The Arc, 1993. (http://www.thearc.org/)

6. Matilainen R, Airaksinen E, Monomen T, et al. A population-based study on the causes of mild and severe mental retardation. Acta Paediatr 1995;84:261–266.

7. Scriver C. The metabolic and molecular bases of inherited disease. 7th ed. New York: McGraw-Hill, 1995.

8. Genetic Causes of Mental Retardation. Arlington, TX: The Arc, 1996. (http://www.thearc.org/)

9. Kaplan H, Sadock B, Grebb J. Synopsis of Psychiatry. 7th ed. Baltimore: Williams & Wilkins, 1994.

10. Rogers B, et al. Neurodevelopmental outcome of infants with hypoplastic left heart syndrome. J Pediatr 1995;126:496–498.

11. Reuss M, Paneth M, Pinto-Martin J, Lorenz J, Susser M. The relation of transient hypothyroxinemia in preterm infants to neurologic development at two years of age. N Engl J Med 1996;334:821–827.

12. Jardim L, Palma-Dias R, Silva L, et al. Maternal hyperphenylalaninemia as a cause of microcephaly and mental retardation. Acta Paediatr 1996;85:943–946.

13. Gror M, Shekleton M. Basic pathophysiology, a conceptual approach. St. Louis: CV Mosby, 1979.

14. Harris S, Tada W. Genetic disorders. In: Umphred D, ed. Neurological Rehabilitation. St. Louis: CV Mosby, 1990.

15. Baraff L, Lee S, Schriger D. Outcomes of bacterial meningitis in children: a meta-analysis. Pediatr Infect Dis J 1993;12:389–394.

16. Frayers T. Epidemiological thinking in mental retardation: issues in taxonomy and population frequency. Int Rev Res Ment Retard 1993;19:97–133.

17. Hauser M, Ratey J. The patient with mental retardation. In: Hyman S, Tesar G, eds. The Manual of Psychiatric Emergencies. Boston: Little Brown & Co, 1994:104–109. (http://www.psychiatry.com/)

18. Silka V, Hauser M. Psychiatric assessment of the person with mental retardation. Psychiatr Ann 1997;27:3. (http://www.psychiatry.com/)

19. Reiss S, Goldberg B, Ryan R. Mental illness in persons with mental retardation. Arlington, TX: The Arc, 1993. (http://www.thearc.org/)

20. Zigman W, Schupf N, Zigman A, et al. Aging and Alzheimer disease in people with mental retardation. Int Rev Res Ment Retard 1993;19:41–70.

21. Behrman R, Kliegman R, Nelson W, et al, eds. Nelson's Textbook of Pediatrics. 14th ed. Philadelphia: WB Saunders, 1992.

22. Berkow R, Fletcher A, eds. The Merck Manual of Diagnosis and Therapy. 15th ed. Rahway: Merck Sharp & Dohme Research Laboratories, 1987.

SUGGESTED READINGS

Behrman R, Kliegman R, Nelson W, et al, eds. Nelson's Textbook of Pediatrics. 14th ed. Philadelphia: WB Saunders, 1992. *Good medical reference for common and rare conditions found in childhood. Expensive, but available in reference section of most libraries.*

Case-Smith J, Allen A, Pratt P. Occupational Therapy for Children. 3rd ed. St. Louis: Mosby, 1996. *Good overall reference for occupational therapy practice with children. Has separate chapters dealing with many issues and performance problems faced by children with mental retardation.*

American Association on Mental Retardation. Mental Retardation: Definition, Classification, and Systems of Support. 9th ed. Washington DC: 1992. *Good overall reference on mental retardation that looks at performance in a functional manner.*

CHAPTER 5

SCHIZOPHRENIA

Yvonne Russell Teske

CRITICAL TERMS

Agranulocytosis
Akathisia
Akinesia
Alogia
Anhedonia
Antiadrenergic
Anticholinergic

Avolition
Blunt affect
Catalepsy
Delusion
Echolalia
Echopraxia
Neuroleptic

Parkinsonism
Psychosis
Sensory gating deficit
Tachycardia
Tardive dyskinesia
Volition
Waxy flexibility

Today is Susan's first day as an occupational therapy student at the community mental health living skills center. In the coffee room, she notices a tall, slender young man leaning against the wall. Like the other men in the room, he wears layers of shirts and sweaters under a well-worn down vest. Over the vest, he wears a large jacket.

"Hello, my name is Susan. I'm an occupational therapy student just starting here today." The man looks at Susan, looks away, and then looks again while shifting his balance from side to side.

"Hi, who?" He answers and laughs as if something is funny.

"Susan."

"Jake, I'm Jake; I like Venus, you too?" He laughs and restlessly paces the floor.

"Mmm, I guess so. What do you like to do?"

"Do, do, hmm, sing?" Jake slides along the wall toward the door.

"Great, it must be great to sing. Do you like rock?" Susan asks as she follows Jake from the room.

"Rock, what rock, rock, lock. I have to go now." Jake laughingly repeats the words.

As Jake starts moving away, the occupational therapist approaches and asks him if he would like to shoot pool with Susan. Jake stops laughing, sighs deeply, and heads toward the pool table with Susan following. Later, Susan's supervisor describes Jake's inability to follow the pace or meaning in normal conversation and his frequent grinning and laughter. She says that these problems are more noticeable after nights when the shelter where he stays has been full and noisy. She tells of his first episode of schizophrenia, when he was a music student at the local university.

INTRODUCTION

Schizophrenia is a psychiatric disorder that can affect all areas of occupational performance. The natural course of the disorder often leads to disintegration of sensorimotor, cognitive, and psychosocial abilities. Because of the apparent disintegration, Emil Kraepelin, almost 100 years ago, called the disorder dementia praecox. He described the clinical picture of early dementia he saw in young adults admitted to nineteenth century mental hospitals (1).

Eugene Bleuler used the word schizophrenia to communicate a lack of integration among the mental functions of thought, perception, and emotion. Patients showed an absence of will, interest, attention, facial expression, and emotion. They showed diminished movement in response to stimulation and feedback from the environment. Their peculiar speech, movements, and habits showed a focus on themselves. Bleuler called the unusual absences of behavior and diminished responsiveness negative symptoms (1).

Later psychiatrists observed language and motor behavior they believed was excessive and unrelated to environmental demands. Psychiatrists called the patients' peculiar sensory perceptions, hallucinations, and the highly personal and rigid thoughts, delusions. The two patterns—one describing an absence of normally expected behavior called negative symptoms and another describing an excess of normally expected behavior called delusions and hallucinations—remain key concepts psychiatrists use to diagnose schizophrenia.

ETIOLOGY

Because so much remains unknown about schizophrenia, questions arise about the link between the observable symptoms and the abnormalities that cause them.

Three approaches to etiology and pathophysiology attempt to link symptoms and cause. The first approach views schizophrenia as one homogeneous disorder—a single disorder from a single abnormality. In this approach, one abnormality leads to many groups of symptoms. The second approach says that schizophrenia is a syndrome consisting of several disorders, each with its own abnormality and related symptoms. The third approach describes schizophrenia as a homogeneous disorder with widely varying symptoms. This approach organizes the varied symptoms into groups, each with its own etiology and pathophysiology (2). Although international advances in data collection and analytic methods have improved research quality, extensive research shows no single cause of schizophrenia. No single theory is supported by sufficient data to explain a cause, and no single abnormality consistently identifies schizophrenia as separate from other disorders. In this chapter, a discussion of etiology will include information on neuroanatomy, genetics, and other risk factors.

Neuroanatomy

No one abnormality is common to most patients with schizophrenia, even though extensive research indicates several sites of brain abnormalities. Brain anatomy and physiology are being studied, both in individuals who currently have schizophrenia and in postmortem examinations. Imaging methods such as positron emission tomography are expanding research opportunities, while at the same time increasing the possibility of study error because of their complexity (2).

The most consistent finding from both postmortem and imaging studies is enlargement of the lateral and third ventricles of the brain in 15 to 30% of those with schizophrenia when compared with controls (3). Ventricular enlargement usually means brain tissue has been lost after the skull has completed growth. So far, no relationship has been found between ventricular enlargement and brain tissue atrophy. In addition, comprehensive studies have shown no consistent relationship between enlarged ventricles and potential factors such as obstetrical complications, social function before illness, genetics, or the age of the person at the onset of schizophrenia. Several studies do show enlarged ventricles in persons with chronic schizophrenia. Other health conditions involving the brain also show enlarged ventricles, and so the anatomical finding is not unique to schizophrenia (3).

In about 25% of schizophrenic patients, computerized tomography (CT) scans show mild cerebral atrophy, both in those newly diagnosed and in chronic patients (4). The atrophy is not unique to schizophrenia; it is not progressive but may be evidence of earlier brain injury. According to researchers, earlier brain injury may leave a person vulnerable to many risk factors connected with schizophrenia. However, patients who have schizophrenia and mild cerebral atrophy often show mild neurological signs of impairment and severe negative symptoms. These include apathy, withdrawal, and a poor level of function before diagnosis. This group of patients shows a poor response to treatment (4).

Current research appears to be moving toward the idea that brain etiology and pathophysiology in schizophrenia take place in the complex interconnections among several locations in the brain. Researchers call the interconnections "neuronal circuits." For example, studies have focused on neuronal circuits that involve the prefrontal cortex and the limbic system, as well as those that involve the temporal cortex, the hippocampus in the limbic system, and the anterior cingulate of the basal ganglia. The concept that abnormalities in brain anatomy and physiology could be located in neuronal circuits linking several areas of the brain could explain the diverse sensorimotor, cognitive, and psychosocial disabilities seen in persons with schizophrenia (5, 6).

Genetics

A close genetic link with someone who has schizophrenia increases a person's risk of schizophrenia. An individual who has an identical twin with schizophrenia has a 48% risk of becoming schizophrenic too (4). The twin with schizophrenia is more likely to have a history of obstetric complications. From this primary risk, the risk declines according to the genetic closeness of family members: children with both parents who have schizophrenia, then immediate relatives including aunts, uncles, and grandparents. The risk declines to 1% in the general population. Children with one parent who has schizophrenia do not have an increased risk of having the disorder. Approximately 85 to 90% of cases of schizophrenia show no family history of the disorder (4).

To study genetic factors in the etiology and pathophysiology of schizophrenia, researchers look for measurable irregularities that appear to be associated with schizophrenia in families. Some, but not all, family members may inherit the irregularities. The discovery of a link between unique irregularities and schizophrenia is important because genetic linkages do not change over time, as do behavioral symptoms. The consistent and stable irregularities are called "markers." Some genetic markers are found in about 50% of immediate family members of persons with schizophrenia. Deficits in smooth-pursuit eye movements (SPEM) and in the ability to screen out irrelevant stimuli are two examples.

Most people can follow moving objects across their visual field with slow, coordinated eye movements called SPEM (7). Slow and fast eye movements work together. Once the object starts to move, a short, fast eye movement helps the retina catch up. While the object crosses the retina, the fast movements are inhibited and slow pursuit of the object takes over. In schizophrenia, rapid eye movements are not inhibited, and they interrupt slow eye pursuits. People without SPEM can neither pursue a moving object smoothly nor move their heads across a line of print. The abnormal genetic marker also appears in nonschizophrenic family members of persons who have schizophrenia.

The capacity to discriminate and attend is the result of the limbic system's gating function. A deficit in the ability to screen out irrelevant stimuli is called the "sensory gating deficit." Persons who have the deficit are unable to filter out background sounds in the environment, for example people talking, appliance noise, or traffic sounds. Normal individuals can prevent themselves from reacting to sounds not relevant to the task at hand. They "close the gate," not allowing themselves to respond. The presence of a sensory gating deficit leads to hypervigilance. These people are unable to prevent themselves from responding. They become disturbed and distracted by the stimuli (8).

Because individuals who have schizophrenia, as well as their close relatives who do not have schizophrenia, show the sensory gating deficit, a link may exist between abnormalities in the limbic system and genetic variations. Persons who become schizophrenic and have the sensory gating deficit have a smaller hippocampus—part of the limbic system—than healthy siblings who also have the gating deficit (4).

Other Risk Factors

Risk factors for getting schizophrenia, such as the time of year a person is born or whether they are single or married, are based on studies of groups of people and cannot be used to determine the chances of an individual becoming schizophrenic. However, researchers who are pursuing answers to questions about etiology are investigating relationships between population risk factors, genetics, and neuroanatomy, hoping to improve their ability to predict who might be stricken with schizophrenia.

One risk factor is the season of birth. About 10% of those treated for schizophrenia were born in the late winter or early spring season. Although an extensive number of research studies show no theory or explanation for the pattern, several factors may play a part. Nutritional, infectious, or other unknown factors associated with cool weather may affect the second trimester of fetal development. In the month of March, premature births, which are associated with minimal brain damage, are more common. Minimal brain damage may increase a person's risk for schizophrenia. The link between birth complications and winter births is seen in mental retardation, depression, and other mental illnesses. Older mothers may be vulnerable to nutritional deficits

or infectious illnesses associated with winter births. Schizophrenia is more likely to be diagnosed in children born to older mothers, according to studies conducted in several countries. Births to older women are more frequent in the winter months from January through March (4).

Schizophrenia is more common in lower socioeconomic groups in developed countries. Higher rates of mental disorders, particularly schizophrenia, are concentrated in central, urban, and low-income areas of major American and European cities. Increased stress from daily life events and neurological impairment from infectious diseases and childhood head trauma, all more common in cities, are believed to be possible risk factors (4).

When looking at results of international studies of incidence of schizophrenia, men and women have an equal risk of having schizophrenia; men, however, have earlier onset. For men, the first episode of symptoms often happens in late adolescence or the early 20s. For women, the first episode usually occurs when they are in their late 20s or early 30s (9). Unmarried people show a greater risk of schizophrenia. Some studies suggest that the symptoms and problems associated with schizophrenia may act as a barrier to getting married (4).

Other studies cite stress as a cause of schizophrenia. According to data collected from both developing and developed countries, persons with schizophrenia experience about the same levels of stress before their episodes of illness as those with other psychiatric disorders. Stress is not a risk factor unique to schizophrenia (4).

Studies of the relationship between migration from one country to another and onset of schizophrenia show an inconsistent pattern. In fact, being born in a country as a second-generation immigrant increases the likelihood of schizophrenia. According to some studies of etiology, children born to immigrant mothers have a higher risk of schizophrenia, possibly related to the combination of increased maternal viral infections, obstetric factors, and changing responses of the maternal immune system (4).

INCIDENCE AND PREVALENCE

Standardized international measurement methods and diagnostic criteria are reducing the variability of incidence and prevalence across countries. In the United States, fewer than 1 adult in 100, age 15 to 54, will have schizophrenia in a lifetime. Childhood schizophrenia is rare. Although schizophrenia is a severe psychiatric disorder, its prevalence is considered low. In the United States, the direct costs of treating individuals with schizophrenia and the indirect costs of losses, such as fewer workers, amounted to $33 billion in 1990 (10).

Some comparisons of the prevalence of physical illnesses among persons with schizophrenia, mood disorders, and normal individuals show that those with schizophrenia have about the same incidence of such major physical illnesses as cancer, cardiovascular disease, diabetes, and others (11). However, according to World Health Organization data, those with schizophrenia have increased chances of dying of most other serious medical problems, except cancer (4). Internationally, the incidence of lung cancer is lower for patients with schizophrenia, even with their heavier-than-average smoking. One possible explanation is the presence of a gene to suppress lung cancer; another is the possible protective effect of medications used to treat schizophrenia. Persons who have schizophrenia are less likely to have rheumatoid arthritis than the general population, but the reason is unknown (4, 11).

SIGNS AND SYMPTOMS

The symptoms of schizophrenia include diverse sensorimotor disabilities. Some examples are the inability to interpret sights, sounds, and touch, irregular eye movements, and orientation to space and the environment. The symptoms also include a variety of cognitive and psychological disabilities in inferential and abstract thinking, language, attention, social interaction, emotional expression, and volition. Based on data from large-scale, longitudinal studies of persons with schizophrenia, major symptoms considered typical of schizophrenia are grouped together according to whether they are associated with psychosis, disorganization, or negative symptoms. Psychosis is associated with the major observable symptoms of delusions and hallucinations. A person can be called psychotic when delusions and hallucinations are present (12–14).

Disorganization includes the observable behaviors of disorganized speech, disorganized behavior, and affect that appears inappropriate for the situation. The emphasis on observable behavior is a move away from drawing conclusions about unobservable mental processes. The move to observable behavior recognizes the complexity of sensorimotor, cognitive, and psychosocial performance.

Negative symptoms may not be noticed. They represent diminished function or the absence of normally present behavior. They include avolition, anhedonia, blunt affect, short attention, and alogia. Alogia and attention impairment usually appear with negative symptoms but can be part of disorganization (12) (Table 5.1).

COURSE AND PROGNOSIS

The course of schizophrenia and the prognosis for persons who have it show tremendous variability. A person's symptoms, the subtype of schizophrenia, response to treatment drugs, and acceptance of treatment approaches are some of the factors that play a part. In the time of Kraepelin and Bleuler, course and prognosis were negative, with patients showing very poor outcomes. Now, the combination of medications, shorter periods of hospitalization, and new treatment approaches means fewer people experience long-term hospitalization.

According to Stevens, persons with schizophrenia experience one of three possible courses of illness: a single episode of symptoms with almost total recovery, repeated episodes with moderate recovery in between, and a progressive slide into long-term disability (3). Estimates are that about one-third make significant and lasting

TABLE 5.1 Symptoms of Schizophrenia	
SYMPTOM GROUP	**SYMPTOMS**
Psychosis	Delusions, distortion of inferential thinking Hallucinations, distortion of perception
Disorganization	Disorganized speech Disorganized behavior Affect regulation, inappropriate affect
Negative Symptoms	Avolition, lack of will and purposeful activity Anhedonia, lack of pleasure Blunt affect, lack of emotional expression Attention impairment Alogia, decrease in speech fluency

improvement; one-third show some improvement with periodic episodes of symptoms; and one-third become permanently incapacitated (15).

Some studies investigating the course of schizophrenia show periods of increased rehospitalizations up to about 2 years after initial onset, followed by a decline in rehospitalization (16). With repeated hospitalizations, patients and families expect fewer positive results from the hospital stays; a cure is not expected. Unless the person becomes unmanageable, the family copes alone or with community support. Less frequent rehospitalizations may mean a decline in dramatic symptoms after treatment or may be a result of the natural course of the disorder.

Individuals with schizophrenia may not deteriorate over time. They fluctuate between severe and moderate disability, with some experiencing moderate periods of remission (16). Although not continually hospitalized, most people do fail to return to normal function in work and social skills. About 5 to 10 years after onset and disability, some people show symptom stability and improved abilities (15).

When compared with other patients with psychosis, persons with schizophrenia recover more slowly and are less likely to show improvement in follow-up periods. Individuals with schizophrenia show a poorer outcome than those with other psychoses, such as mood disorders (16).

The presence of medical disorders and substance abuse has some effect on the course and prognosis of schizophrenia. The death rate in schizophrenia is two to four times greater than that in the general population and the life span is about 10 years shorter. The shorter life span result from several factors, including higher rates of suicide, deaths from traumatic injuries, and deaths from unknown causes (11). Hallucinations and suicidal tendencies dramatically increase the risk of death in schizophrenia, and 10% of patients do commit suicide (17). Persons with schizophrenia also are at risk from injury during repeated episodes of symptoms and from adverse reactions to medications.

Individuals with schizophrenia are more likely to abuse multiple substances than the general population. Substance abuse increases the chances that those with schizophrenia will refuse medications and other treatment. Their prognosis is poor. The odds of alcohol abuse or dependence are 3.3 times higher, and drug-abuse disorder is 6 times higher (11). Recent studies of addiction show that persistent drug use modifies brain function. Drug addiction especially influences neuronal circuits to the limbic and prefrontal areas of the brain (18). Substance abuse increases the severity of symptoms, behavioral problems, and the number of rehospitalizations.

According to the American Psychiatric Association, homelessness and schizophrenia are linked, with about one-third of homeless people having mental illness, primarily schizophrenia (17). Estimates of the prevalence of schizophrenia over a lifetime for those who are homeless range from 1.4 to 30.3%, higher percentages than in the general population (4). Homelessness is one outcome of substance abuse, and substance abuse is a major factor in homelessness of persons with schizophrenia (11).

Negative symptoms are associated with poor premorbid adjustment, before the onset of schizophrenia, possibly as a result of brain structure and neurodevelopmental abnormalities. Individuals who have negative symptoms show a poorer response to treatment, including medications, and a poorer treatment outcome. Negative symptoms can prevent people from working, returning to school, or performing critical life roles (15).

DIAGNOSIS

The process of making a comprehensive and accurate clinical diagnosis to guide treatment is complex. Unlike many other chronic health conditions, no useful laboratory or imaging markers guide diagnosis and treatment (1). Accuracy depends on patient cooperation, medication status, medical reports regarding health problems, family interviews, case history, and scores from structured assessments. If the patient is disruptive, violent, or withdrawn, accurate information may be impossible to gather. Observable behavior gives some information. However, by the time the individual sees a psychiatrist, he or she may show symptoms greatly diminished by medications prescribed by a primary care physician. Psychiatrists may conduct interviews with the patient and family over time and may use information from case conferences to increase the accuracy of assessment and treatment.

Several well-studied assessments can contribute to diagnosis and treatment. Andreasen developed two extensive assessment scales that lead to a rating of positive symptoms in the scale for the assessment of positive symptoms (SAPS), and a rating of negative symptoms in the scale for the assessment of negative symptoms (SANS) (19, 20).

In the United States, the *Diagnostic and Statistical Manual IV (DSM IV)* (9) provides standard criteria for psychiatric diagnosis. The *DSM IV* presents specific criteria to distinguish between schizophrenia and conditions like mood disorders, substance abuse, and medical conditions. The *DSM IV* aims to improve diagnosis, treatment, and communication among mental health professionals. The system resulted from extensive review of literature, reanalyses of research data and results, and field studies of psychiatrists using the *DSM IV* to assess patients. This manual is also used to collect standard data for research about psychiatric disorders (1).

The *DSM IV* includes six criteria, A through F, covering characteristic symptoms, duration, and the extent of dysfunction in major life areas such as work, interpersonal relationships, and self-care. The criteria also include guidelines for differentiating between schizophrenia and diagnoses of mood disorders, substance abuse, general medical conditions, autism, and pervasive developmental disorders (9).

Criterion A requires two or more of the symptoms of delusions, hallucinations, disorganized speech, disorganized behavior, and negative symptoms to make a diagnosis of schizophrenia. The person must have the symptoms for most of a 1-month period. Criterion B requires functional decline in one or more areas of work, interpersonal relations, or self-care for much of the time since the beginning of symptoms. Criterion C requires that some disruption and some level of symptoms be present for at least 6 months (9). All three criteria are important in making a diagnosis of schizophrenia.

Criteria D, E, and F attempt to exclude other disorders as primary or coexisting diagnoses. Criterion D asks the psychiatrist to rule out mood disorders as an explanation for the present symptoms and performance problems. Criterion E excludes substance abuse and general medical disorders as the primary cause of the present symptoms and problems. Criterion F refers to pervasive developmental disorders usually diagnosed in childhood. If a diagnosis of pervasive developmental disorder had been made previously, then at the current time, prominent delusions and hallucinations must have been present for at least 1 month (9).

Beyond the initial diagnoses of schizophrenia, the *DSM IV* uses symptoms to further define subtypes of schizophrenia: disorganized, catatonic, paranoid, residual, and undifferentiated. This helps psychiatrists and mental health professionals to match treatment more closely with symptoms.

Disorganized Type

The person shows a mixture of disorganization and negative symptoms with disorganized speech and behavior, blunt or inappropriate affect like silliness and laughter, and grimacing. Onset is slow and almost undetectable. Personality and social problems before onset gradually lead to a diagnosis. The course of the disorganized type of schizophrenia is continuous and steady without dramatic remissions or exacerbations (9).

Catatonic Type

Catatonia, although rarely seen today in the United States, is still present in developing countries. The dominant symptoms of the catatonic type are sensorimotor. The person may be immobile and stuporous, showing catalepsy and waxy flexibility. When a person is in a cataleptic or trance-like state, the arms or legs will retain the position in which they are placed. The limbs, once placed, hold their form like wax. Conversely, the person may show excessive, purposeless, or odd movements and unusual facial mannerisms like grimacing. He or she may be mute and extremely negative. The unusual speech and movements of echolalia and echopraxia may accompany these symptoms. Echolalia involves repetition of a word or phrase just said by another person in a way that shows no understanding of the meaning, like a parrot. Echopraxia is the involuntary repetition of another person's movement. Safety is an important concern when a person shows the wide range of symptoms of catatonia. Some areas of danger are self-injury, malnutrition, exhaustion, and excessively high body temperature (9).

Paranoid Type

In this subtype, cognitive and sensorimotor abilities are normal. Paranoid schizophrenia shows a later onset and better prognosis for role function, including self-care and work. The person shows obvious and often dramatic delusions and hallucinations while affect and mental ability usually are normal. The themes of delusions and hallucinations often are coherent and well organized. Common themes are jealousy, religion, and physical issues or problems (9).

Those who have delusions of persecution believe they are being harassed, cheated, and persistently ill treated in several ways. They may feel harassed by people they know, like relatives and neighbors, as well as politicians, political parties, and the government. They may take legal action against the persecutors in cases that last for years. Although individuals who feel persecuted may feel isolated, they also seek isolation.

Persons who have delusions of grandeur believe their worth, value, or importance to be greater than the evidence shows. For example, one patient had a well-organized belief that everyone existed on one of seven levels. He believed that most people were on the first, second, or third level, but he was on the seventh level close to God. He said he felt protected, that personal criticism did not matter.

Persons who have delusions of reference strongly believe they are the focus of events, objects, and the behavior of other people. The comments of others and daily events take on unusual and personal, often negative, meaning. For example, one young woman felt that other people were calling her a whore. She believed that she heard the telephone ring, most likely an hallucination, and when she went to answer it, she said the caller called her a whore. She did not express feeling persecuted by the world or the caller, but was certain the call was for her.

Residual Type

This diagnosis is made when a person has had at least one episode of symptoms in the past but currently does not show delusions, hallucinations, or disorganization. Alternatively, the person can have negative symptoms or two or more mild psychotic symptoms. The episodes can be time limited, part of a transitional period in a person's life, or continuous (9).

Undifferentiated Type

The person has psychoses with delusions, hallucinations, disorganized speech and behavior, but symptoms either overlap other diagnostic types or do not match any one type. Symptoms usually are observed early in life in childhood behavior problems resembling attention deficit disorder. The outcome is varied, but often symptoms are quiet (9).

MEDICAL/SURGICAL MANAGEMENT

Treatment involves developing a plan for a person with schizophrenia who may require years of comprehensive and continuous care. For most patients, schizophrenia is a chronic health problem. The treatment team aims to reduce the number and length of recurring episodes of disruptive symptoms and the occupational dysfunction the symptoms cause. At the same time, the team enables optimal function between episodes, working to even out the cycles of function and dysfunction. The treatment team, patient, and family must make important decisions about medications, living situation, and support treatments. The fact that treatment may continue for years, even a lifetime, poses a great challenge to providing continuous care. The patients will receive mental health care longer than staff members who provide that care may be in their helping positions.

From onset, the patient receives treatment in three phases: acute, stabilization, and stable (17).

Acute-phase goals emphasize safety, symptom reduction, and behavior control. Quickly, team members begin a supportive relationship with the patient and family that will lead to the care network tailored to return the person with schizophrenia to optimal function. Comprehensive yet rapid assessment helps determine threats to safety like hallucinations and delusions. In addition, it helps determine what substance abuse and medical conditions are complicating factors requiring referral to appropriate treatment.

A primary psychiatric goal of the acute phase is matching medications to the symptoms the person presents. To be both acceptable to the patient and effective in diminishing symptoms, the medication must offer the greatest behavior and symptom control with the least discomfort.

The psychiatrist and team structure a low-stress, protective environment aimed at the safest yet least restrictive setting. If the patient is dangerous to self or others and requires careful monitoring of medications to avoid adverse reactions, the hospital is often the placement in the acute phase. However, placement also depends on the availability of alternative treatment settings and the patient's acceptance of voluntary treatment, including medications. Alternative settings might include crisis centers, partial hospitalization, day hospitals, and home care.

During the stabilization phase, many approaches are combined to prevent patient relapse and recurring episodes and to ease transition to community life. The treatment team aims to reduce both the amount of stress the person feels and unrealistic expectations from family members and others. Treatment activities help the patient in the difficult process of self acceptance. Psychiatrists may adjust medications to continue symptom reduction.

In the stable phase, treatment goals are to maintain or improve occupational performance and to monitor the patient for symptoms of schizophrenia and treatment side effects. Patients are ready for increased psychosocial treatment, including living skills education, social skills training, cognitive rehabilitation, and beginning vocational rehabilitation. Long-term medication management consists of balancing the risk of relapse with side effects.

Medications

Almost all people with schizophrenia can benefit from medications (21). Medications can reduce the initial disturbing symptoms, improve symptoms between episodes, and prevent future episodes. The advent of drug treatment has reduced the need for long-term care in mental institutions and has returned the treatment environment to community settings. Drugs have allowed people to maintain and establish new social relationships shown to be important in maintaining occupational performance. Drugs allow individuals to perform valued roles in activities of daily living (ADL), work, and leisure.

Physicians administering medications weigh several factors when deciding on the best dose for a particular person. People vary greatly in their tolerance and sensitivity to medications. Considerations include age, phase of treatment, method of taking the medication, patient willingness to comply with the medication regimen, and manageability of side effects (17). The elderly show more sensitivity to drug dosage and side effects.

For all of the benefits of drugs, patients and families resist drug treatment. Resistance may come from family and cultural beliefs about the use of medications in treating health problems. Drugs used in acute illnesses reduce symptoms and cure problems in a short time. When used to treat chronic health problems, drugs can diminish symptoms and prevent relapse over the long term. During a period when an ill patient is symptom-free, the patient does not actively experience the preventive effects of the drugs. Persons who have chronic illnesses often stop taking even the most powerful drugs when they have no symptoms. People expect drugs to help an illness. With symptoms reduced, patients with schizophrenia may believe they no longer need the drug or that the drug can no longer do them good. They stop taking their medication.

When drugs focus on major body systems, they often have side effects on other, unrelated parts of the body. Drugs for schizophrenia are no exception. Patients may experience uncomfortable and even disabling side effects. Drug treatment requires careful monitoring and assertive outreach to patients who fail to keep appointments. Depending on the age of onset, patients may require monitoring for more than 40 years. Patient resistance, and other factors that may cause compliance problems with drug regimens, increase the importance of patient and family education. When a patient with active symptoms is unable to understand the drug's effects on reducing and preventing symptoms, the family can encourage the patient to continue medications.

Antipsychotic medications refer to conventional neuroleptic medications, such as haloperidol and fluphenazine, as well as clozapine and risperidone. Conventional antipsychotic drugs have been used for more than 40 years to reduce symptoms of psychoses, disorganization, and negative symptoms for patients with schizophrenia. Neuroleptic drugs are dopamine antagonists because they oppose the excessive activity of the neurotransmitter, dopamine, which projects to the cortex. Several large studies show that antipsychotic medications reduce hallucinations, lack of cooperation, hostility, paranoia, and disorganized thinking. At the same time, affect, motor responses, and social contact improve. Within weeks of antipsychotic drug treatment, patients may show mild or absent symptoms when compared to those receiving a placebo (17).

Side effects can obscure an accurate assessment of medication effectiveness. The primary side effects are sedation, anticholinergic and anti-adrenergic effects, and neurologic effects. Less common side effects include seizures, weight gain, endocrine effects, sexual dysfunction, allergies, jaundice, visual changes, and changes in blood chemistry (17).

Sedation, the most common side effect, produces a feeling of sleepiness. During the day, sleepiness can interfere with daily living tasks but can benefit individuals who have disruptive behaviors and agitation. Often, sedation from medication decreases over time.

Anticholinergic effects are caused by drug action at several locations in the parasympathetic nervous system. As a result, patients may experience a variety of side effects, such as dry mouth, blurred vision, constipation, and urine retention. Whereas some side effects seem mild, others are life threatening. Intestinal obstruction can lead to death if not treated quickly. The body may be unable to regulate temperature, especially in warm weather, resulting in hyperthermia. Tachycardia can result from anticholinergic side effects or from the antiadrenergic effects of hypotension.

Potentially all antipsychotic medications can cause undesirable neurological side effects. Patient reactions may show immediately and medications may be reduced, or reactions may show with long-term use of medications. About 60% of persons using conventional antipsychotic drugs show fairly immediate extrapyramidal side effects (17). The extrapyramidal system contributes to control and coordination of motor performance, especially the mechanisms responsible for postural support and movement. Immediate, common responses included dystonia, parkinsonism, and akathisia. Dystonic movements are slow muscle contractions or spasms that involve the neck, jaw, tongue, eyes, and the entire body. The involuntary movements can be frightening and painful.

Parkinsonian reactions include motor rigidity, tremor, akinesia, and bradykinesia. Akinesia describes the amount of movement; movement is absent or reduced. Bradykinesia describes the speed of movement and thinking; mental and physical responses become slow and sluggish. Akinesia and bradykinesia can look like negative symptoms.

Patients who have akathisia feel physically uncomfortable. They move and adjust their bodies constantly to relieve the feeling of muscle discomfort. Observers note the agitation, restlessness, pacing, and repeated sitting down and standing up.

Less than 1 to 2% of patients may have the potentially fatal extrapyramidal side effect, neuroleptic malignant syndrome, that may occur when antipsychotic medications are used to treat acute symptoms (17). The often-rapid onset includes symptoms of rigidity, hyperthermia, hypertension, and tachycardia, especially in young male patients. Psychiatrists manage any immediate adverse effects of antipsychotic medications on the extrapyramidal system by giving drugs to treat the reaction. Then they may change the medication and dosage after the acute effects diminish.

Symptoms of tardive dyskinesia usually occur after 6 months of drug treatment. Movements are involuntary. Patients have repetitive, rapid, jerky, and writhing movements in the limbs, trunk, and head. Mouth, tongue, and jaw movements are most common. One of the challenges of identifying tardive dyskinesia is distinguishing between the chronic changes in schizophrenia and the effects of antipsychotic medications. Risks of tardive dyskinesia are greater for persons who are older and for women who are postmenopausal with mood disorders along with general medical conditions such as diabetes. Because no medication has yet proven effective to treat tardive dyskinesia, psychiatrists change medications and dosage.

The highly potent antipsychotic drugs, haloperidol and fluphenazine, require lower dosages but are more likely to cause extrapyramidal side effects (17). Intermediate potency medications like loxapine and perphenazine have fewer tendencies to cause side effects. The low potency medication, chlorpromazine thioridazine, causes mild to moderate extrapyramidal side effects (17). Patients who have schizophrenia also may have symptoms of other psychiatric disorders, such as bipolar disorder and depression, and serious chronic medical conditions. Medications taken to manage these conditions can complicate side effects.

Two other widely used antipsychotic drugs, clozapine and risperidone, do not cause extrapyramidal side effects. Clozapine was developed to treat the 20% of patients with schizophrenia who do not respond to or tolerate other antipsychotic medications. It can reduce psychoses, disorganization, and negative symptoms, but it is expensive. Patients who use clozapine must be closely monitored because the drug causes agranulocytosis in about 1% of patients. Agranulocytosis is the marked decrease of granular leukocytes or white blood cells, and patients may die of infections. Lesions appear in the throat and other mucous membranes, gastrointestinal tract, and skin. Because correct dosage and white blood cell counts are critical, the initial period of clozapine use may require hospitalization for the patient. Patients must be willing to have weekly white blood cell checks and must monitor themselves for side effects. Most patients taking clozapine gain weight and salivate excessively, especially when beginning the medication. Other less common side effects are tachycardia, hypotension, and fever (17).

Risperidone is a drug that works as an antagonist to neurotransmitters other than dopamine, including serotonin. Large-scale studies conducted in the United States and Canada show the effectiveness of risperidone in treating psychoses and disorganization. There is some evidence that risperidone is more effective than conventional antipsychotic medications for treating negative symptoms (17). Risperidone does cause extrapyramidal side effects but some studies show them to be less than with conventional antipsychotic medication. Sedation, hypotension, and weight gain occur in less than one-third of patients. Patients may experience loss of interest in sex, problems with erections, breast secretions, and menstrual changes. Long-term side effects are unknown at this time.

Three newer medications, olanzapine, sertindole, and quetiapine have been developed. According to the American Psychiatric Association (APA), at this time little information on effectiveness and side effects is available for these drugs. However, drug development studies report less severe and fewer extrapyramidal side effects (17).

It is hard to determine the clinical usefulness of a drug from the results of large-scale studies of its effectiveness. Studies involving large numbers of people may show statistically significant results, leading to the conclusion that the drug is effec-

tive. Psychiatric assessment measures of the person on the drug may show statistically significant change in symptoms. However the patient, family, and psychiatrist may observe very little behavioral change. Also, patients who have chronic schizophrenia are less responsive to some medications than newly diagnosed, acutely ill patients.

Electroconvulsive therapy (ECT) is effective in dramatically reducing symptoms in patients during their first hospital admission, either when used alone or in combination with antipsychotic medications (17). The use of ECT requires careful assessment, including medical history and laboratory tests, to determine risks. Follow-up treatment helps patients manage memory loss, confusion, and disorientation. For a complete description of ECT administration, refer to the chapter on mood disorders in this book.

Treatment Settings

The inpatient hospital setting provides a safe environment for patients who are suicidal or violent to other people. A well-organized milieu with clear expectations, structure, and supervision provides a stress-free environment for adjustment to medications and recovery in the acute phase of treatment. The length of inpatient hospitalization is brief—a matter of days. Long-term hospitalizations are reserved for patients who show no improvement during the acute phase of treatment. The best long-term programs are not custodial but are carefully structured by setting clear expectations and using behavioral approaches.

If, after a few days, the patient still requires structure and supervision, he or she can transfer to a day hospital program instead of being kept longer in inpatient care. The results of day hospitalizations show more improvement in role functioning and less family stress than longer-term hospitalizations. Day hospitalization does not lead to an increase in rehospitalization (17). Day hospitals or crisis treatment residences can be alternatives to hospitalization or may serve as follow-up to inpatient hospitalization. Here, the treatment goals emphasize a safe environment with structure and programs similar to an inpatient program but in a less-restricted setting. The patient keeps close contact with family members with fewer interruptions in family life and greater community acceptance.

During the stabilization phase of treatment, patients may benefit from the support of a day treatment facility. The long-term program can benefit persons with schizophrenia who may continue to have active symptoms and social difficulties. A Veterans' Administration study conducted by Linn compared day treatment with outpatient treatment (17, 22). There were fewer rehospitalizations, and symptoms and social function improved for day treatment patients after 2 years. Successful centers provided a low stress predictable setting, more occupational therapy, and less emphasis on psychotherapy. Day treatment was less effective for anxious and physically or mentally withdrawn patients.

For patients who do not live with their families, several types of housing can provide degrees of support and structure. Communities vary in housing availability for persons with schizophrenia and other mental illnesses. Lengths of stay range from short term in transitional, halfway, and crisis housing to long term in apartments and houses providing room and board.

Psychosocial Intervention

Psychotherapy

Research studies of the value of individual and group psychotherapy for persons with schizophrenia are hard to conduct and show mixed results. In the acute treatment phase, a therapeutic relationship that offers education about the nature of schizophrenia helps increase patient acceptance of treatment and family support. Beyond the acute phase, the most beneficial psychotherapy is reality oriented, emphasizing problem-solving and coping skills. Group therapy is best for patients who do not have severe symptoms of psychosis or disorganization. Those with negative symptoms usually do not respond to psychotherapy but do benefit from other structured and supportive approaches (17).

Case Management

For a person who has schizophrenia, the location of treatment extends from the hospital into the community. Case management helps a treatment team provide continuity of care. A case manager coordinates the services identified in the treatment plan and periodically evaluates the effectiveness of the goals and methods in producing desirable outcomes.

Program for Assertive Community Treatment

Program for Assertive Community Treatment (PACT) provides comprehensive services around the clock, 7 days a week to prevent relapse and rehospitalization. The services combine 24-hour case management and active treatment in places where patients live and work. The PACT teams support the strengths and abilities of individuals who are low functioning in ADL, work, and leisure. Staff members work with persons who have difficulties after treatment routines, family members, employers, and others. Many outcomes studies show decreased lengths of hospital stays and improved living conditions (17, 23).

Clubhouses and Lodges

Clubhouses provide transition from dependence to independence by empowering their members through a variety of supports and self-help programs. Fountain House was the original residential model for empowerment of the mentally ill beginning in the 1960s. Although mental health professionals provide leadership, members increase their independence through programs to improve social, recreation, and work skills. Clubhouses expect their members to function at their highest possible level. Because programs vary from clubhouse to clubhouse, they are hard to study and show uncertain outcomes in meeting their goals (17).

Shortly after World War II, lodge programs began to help patients in state hospitals make a successful transition to community living. The number of lodge programs declined as state hospitals closed their doors, but the ideas and principles transferred to other supervised community living programs. Persons who are compatible with each other in skills and function live together in housing in the community where mental health staff members provide supervision and programs to increase independence and autonomy. Residents lead and participate in self-governing councils within the residences. They discuss issues that arise as people make the adjustment to living with others in community settings. Controlled studies show that lodge programs are effective in helping residents move through the steps from supervised to independent living (19).

Mental health professionals now recognize the long-term nature of schizophrenia and other psychiatric disorders. As a result, new community treatment programs emphasize a person's current occupational performance and enhance that performance by trying to build specific skills. A variety of rehabilitation programs work with individuals with moderate to severe deficits to improve and maintain long-term occupational performance. Social skills training, vocational rehabilitation, and cognitive rehabilitation and cognitive therapy programs are part of this effort.

Social Skills Training

Social skills training programs provide training in social adaptation, self-care, and interpersonal relationships to help the person with schizophrenia fill roles in the community. Inadequate social skills are a major source of stress for some people with schizophrenia, especially those who have negative symptoms. The highly structured training is based on learning theory and behavioral therapy principles such as modeling, feedback, reinforcement, and role play. Homework assignments emphasize practice in the person's environment. Studies show the effectiveness of social skills training and the continued retention of those skills after 1 year. It is

not clear whether persons can generalize skills into their own environment for longer than 1 year, or whether social skills training can prevent repeated schizophrenic episodes.

Vocational Rehabilitation

The worker role combines critical skills essential to adult mental health. Persons with schizophrenia also benefit from paid work. Those who are paid tend to work significantly more hours than those who are not paid (24). Paid workers show fewer symptoms and lower rehospitalization rates than workers who volunteer. Several studies show that although individuals with schizophrenia can obtain jobs, they fail to retain them. Several work programs aim to build skills and support workers on the job.

Sheltered workshops can be a stepping stone to community employment but usually provide long-term placement for persons unable to work otherwise. Whereas workers benefit from the low stress, structured work tasks and supportive environment, the leap to competitive community employment is too great for most to succeed.

Supportive employment helps individuals while they hold jobs in community settings. The most effective programs are part of comprehensive community mental health support programs, able to provide transportation and coaching in self-care and interpersonal skills. Job clubs train participants in job exploration and job search, and then provide support from job search to job acquisition.

Closely linked to clubhouse programs, transitional employment helps move persons from in-house job assignments and industrial contracts to outside jobs. The worker chooses in-house or outside work from a variety of possibilities and can attend clubhouse groups and activities. In transitional employment, as in any other work program, the demands of the job must be close to the abilities of the worker and must increase as the worker becomes more skilled. Job and worker mismatches make long-term employment difficult for persons with schizophrenia. They may lack the specific skills required in the job. Situations causing too much or too little challenge cause people to leave jobs because of anxiety or boredom.

Cognitive Rehabilitation and Therapy

Cognitive rehabilitation methods developed for the treatment of people who have brain injury are being used for patients with schizophrenia to increase their skills in processing and using information. Retraining to increase attention, memory, planning, and decision-making may help patients benefit from other treatment approaches. There is unclear but promising evidence that cognitive rehabilitation methods can improve social and cognitive function for patients with schizophrenia (17).

Another approach to improving cognitive function in those with schizophrenia comes from the work of Beck, who developed cognitive therapy techniques for persons with depression. This approach shows some positive clinical outcomes (17).

Self-Help Groups

Self-help groups aim to empower patients, families, and other community members to advocate for community acceptance, research, treatment, and support. Groups encourage members to take more responsibility for their treatment instead of relying completely on mental health professionals. Persons who are members of some patient organizations may refuse psychiatric treatment. Self-help treatment organization, such as Recovery, Inc., follow the step model familiar in alcohol self-help programs. Organizations of parents and family members of individuals with schizophrenia and other mental disorders form the largest number of self-help organizations. They extend advocacy and education activities to health care policy and legislation, public mental health systems, and private services.

IMPACT ON OCCUPATIONAL PERFORMANCE

Factors such as symptoms of schizophrenia, response to medication treatment and side effects, lifestyle and living conditions, presence of sub- stance abuse and medical problems, and the course of the condition itself affect occupational performance in ADL, work, and leisure activities. Most persons who have schizophrenia fail to meet society's expectations of normal performance, even when symptoms are controlled by medication.

Activities of Daily Living

The occupations included in ADL usually require the ability to initiate and repeat purposeful task performance, so that it becomes habitual or routine. Persons who have schizophrenia may find routine task performance interrupted by symptoms, side effects of medication, and the progression of schizophrenia. On the other hand, they may find occupational performance enhanced when medications diminish symptoms and psychosocial treatments strengthen skills.

Although performance skills and problems vary widely among persons with schizophrenia, they face some challenges in common. Activities of daily living consist of a sequence of tasks carried out in routines. Examples are the series of routines involved in bathing, grooming, and dressing, washing hands before a meal, eating with reasonable table manners, then cleaning up. In schizophrenia, cognitive difficulties like attention, organization, decision-making, and reasoning can sometimes lead to the inability to initiate and complete the routines of daily living in keeping with what is usually considered normal.

The challenge of completing tasks that require perceptual skills like spatial relationships, figure ground, and body position may result in idiosyncratic methods and styles. Auditory or visual hallucinations may interrupt attention, and tactile discomfort with the texture of materials may limit occupational performance.

Many ADL routines become challenging in the presence of motor problems produced by negative symptoms and the neurological side effects of medications. Incoordination, tremors, rigidity, or slow movement may interfere with tasks like replacing caps on bottles, shaving, and using eating utensils.

In the psychological area, major barriers to ADL are apathy, avolition, or extreme withdrawal.

Even persons who show interest in social interaction may not complete the self-maintenance tasks that would increase social acceptance. They are unable to engage themselves in tasks and may depend on others to involve them. Self-management difficulties in schizophrenia influence ADL performance to a great extent. Routines are abandoned when persons are unable to cope with environmental or internal stressors. Time management and self control become tenuous. The comfort and structure of the home environment and compatibility of housemates are important factors in supporting ADL routines and habits, especially during stressful periods. The intelligence of persons with schizophrenia can lead to innovative solutions to ADL problems.

Work

The ability to initiate and complete routines in home management, work, and school performance presents challenges for persons with schizophrenia. Tasks and routines may be unfamiliar and complex, whereas performance expectations may be high. Home management, care of others, educational, and vocational activities require cognitive skills such as attention, organization, sequencing, problem solving, decision-making, abstract reasoning, and generalization. Safety procedures in work and home environments require an appropriate and immediate response. Cognitive and sensorimotor problems may result in an inappropriate or delayed response.

Often persons with schizophrenia have difficulty finding satisfactory housing or keeping a job because of psychological, psychosocial, and self-management performance difficulties. Few hold full-time jobs and a many have considerable difficulty with work-related tasks. In an area critical to most people's self-esteem and self-value, the individual with schizophrenia struggles to hold jobs after long periods of unemployment. Workers with a history of schizophrenia feel anxious when they believe expectations are too high and apathetic when expectations are too low. If they find a job, high employer expectations or inadequate job skills lead to failure, or they may be stuck in jobs that lack appropriate challenge. Negative symptoms such as withdrawal, avolition, substance abuse, neurological impairment, medication side effects, and coexisting medical conditions make work and school performance impossible for many.

Most performance in home management, jobs, or school requires some social interaction, especially if other people organize the specific tasks. Persons with hallucinations or delusions may be unable to interact comfortably with others. The inability to understand or express the symbolism or meaning in language creates barriers to communication. Conversational mannerisms like echolalia especially affect social conversation in unstructured periods at work or school.

Play and Leisure

On the surface, play and leisure would seem to offer persons with schizophrenia the chance to participate in pleasurable and social activity. Instead, many wander aimlessly, unable to re-engage themselves in familiar activities or take up new pursuits. Some find that familiar activities from their lives before schizophrenia lack personal meaning in the current context of daily living. Others may have never found success or satisfaction in occupational performance. They depend on others to initiate occupations and to include them.

The psychological performance components of anhedonia and avolition may combine to reduce satisfaction and participation in leisure activities. If the activity requires routines, attention, organization, fine motor manipulation, symbolic language, and comfort with competition, the person with schizophrenia may withdraw. Card and table games, popular in community drop-in programs, require most of these skills. The person who paces restlessly may not be able to sit and participate in an activity, yet may be too tired for a recreational walk.

The low incomes of unemployed persons curtail spending for recreation and entertainment. Walking, watching television, drinking coffee, and listening to music are frequent activities. The largest expenditure may be for cigarettes (Table 5.2).

TABLE 5.2 Occupational Performance Profile

I. PERFORMANCE AREAS	II. PERFORMANCE COMPONENTS	III. PERFORMANCE CONTEXTS
A. Activities of Daily Living*	A. Sensorimotor Component	A. Temporal Aspects
1. Grooming	1. Sensory	1. Chronological
2. Oral Hygiene	a. Sensory Awareness	2. Developmental
3. Bathing/Showering	b. Sensory Processing	3. Lifecycle
4. Toilet Hygiene	(1) Tactile	4. Disability Status
5. Personal Device Care	(2) Proprioceptive	B. Environment
6. Dressing	(3) Vestibular	1. Physical
7. Feeding and Eating	(4) Visual	2. Social
8. Medication Routine	(5) Auditory	3. Cultural
9. Health Maintenance	(6) Gustatory	
10. Socialization	(7) Olfactory	
11. Functional Communication	c. Perceptual Processing	
12. Functional Mobility	(1) Stereognosis	
13. Community Mobility	(2) Kinesthesia	
14. Emergency Response	(3) Pain Response	
15. Sexual Expression	(4) Body Scheme	
B. Work and Productive Activities	(5) Right–Left Discrimination	
1. Home Management	(6) Form Constancy	
a. Clothing Care	(7) Position in Space	
b. Cleaning	(8) Visual–Closure	
c. Meal Preparation/	(9) Figure Ground	
Cleanup	(10) Depth Perception	
d. Shopping	(11) Spatial Relations	
e. Money Management	(12) Topographical Orientation	
f. Household Maintenance	2. Neuromusculoskeletal	
g. Safety Procedures	a. Reflex	
2. Care of Others	b. Range of Motion	
3. Educational Activities	c. Muscle Tone	
4. Vocational Activities	d. Strength	
a. Vocational Exploration	e. Endurance	
b. Job Acquisition	f. Postural Control	
c. Work or Job	g. Postural Alignment	
Performance	h. Soft Tissue Integrity	
d. Retirement Planning	3. Motor (may be affected)	
e. Volunteer Participation	a. Gross Coordination	
C. Play or Leisure Activities	b. Crossing the Midline	
1. Play or Leisure Exploration	c. Laterality	
2. Play or Leisure Performance	d. Bilateral Integration	
	e. Motor Control	
	f. Praxis	
	g. Fine Coordination/Dexterity	
	h. Visual–Motor Control	
	i. Oral–Motor Control	

(continued)

| TABLE 5.2   Occupational Performance Profile (Continued) | | |

I. PERFORMANCE AREAS	II. PERFORMANCE COMPONENTS	III. PERFORMANCE CONTEXTS
	B. Cognitive Integration and Cognitive Components (may be affected) 　1. Level of Arousal 　2. Orientation 　3. Recognition 　4. Attention Span 　5. Initiation of Activity 　6. Termination of Activity 　7. Memory 　8. Sequencing 　9. Categorization 　10. Concept Formation 　11. Spatial Operations 　12. Problem Solving 　13. Learning 　14. Generalization C. Psychosocial Skills and Psychological Components 　1. Psychological 　　a. Values 　　b. Interests 　　c. Self-Concept 　2. Social 　　a. Role Performance 　　b. Social Conduct 　　c. Interpersonal Skills 　　d. Self-Expression 　3. Self-Management 　　a. Coping Skills 　　b. Time Management 　　c. Self-Control	

*May affect all areas depending upon current symptoms, medications, and the progression of the condition.

CASE STUDIES

CASE 1

R., who has been diagnosed with schizophrenia, paranoid type, is a 35-year-old white male from a Midwestern city. He has been hospitalized for several brief periods. Just prior to hospitalization, R.'s auditory hallucinations increased, telling him to harm his mother and brother. His fears overwhelm him and cause him to lose self control. Currently, R. lives in transitional housing where he has staff supervision and housemates. He thinks he may feel better if he lives alone in an apartment but wants the house to keep his spot open just in case he needs to return.

R. performs all ADL routines safely. Although he can perform the tasks independently, he often relies on prompting from others to get started. He does not like to wash his hair and wears colorful hats to cover it. At times, R.'s voices tell him not to wear or to throw out some of his clothes. Because of the voices, at this time he is unable to wear some of his clothes, including gloves in the coldest weather. According to R., he takes his medications, clozapine and haloperidol, regularly. He says the medications do not help him because they do not stop the voices. R. eats regularly, but he is sedentary and has low endurance. His constant fatigue increases the effort he must expend to complete ADL. R. can solve emergencies, such as knowing when he needs hospitalization, and can use the bus system to get around town. Voices disrupt R.'s performance in all occupations. Even though he shows considerable independence, self management is an area of concern, especially time management and self control.

When he runs out of clean clothes, he will wash them. At his residence, R. prepares hamburgers and onion rings when he takes his turn preparing one meal a week. He does not shop for food but can manage money and has good arithmetic skills.

R. recently renewed contact with his mother and brother through telephone calls and regular visits. Otherwise, he has few good friends but is able to live with his roommate. Depending on the strength of his voices, R. is well mannered and pleasant. After a long period of talking about working, R. joined a transitional employment group at a local clubhouse program. His part time placement was a position as a cashier and attendant in a parking structure. His work performance and his advocacy with the parking lot owners resulted in full-time employment. He works alone in a booth within the structure where he says the voices do not bother him.

R. is unable to balance leisure, work, and ADL. Although he used to like chess, basketball, drawing, and playing the trumpet, now he rarely plans or participates in these activities. Instead, he relaxes by listening to music and smoking cigarettes. Recently, R. joined his occupational therapist in several sessions of a community art class, but he stopped when the threatening voices escalated. Whenever he attempts to engage in meaningful and pleasurable occupations, his auditory hallucinations increase until he quits. R. believes his mental illness is a spiritual experience.

CASE 2

T. is a 44-year-old African American woman who lives in a large urban area. She has a dual diagnosis of schizophrenia, paranoid type, and abuse of multiple substances. Since her first hospitalization 20 years ago, T. now is rehospitalized two to three times a year. Incidents of physical aggression and physical destructiveness follow periods of increased substance use and intensified paranoid delusions. The dual effects of schizophrenia and substance

abuse may impair her brain function. Conventional antipsychotic medication had little effect on her delusions and disorganization but a brief trial of clozapine did. However, T. did not like the weekly blood tests required to monitor the level and safety of the medication. Currently her delusions of persecution and of reference remain unchecked.

In ADL, T.'s occupational performance fluctuates with the intensity of her delusions and substance use. During periods when she can screen out the irrelevant delusional thoughts, she independently creates and follows rather rigid routines to complete her self-care tasks. She holds high standards for personal appearance, which she believes she is unable to meet because she doesn't have enough money. Whereas money is a realistic worry, she spends her money for alcohol and eating meals out. Her lack of trust in other people and her isolation make it impossible for her to use public transportation and the group home van. She used to ride her bicycle for transportation. When it was missing, she said it was stolen because of something bad she had done. When delusions and substance use increase, she becomes dependent in most ADL routines but resists assistance. Her appearance becomes unkempt and disheveled.

The occupational performance area of work is a priority for T. In the large group home she shares with other persons who are mentally ill, T. prepares her own food or eats out. She says the staff who cook don't know what they're doing and anyway, she doesn't know them well enough to eat their food. Restaurant meals strain her limited welfare funds. Her meals often lack nutritional balance. She does her own laundry.

T. is unable to carry out her roles of mother and family member. She has no contact with her daughter, former husband, or other relatives. Her main support came from an aunt who died 3 years ago during a time when T. was hospitalized. The disruption of cognition in the form of threatening and rigid delusions leads to T.'s social isolation. Her need to protect herself by remaining isolated limits the amount of support from other people, even though she needs support.

In the future, T. hopes to get a job in the community but now works in a supported employment setting as a janitor. Before this job, she worked with a janitorial crew, performing tasks safely and efficiently. On the job, she was thorough, precise, and persistent. However, she could not tolerate changes in her work routine and blamed others for trying to trick her. In response to direction or criticism from her supervisor, T. would leave the job site. In her current job, she is able to work with her job coach and is appropriate in her minimal interaction with other workers.

T. is unable to balance ADL, work, and leisure seen in a complete lack of any avocational or recreational activities. She rarely initiates or participates in spontaneous or planned leisure, either alone or with other people. She used to enjoy competitive sports and physical activities like jogging. Church attendance was an important part of her routine. Now, anhedonia, delusions, isolation, the lack of money, and substance abuse lead to aimless and solitary wandering in her leisure time.

Acknowledgments

I want to thank Valerie Howells, Ph.D., OTR, Ypsilanti, MI, for her contributions to this chapter.

POINTS FOR REVIEW

1. What are negative symptoms? What is the difference between negative symptoms and delusions and hallucinations?

2. What are three major theories about the etiology of schizophrenia?

3. What are the major risk factors for getting schizophrenia?

4. What are the three major symptoms groups for schizophrenia? What are symptoms within each group?

5. What are the four types of schizophrenia? What are the diagnostic criteria for each?

6. Why are the death rates for individuals with schizophrenia so much greater than the general population?

7. Explain the correlation between schizophrenia, substance abuse, and homelessness.

8. What are the three phases of treatment? Describe each.

9. What categories of medications are used to treat schizophrenia? What are the side effects of each group?

REFERENCES

1. McGee M, Swanson C, Jones C, et al. Diagnosis: The DSM IV approach to schizophrenia. In: Moscarelli M, Rupp A, Sartorius N, eds. Handbook of Mental Health Economics and Health Policy, Volume I: Schizophrenia. New York: John Wiley and Sons, 1996.

2. Buchanan RW, Carpenter WT. The neuroanatomies of schizophrenia. Schizophr Bull 1997;23:367–372.

3. Stevens JR. Anatomy of schizophrenia revisited. Schizophr Bull 1997;23:373–383.

4. Warner R, deGirolamo G. Schizophrenia. Epidemiology of mental disorders and psychosocial problems. Geneva: World Health Organization, 1995.

5. Buchanan RW, Stevens JR, Carpenter WT. The neuroanatomy of schizophrenia: editor's introduction. Schizophr Bull 1997;23:365–366.

6. Weinburger DR. On localizing schizophrenia neuropathology. Schizophr Bull 1997;23:537–540.

7. Holzman PS. Basic behavioral sciences. Schizophr Bull 1988;14:413–426.

8. Leonard S, Adams C, Breese CR, et al. Nicotinic receptor function in schizophrenia. Schizophr Bull 1996;22:431–435.

9. American Psychiatric Association. Diagnostic and Statistical Manual of Mental Disorders, 4th ed. Washington, DC: American Psychiatric Association, .

10. Norquist GS, Regier DA, Rupp A. Estimates of the cost of treating people with schizophrenia: contributions of data from epidemiologic surveys. In: Moscarelli M, Rupp A, Sartorius N, eds. Handbook of Mental Health Economics and Health Policy, Volume I: Schizophrenia. New York: John Wiley and Sons, 1996.

11. Jeste DV, Gladsjo JA, Lindamer LA, et al. Medical comorbidity in schizophrenia. Schizophr Bull 1996;22:413–430.

12. Andreasen NC, Arndt S, Alliger R, et al. Symptoms of schizophrenia. Arch Gen Psychiatry 1995;52:341–351.

13. Liddle P, Carpenter WT, Crow T. Syndromes of schizophrenia. Br J Psychiatry 1994;165:721–727.

14. Liddle PF, Barnes TRE. Syndromes of chronic schizophrenia. Br J Psychiatry 1990;558–561.

15. Fenton WS. Longitudinal course and outcome of schizophrenia. In: Moscarelli M, Rupp A, Sartorius N, eds. Handbook of Mental Health Economics and Health Policy, Volume I: Schizophrenia. New York: John Wiley and Sons, 1996.

16. Harrow M, Sands JR, Silverstein ML, et al. Course and outcome for schizophrenia versus other psychotic patients: a longitudinal study. Schizophr Bull 1997;23:287–302.

17. American Psychiatric Association. Practice Guideline for the Treatment of Patients with Schizophrenia. Washington DC, American Psychiatric Association, 1997.

18. Leshner AI. Addiction is a brain disease and it matters. Science 1997;273:45–47.

19. Andreasen NC. The Scale for the Assessment of Negative Symptoms (SANS). Iowa City: The University of Iowa, 1983.

20. Andreasen NC. The Scale for the Assessment of Positive Symptoms (SAPS). Iowa City: The University of Iowa, 1984.

21. Kane JM. Drug treatments. In: Moscarelli M, Rupp A, Sartorius N, eds. Handbook of Mental Health Economics and Health Policy, Volume I: Schizophrenia. New York: John Wiley and Sons, 1996.

22. Linn MW, Caffey EM, Klett CJ, et al. Day treatment and psychotropic drugs in the aftercare of schizophrenic patients. Arch Gen Psychiatry 1979;36:1055–1066.

23. Test MA, Knoedler WH, Allness DJ, et al. Comprehensive community care of persons with schizophrenia through the programme of assertive community treatment (PACT). In: Brenner HD, Boker W, Genner R, eds. Towards a Comprehensive Therapy for Schizophrenia. Seattle: Hogrefe and Huber, 1997.

24. Bell MD, Lysaker PH. Clinical benefits of paid work activity in schizophrenia: 1-year follow-up. Schizophr Bull 1997;23:317–328.

CHAPTER 6

MOOD DISORDERS

Virginia Allen Dicke

CRITICAL TERMS

Affect	Episode	Paradigm
Affective	Hallucinations	Psychomotor agitation
Antidepressant	Mood	REM (rapid eye movement)
Cognition	Neuroendocrine	Serotonin
Dementia	Neurotransmitter	Syndrome
Disorder	Norepinephrine	

Betsy is at the door waiting for the occupational therapist to arrive on the unit. "I want to go to the O. T. shop right now. I have to make presents for all of my nieces and nephews and for my two sisters. I want to make some pillows like my roommate made, but I want mine to be larger, and I need lots more colors, and. . ." The occupational therapist interrupts Betsy as she pauses to catch her breath. He explains that he will have to check to see if she has been referred for O.T. He adds that, in any case, the occupational therapy group session will not begin for another 10 minutes.

As he walks down the hall, the therapist thinks to himself that most of that 10 minutes will be spent in Elizabeth's room, encouraging her to leave her bed and "try out" occupational therapy. As he predicted, Elizabeth is curled up on her bed and refuses the therapist's request that she get up and join the group. At first she doesn't say anything. Then she responds to the therapist's gentle encouragement with short statements: "I don't feel good," "I didn't sleep last night," "I'm not good at making things," "Nothing I do ever turns out," "I just don't feel like doing anything." Only after considerable persuading does Elizabeth consent to come to the clinic and "only to watch." She joins the therapist as he approaches the door. Betsy is waiting there impatiently, telling everyone who is near of her plans to make a set of pillows for each of her relatives.

Betsy and Elizabeth have both been admitted to a psychiatric ward because a mood disorder has caused each of them to be unable to function in her normal environment. As different as their problems seem in this brief description, they could in fact be the same person at different times in the course of a bipolar disorder: Betsy in a manic episode and Elizabeth in a depressed episode; or Elizabeth might be suffering with a major depression. In either case, each of these women is severely incapacitated in all occupational performance areas.

This chapter discusses mood disorders: how they are classified and diagnosed, how they differ from the "moods" we all feel normally, and research and theories regarding their etiology. Standard treatment approaches are reviewed. The impact of mood disorders on occupational performance is described and then examined in more detail in two case studies.

WHAT IS A MOOD DISORDER?

Mood disorders always involve a disturbed mood, which may be either depressed or manic (1). Each of us has had many disturbed moods. How then do mood disorders differ from the normal experience of being "down," "having the blues," or feeling elated? Stated simply, mood disorders differ from normal mood variations in apparent cause, severity, duration, and impact on functioning. Our personal experiences of emotional "ups and downs" can help us to understand a little bit about how a person with a mood disorder might be feeling. However, to even begin to comprehend clinical depression or bipolar disorder, we must multiply the feelings we have experienced. Imagine feeling so bad that there is no reason to get out of bed day after day, or always feeling as if there is a heavy weight on your shoulders, or feeling "high" for several weeks. The novelist William Styron described his own depression as a "smothering" illness (2). Others refer to the "pain" of depression.

It is possible to misunderstand mood disorders, though, if we use only our own experiences

with mood changes to try to comprehend these problems. We have developed methods to handle our ups and downs; for example, we get together with a friend, take a walk, help someone else, take on a nasty clean-up job, or exercise. Because we can manage unpleasant moods, we may feel that everyone else should be able to do the same thing. Unfortunately, it is not that easy for people who have a mood disorder. Their disturbed moods do not respond to such "do-it-yourself" approaches.

We must also avoid thinking that these disorders are unimportant because they are somewhat like our normal feelings. Mood disorders disrupt occupational functioning, destroy family and social supports, and can result in serious consequences, including death, if they are not treated. The good news is that treatment for mood disorders is usually successful (3). The bad news is that only a fraction of the people with depression (by far the more common of the two broad types of mood disorders) receives treatment (4, 5). Furthermore, mood disorders often are chronic, even when a person experiences periods of normal moods between episodes of the condition.

The economic cost of depression is staggering. In the United States the annual cost is calculated to be $43 billion, almost three-fourths of which relates to absenteeism and lost productivity (5).

CLASSIFICATION OF MOOD DISORDERS

The *Diagnostic and Statistical Manual of Mental Disorders (DSM-IV)* sets forth criteria that must be met for the mood disturbance to be considered pathologic (1). These criteria include both symptoms and minimum duration, as well as the necessity of ruling out other physical or mental disorders as the cause. The *DSM-IV* organizes mood disorders into *depressive disorders, bipolar disorders,* and *other mood disorders.* Depressive disorders include *major depressive disorders, dysthymic disorders,* and *depressive disorders not otherwise specified.* The types of bipolar disorders are *bipolar I disorder, bipolar II disorder, cyclothymic disorder,* and *bipolar disorders not otherwise specified.* Other mood disorders include *mood disorders due to a medical condition, substance-induced mood disorders,* and *mood disorders not otherwise specified* (1).

This chapter focuses on major depressive disorders and bipolar I and II disorders. These are the conditions seen most frequently as a primary diagnosis in the mental health settings where an occupational therapist is likely to work. Keep in mind, however, that any of the mood disorders may be part of the clinical picture of a client in any type of setting.

For a person to receive a diagnosis of major depressive disorder or bipolar I and II disorders, he or she must be experiencing a *mood episode.*

Mood episodes include *major depressive episodes, manic episodes, mixed episodes, and hypomanic episodes* (1). Major depressive disorders are "characterized by one or more major depressive episodes without a history of manic, mixed, or hypomanic episodes" (1). Bipolar I disorder is diagnosed when an individual has experienced one or more manic or mixed episodes. Bipolar II disorder presents with major depressive and hypomanic episodes (1). To remember the distinctions between the three disorders, note that major depressive disorder has only depressive episodes (Table 6.1); bipolar I disorder must have either manic (Table 6.2) or mixed episodes

---

TABLE 6.1   Criteria for Major Depressive Episode

A. Five (or more) of the following symptoms have been present during the same 2-week period and represent a change from previous functioning; at least one of the symptoms is either (1) depressed mood or (2) loss of interest or pleasure.
   Note: Do not include symptoms that are clearly due to a general medical condition or mood-incongruent delusions or hallucinations.
   (1) Depressed mood most of the day, nearly every day, as indicated by either subjective report (e.g., feels sad or empty) or observation made by others (e.g., appears tearful). **Note:** in children and adolescents, can be irritable mood.
   (2) Markedly diminished interest or pleasure in all, or almost all, activities most of the day, nearly every day (as indicated by either subjective account or observation made by others).
   (3) Significant weight loss when not dieting, or weight gain (e.g., a change of more than 5% of body weight in a month), or decrease or increase in appetite nearly every day. **Note:** in children, consider failure to make expected weight gains.
   (4) Insomnia or hypersomnia nearly every day.
   (5) Psychomotor agitation or retardation nearly every day (observable by others, not merely subjective feelings of restlessness or being slowed down).
   (6) Fatigue or loss of energy nearly every day.
   (7) Feelings of worthlessness or excessive or inappropriate guilt (which may be delusional) nearly every day (not merely self-reproach or guilt about being sick).
   (8) Diminished ability to think or concentrate, or indecisiveness, nearly every day (either by subjective account or as observed by others).
   (9) Recurrent thoughts of death (not just fear of dying), recurrent suicidal ideation without a specific plan, or a suicide attempt or a specific plan for committing suicide.
B. The symptoms do not meet criteria for a Mixed Episode (see p. 335).
C. The symptoms cause clinically significant distress or impairment in social, occupational, or other important areas of functioning.
D. The symptoms are not due to the direct physiological effects of a substance (e.g., a drug of abuse, a medication) or a general medical condition (e.g., hypothyroidism).
E. The symptoms are not better accounted for by Bereavement, i.e., after the loss of a loved one; the symptoms persist for longer than 2 months or are characterized by marked functional impairment, morbid preoccupation with worthlessness, suicidal ideation, psychotic symptoms, or psychomotor retardation.

TABLE 6.2   Criteria for Manic Episode

A. A distinct period of abnormally and persistently elevated, expansive, or irritable mood, lasting at least 1 week (or any duration if hospitalization is necessary).

   During the period of mood disturbance, three (or more) of the following symptoms have persisted (four if the mood is only irritable) and have been present to a significant degree:

   (1) Inflated self-esteem or grandiosity.
   (2) Decreased need for sleep (e.g., feels rested after only 3 hours of sleep).
   (3) More talkative than usual or pressure to keep talking.
   (4) Flight of ideas or subjective experience that thoughts are racing.
   (5) Distractibility (i.e., attention too easily drawn to unimportant or irrelevant external stimuli).
   (6) Increase in goal-directed activity (either socially, at work or school, or sexually) or psychomotor agitation.
   (7) Excessive involvement in pleasurable activities that have a high potential for painful consequences (e.g., engaging in unrestrained buying sprees, sexual indiscretions, or foolish business investments).

D. The mood disturbance is sufficiently severe to cause marked impairment in occupational functioning or in usual social activities or relationships with others, or to necessitate hospitalization to prevent harm to self or others, or there are psychotic features.

E. The symptoms are not due to the direct physiological effects of a substance (e.g., a drug of abuse, a medication, or other treatment) or a general medical condition (e.g., hyperthyroidism).

   Note: Manic-like episodes that are clearly caused by somatic antidepressant treatment (e.g., medication, electroconvulsive therapy, light therapy) should not count toward a diagnosis of bipolar I disorder.

(Table 6.3) but also may have depressive episodes; and bipolar II disorder has major depressive episodes and hypomanic episodes (Table 6.4), but not manic or mixed episodes. Tables 6.1 through 6.4 give the criteria for each type of episode.

Scientists and clinicians continue to argue about whether bipolar disorders and depressive disorders are part of one continuum, whether there are distinct subtypes of both, and what these might be (4). Both syndromes are expressed in a wide variety of ways, both by different individuals and at different times by the same person. This chapter will adhere to the *DSM-IV* classification system, generally ignoring questions of subtypes, but adding information from other sources as pertinent. The *DSM-IV* system will continue to be modified in further revisions and editions based on research and clinical experience that supports or refutes existing classification criteria. For example, in the fourth edition, bipolar disorders have been newly categorized as bipolar I and bipolar II. As changes occur in the future, compare new editions with previous systems for clarification.

A wide variety of terms are used to describe mood disorders within clinical settings. Many are derived from past classification systems or from particular theoretical perspectives. If you find yourself in a situation where terms other than those from *DSM-IV* are used, it is best to seek clarification of their meaning within that setting. The *DSM-IV* is currently used nationwide to code psychiatric disorders for reimbursement and reporting purposes and to ensure consistency in research. Thus, when other terminology is used, it usually supplements the *DSM-IV* diagnosis. The codes for diagnoses in *DSM-IV* are compatible with those of the *International Statistical Classification of Diseases and Related Health Problems* (ICD-9 and ICD-10) (1).

It is easiest to discuss depressive disorders and bipolar disorders separately because their etiology and treatment are different and because they are very different in clinical manifestations when the person with a bipolar disorder is in the manic

TABLE 6.3 Criteria for Mixed Episode

A. The criteria are met for a Manic Episode and for a Major Depressive Episode (except for duration) nearly every day during at least a 1-week period.
B. The mood disturbance is sufficiently severe to cause significant impairment in occupational functioning or in usual social activities or relationships with others, or to necessitate hospitalization to prevent harm to self or others, or there are psychotic features.
C. The symptoms are not due to the direct physiological effects of a substance (e.g., a drug of abuse, a medication, or other treatment) or a general medical condition (e.g. hyperthyroidism).
   Note: Mixed-like episodes that are clearly caused by somatic antidepressant treatment (e.g., medication, electroconvulsive therapy, light therapy) should not count toward a diagnosis of bipolar I disorder.

TABLE 6.4 Criteria for Hypomanic Episode

A. A distinct period of persistently elevated, expansive, or irritable mood, lasting throughout at least 4 days, that is clearly different from the usual nondepressed mood.
B. During the period of mood disturbance, three (or more) of the following symptoms have persisted (four if the mood is only irritable) and have been present to a significant degree:
   (1) Inflated self-esteem or grandiosity.
   (2) Decreased need for sleep (e.g., feels rested after only 3 hours of sleep).
   (3) More talkative than usual or equalize pressure to keep talking.
   (4) Flight of ideas or subjective experience that thoughts are racing.
   (5) Distractibility (i.e., attention too easily drawn to unimportant or irrelevant external stimuli).
   (6) Increase in goal-directed activity (either socially, at work or school, or sexually) or psychomotor agitation.
   (7) Excessive involvement in pleasurable activities that have a high potential for painful consequences (e.g., unrestrained buying sprees, sexual indiscretions, or foolish business investment)
C. The episode is associated with an unequivocal change in functioning that is uncharacteristic of the person when not symptomatic.
D. The disturbance in mood and the change in functioning are observable by others.
E. The episode is not severe enough to cause significant impairment in social or occupational functioning, or to necessitate hospitalization, and there are no psychotic features.
F. The symptoms are not due to the direct physiological effects of a substance (e.g., a drug of abuse, a medication, or other treatment) or a general medical condition (e.g., hyperthyroidism).
   Note: Hypomanic-like episodes that are clearly caused by somatic antidepressant treatment (e.g., medication, electroconvulsive therapy, light therapy) should not count toward a diagnosis of bipolar II disorder.

phase. Keep in mind that this distinction may not be nearly so clear in reality.

You may see patients with any of these conditions in any setting. If a mood disorder coexists with other conditions, treatment of problems relating to those conditions may be seriously affected by the mood disorder.

DEPRESSIVE DISORDERS
Etiology

People suffering from depression, their friends and families, and many professionals working with them tend to look for external causes or environmental events to explain the terrible suffering this disease creates. When a person commits suicide, it is rare to see the act attributed to depression without some additional cause given for the mood disorder. Explanations over centuries have included mysterious changes in body "humors," unusual amounts of stress, real or perceived losses of important people at an early age, recent losses or bad luck, anger turned inward, and on and on. A "melancholic" mood was once thought desirable in artistic individuals as a sign of sensitivity (6); by extension, people who are highly sensitive may be perceived of as vulnerable to depression.

Today we are much closer to understanding possible causes of depression, although the exact mechanisms of the disease are unclear. What is clear is that there is no simple or single answer. Depression appears to be a biopsychosocial phenomenon in both cause and expression. It may be a clinical picture that can be caused by a variety of factors, or it may be a number of different disorders.

Problems in Research

When you read research reports about the cause of depression, you must look carefully at the way investigators have conducted their studies. What condition(s) are they studying? What questions are they asking? What are their methods?

It is often difficult to sort out cause from effect for an existing problem. Much depression research has been conducted with people after they have been diagnosed as depressed; thus the psychosocial antecedents are seen through the lens of the illness and may be distorted. This illness alters individuals' functioning in life roles and relationships. Even the biological differences that are supported in many studies could be a result rather than a cause of the depression. Longitudinal studies of a population from birth to death would help us to understand who becomes depressed and why. Medical records in countries (such as Denmark) that have socialized medicine are helpful in this regard. Research may study people with true depressive disorders or those who are more inclined than the controls to express a depressed mood on some test or scale.

For example, studies are often done with groups of medical students or college students enrolled in psychology courses. The results may say more about different personality types than about depression as a psychiatric disorder. (They also focus on a very limited population.) These studies do not look at clinical depression, but many are very interesting and may help us understand how people with depressed moods think and function. Use caution, however, in applying the findings in such studies to people with major depressive disorder.

Research on depression is further complicated by the possibility that depression is not a single entity. The clinical syndrome may be the outward manifestation of a variety of processes. Investigators also disagree as to whether there are subtypes of depression, what they might be, and if they represent different syndromes. Look carefully at studies to see what criteria have been used to group the subjects. Different subtypes of depression are not yet clearly linked to different causes, but failure to distinguish subtypes or patterns of variation may flaw research results.

Biological Theories of Etiology

Medications are very effective in alleviating symptoms of major depressive disorder in most people. This is one of the most obvious indicators that depression has biological components. Antidepressant medications affect the neurotransmitters, serotonin and norepinephrine. Simply stated, antidepressants cause an increased availability of these neurotransmitters for transmission of nerve impulses. Because of this, we can assume that there is some decreased level or blockage of serotonin or norepinephrine in the brains of depressed individuals (or at least in those who respond well to drug treatment). Dopamine disorders may also contribute to mood disorders (7).

Neuroendocrine studies of patients with depression show irregularities related to the limbic-hypothalamic-pituitary-adrenal axis (7). Disorders of the thyroid and of growth hormones also may be associated with mood disorders (7).

Other research areas that support a biological factor in depression include sleep studies that show depressed persons having disrupted sleep and decreased REM latency (7, 8) and studies of immune function that show changes of cellular response in persons who are depressed. Additional evidence for a biological cause or component of depression comes from the similarity of symptoms in people with known brain lesions and our knowledge of the functions of specific areas of the brain. Some physiological symptoms of depression (e.g., lack of sexual interest, sleep difficulties, and decreased appetite) occur with dysfunction of the hypothalamus (7). Problems such as slowness, lack of energy, and difficulty thinking are similar to problems seen in people with basal ganglia lesions.

Genetics

A number of studies show increased rates of depression in biological family members of depressed persons and in monozygotic (identical) twins. These associations are significant but not nearly as strong as they are for bipolar disorder.

Seasonal Disorders

Ancient writing about depression ascribed a depression-like state to seasonal patterns that modern research has confirmed exist for some individuals. The *DSM-IV* provides criteria for specifying a seasonal pattern (1). Winter depression has distinct symptoms in addition to the time that it occurs. These include overeating, oversleeping, and craving for carbohydrates (9). Light deficiency is implicated as the cause of winter depression, and people with this diagnosis respond well to phototherapy (prescribed exposure to light). (Records of the use of light to treat depression date back 2000 years!) The cause of summer depression is less clear, but it may be related to heat (9). In addition to clear seasonal disorders, data on suicides and on onset of depressive episodes (nonseasonal) also reveal seasonal patterns. Suicide rates peak in late spring and

early summer with a smaller peak in late fall and early winter, and the onset of mood disorders peaks in both spring (March through May) and fall (September through November) (9).

Depressive disorders are sometimes linked to stressful events in a person's life. Unusual stress does appear to be linked to the first major depressive episode for many individuals. It is less evident in subsequent episodes.

Psychosocial Theories of Etiology

The psychosocial theories and explanations of the etiology of depression have varying degrees of support from research but have major impact on the psychotherapy methods clinicians use for depressed persons. Many theories exist. Four theoretical perspectives are discussed here.

Psychodynamic theories characterize depression as evolving from an internal state often involving extreme emotional dependence on others. Many different psychodynamic theories have been proposed over many years, most rooted in Freud's theories of psychosexual development and intrapsychic conflict. Depression is seen as the "consequence of underlying conflict" (10). The following description is my somewhat simplistic version of a psychodynamic approach to explaining how depression occurs.

Depressed individuals never developed the ability to find meaning in life except through other people. They probably experienced some early childhood loss or deprivation from mother or another significant person. They depend on others to make choices and only know that a job is well done if told so by an important person. Their lives are defined totally by significant others. (In psychodynamic terms, this person is referred to as the *object*.)

Now, imagine yourself as a significant other—could you possibly be all things to another person, someone who depended on you exclusively? Even if you tried, inevitably you would fail as you acted to meet your own needs and those of the social system. Unless you were acting from your own pathological needs, you would probably grow to feel burdened by the other person's extreme dependency and would try to encourage him or her to rely upon you less. The person who has this dependency sees these attitudes and actions of the significant other as losses, failures, rejections, or betrayals. These perceived "losses" might range from outright rejection (e.g., a spouse leaving) to more symbolic losses (birth of a sibling and consequent need to share mother's time and attention). The loss "event" may be a sharing of affection with an additional person (best friend gets a boyfriend) or a lack of availability of the other caused by a life event (hospitalization, move to another part of the country). It may simply be perceived indifference to the person's concerns, a sharp word, or a lack of response.

The spiral into depression starts with the loss. The individual is faced with a terrible problem—he or she relies totally on a special person who has let him or her down. Becoming angry with that person only increases the chance that the person will not come back or will continue to be less available. Thus it is not safe to show this anger, and angry feelings generate both fear and guilt. At this point the anger is turned inward. The individual feels responsible for the loss or letdown. Anger with oneself seems safer, but it results in depression, which is destructive to self.

This description of a psychodynamic theory of depression does not begin to cover the multiple and complex approaches that have been put forth over the years. There are many theories in the literature. In his review of psychotherapies for depression, Karasu summarizes modern dynamic theory as combining "such psychoanalytic formulations as early childhood disappointment and loss, damaged self-esteem, persistence of narcissistic rage beneath an unloved and punished self, a sense of helplessness and hopelessness, and difficulties in autonomy and intimacy" (10).

Psychodynamic theories are not well supported by research but are often cited when postulating possible causes for a person's depression. These theories form the basis of psychodynamic therapies for depression. Today such therapy takes many forms other than traditional Freudian psychoanalysis—most notably it is shorter term, and the therapist takes a more active role in treatment.

Existential explanations of depression look at the correlation of depression with the person's life and see the relationship of depression to prolonged periods when it is difficult to find meaning in life, or to major life changes, often the attainment of long-sought goals.

Many of us find meaning in life by striving toward achieving something (e.g., job promotion, graduation from college, marriage, retirement). We expect that when we reach this goal we will be very happy (or at least content), will be able to do what we want to do, or will be recognized by others. But two things happen when you reach your goals. The first is that you no longer have the goal. You have lost something that has been important in guiding your life over a long period. The second is that reaching the goal may not have the expected effects. Happiness is not a guaranteed result. Other things may be going wrong. The promotion may mean more work, longer hours, and loss of friends from the old office. Graduation may decrease exciting intellectual stimulation. Marriage entails a great deal of adjustment. Retirement may exchange a hated job for boredom. The loss of goals or the failure of achievements to meet expectations may result in depression.

Again we have a theoretical perspective that lacks significant research support, but the existential view may be helpful in understanding some of the reactions we have to our successes—there may be a reason for feeling letdown or blue when we and the world around us expect a happy response.

Cognitive Theory

A number of theorists have contributed to the cognitive view of depression, but Aaron Beck and his associates are the ones most associated with this approach today. Beck developed a paradigm to explain the relationship of cognitive patterns to the characteristic symptoms of depression

(11). Depression is caused by problems in thinking. He described three cognitive patterns that differentiate depressed people from others in the way that they think.

First, depressed individuals have a negative view of the world. They consistently interpret their experiences in the worst light or distort events in a negative direction. Less than total success may be seen as failure (e.g., getting a grade of 95 instead of 100 may be seen as defeat). Depressed persons may consider themselves deprived over minor things (e.g., having less money to spend on clothes than a friend has). They tend to overreact to feedback from others, interpreting neutral signs in a negative way (e.g., when her husband doesn't say anything about her new dress, the woman interprets this to mean that he thinks it is ugly).

The second area of cognitive distortion is in individuals' view of themselves. A negative view of self is displayed in a tendency to blame oneself for anything that goes wrong and to view this as a major shortcoming in one's character. The student is convinced that he is stupid because he didn't get a good grade on a test. The woman "knows" she is a terrible mother because her son misbehaves in nursery school. When a girl turns him down for a date, the boy knows it is because he is totally unattractive to the opposite sex. Depressed persons simply do not like, nor see any reason to like, themselves.

The third cognitive distortion is a negative view of the future. Not only is the world a terrible place and the self a terrible person, but there is no reason to expect things to get better in either the short or the long run. The future is seen as a continuation of the current unpleasantness, and this continuity with the present differentiates the depressed person's view of the future from normal anxiety about the future.

In addition to these three cognitive distortions, depressed people have deeply felt silent assumptions that distort the conclusions they draw from events, and they exhibit illogical thinking (11). For example, an isolated event

such as a critical comment will be used to make broad generalizations about one's own worth or others' attitudes toward oneself. Depressed persons may hold themselves responsible for events, even when this could not possibly be the case.

In Beck's view, the symptoms of depression are a result of distorted thinking. Beck further elaborated his theories and developed a treatment approach that helps patients to identify the way in which they develop negative cognitions. Errors in thinking are identified, and alternate patterns are developed and practiced in short-term and time-limited therapy. This treatment approach has been effective for many people, but it must be used in conjunction with medications when a person has a major depressive episode.

Some of Beck's statements about distorted cognitions may be questioned in light of research that shows that depressed persons may *accurately* assess their own role in success and failure in laboratory test situations, whereas "normals" tend to distort their responsibility for negative results, to place themselves in the best light (12, 13). This research does show that depressed persons place more emphasis on their failures than on their successes. Beck's theory is reasonably supported by research in its ability to describe the differences between depressed and nondepressed persons. It is not clear, however, that negative or distorted cognitions cause the clinical entity called "depression." Again it is the question of which came first.

There are a number of other cognitive theories of depression, as well as elaboration of Beck's work by others. Two theories that are frequently cited are Ellis' theory of *irrational beliefs* (14), and Seligman's theory of *learned helplessness* (15).

Behavioral Theories of Depression

Lewinsohn correlates depression with a lack of reinforcement from the environment. Reinforcement must follow behavior, and when it makes the person feel good, Lewinsohn calls it positive reinforcement. If people behave in a way that does not result in positive reinforcement or if they live in an environment that does not provide positive reinforcement, they become depressed (16, 17). A high level of punishing or negative reinforcement (in other words, effects that make the person feel bad) also causes depression.

Based on his theoretical formulation of depression, Lewinsohn developed a short-term, time-limited treatment approach that focuses on increasing the amount of positive reinforcement a person receives by changing behaviors. One central element to his approach is the "Pleasant Events Schedule," which is a listing of several hundred events in which a person might find pleasure (16). Patients go through this list and identify those items that they find pleasurable. Next the frequency of participation in these events is charted (it is usually very low in depressed persons), and a plan is developed to incorporate some of them into the regular daily schedule. This is carried out as a homework assignment that includes monitoring and recording feelings. Lewinsohn incorporates a number of cognitive and behavioral assignments into his treatment, which is usually conducted in an educational (classroom) manner. He also has published a self-help version of his treatment approach (18).

Lewinsohn has supported both his theory of depression and the efficacy of this treatment approach with research. Once again, the research is looking at people who are already identified as being depressed, so cause and effect are hard to sort out. Because his subjects can be treated as outpatients, it is possible that their symptoms are less severe than those of a person hospitalized with major depression.

This discussion has not begun to cover all theories of depression, nor does it provide any detail or depth for those discussed. It is meant to illustrate the many ways this disease is conceptualized and to give some exposure to leading theoretical perspectives. Other perspectives and approaches in use include the interpersonal approach and approaches based on stress. Many of the therapeutic approaches in use today combine aspects of several of these perspectives.

INCIDENCE AND PREVALENCE

Depression is the most common psychiatric disorder. In a study of more than 20,000 adults, the National Institute for Mental Health (NIMH) found an incidence of major depression of 3.0% in a 6-month period and a lifetime incidence of 5.8% (19). When people with bipolar disorders and dysthymia are included, 5.85% of the population can be expected to have mood disorders in a 6-month period and 8.3% during their lifetime (19). Depression often goes unrecognized and untreated, and thus mental health statistics may underrepresent actual occurrences. Various studies give a range of 2 to 20% for lifetime prevalence for mood disorders (7).

Depression cuts across all social, racial, and economic groups. Studies differ on whether rates differ between socioeconomic groups, but rates between racial groups are similar. Physicians may underdiagnose mood disorders in people of a different race from their own (7). (Psychiatric diagnosis requires relating behaviors and symptoms to the individual's own life and situation. This increases the risk of misdiagnosis when there is significant difference between physician and patient.) Women have twice the risk of men for developing depression during their lifetime (7). Depression is more common in people who are single than in those who are married (7). Epidemiological studies may give different rates, which may reflect use of different reporting systems or different protocols for identification and diagnosis. Depression affects people of all ages, from infancy to old age, with the highest rate of occurrence in the 25- to 44-year age range (19). Recently there has been concern about the growing rate of depression in children and adolescents. It is not clear if this is because of a true change in rate or improved diagnostic procedures and increased awareness that depression is common in younger persons.

Signs and Symptoms

Depression is defined by its symptoms. There is no blood test or other laboratory means to determine whether a person has depression. The *DSM-IV* establishes a minimum of five of nine possible symptoms to diagnose a major depressive episode (which then becomes a major depressive disorder if the person has never had a manic episode and if other causes of the depressive episode are ruled out). These symptoms are listed in Table 6.1. There is also a group of associated symptoms that may be exhibited by depressed persons. Cross-cultural studies of depression suggest that the symptoms for depressive disorders vary according to cultural norms of behavior and expression of emotions (20).

As you would expect, a depressed or sad mood is one of the major symptoms of depression. This obvious change in mood does not always occur in patients, and children and adolescents may display an irritable, rather than depressed, mood (1). People may say that they feel sad all the time or hopeless. They may say they are "down" or "feeling blue," or they may complain of always feeling tired. Children may not be able to describe their feelings very clearly.

Another major, and more frequent, indicator of depression is a loss of interest or pleasure in most activities (1, 21). People who are seriously depressed do not want to do the things that they normally enjoy. If they do engage in these activities, it is without pleasure. Bowling with friends may seem more obligation than fun. The garden grows weeds as its owner neglects what was her major source of leisure enjoyment for the past 5 years. A grown daughter may no longer be able to convince her widowed mother to go on their monthly antique hunting and lunch expedition. Grandfather may not feel any joy in a fishing trip with his grandson. Even in the absence of any identified depressed feelings, the loss of interest and pleasure should be a strong indicator that a person may be depressed (21).

Decreased appetite is another common symptom of depression. This may not be evident until the person shows a notable weight loss without having consciously cut back on food. Conversely, a depressed person may overeat, although this is less common.

People who are depressed frequently complain of problems with sleeping. They may have difficulty falling asleep at night or will report not sleeping at all, although the latter usually is not true. When sleep comes late in the night, depressed people have a great deal of trouble getting out of bed in the morning. Sometimes depression is characterized by awakening very early and not being able to return to sleep. Occasionally, people who are depressed sleep much more than normal.

Family and friends may notice that the person moves much more slowly than usual or that he or she seems agitated and may pace or have trouble sitting still. These psychomotor symptoms are often accompanied by extreme fatigue. A man who routinely jogs may report that he just doesn't have the energy to do it anymore. Physical symptoms often cause the individual and concerned family members to look for physical causes and may be the reason for a visit to the family doctor. A focus on physical symptoms may obscure the diagnosis of depression.

People who are depressed often feel useless and unworthy. They may be preoccupied with guilt over some real or delusional occurrence in the past. Having others worry about them or do kind things for them increases their sense of guilt or worthlessness. They may often think of death or suicide, and frequently plan or attempt suicide. William Styron writes of the relentlessness of depression, the lack of hope, and the physical pain. "And so, because there is no respite at all, it is entirely natural that the victim begins to think ceaselessly of oblivion" (2). Ann's failed suicide attempt may be the factor that brings her into treatment. Joe's suicide may be the first indication to his family and friends that he was experiencing depression, and it may forever leave them trying to understand what happened. Sometimes the individual's preoccupation with death is focused on others (e.g., the woman who reads obituaries and recites the recent deaths of all her friends as the major content of her conversation).

Depressed people often have difficulty thinking and problem solving, even in areas in which they are usually skilled. In children this may show up in school performance: Amy "daydreams" and doesn't get her work done, and she no longer "tries" in math. Adults may start to have difficulty handling their work. Making decisions is often extremely difficult. Mrs. Smith agonizes over whether to shop before or after lunch, and it takes her half the day to select a menu for dinner.

A number of symptoms may occur with depression that are not central to its diagnosis. These include such things as crying a great deal, having high levels of anxiety, being preoccupied with the state of one's health, brooding over minor incidents, and experiencing panic attacks. People who are depressed may be delusional or experience hallucinations, usually related to their unworthiness or to being persecuted or punished for something they have done.

People who have depressive disorders exhibit these symptoms to varying degrees. Although not symptoms per se, the feelings of family and friends may also help identify people with depression. Families may worry and feel that they need to take care of the individual. The family may be angry because people who are depressed are no fun to be around and resist all attempts by the family to cheer them.

Some symptoms vary according to age. In addition to school problems, children may show more psychomotor agitation and hallucinations than adults. Adolescents may engage in antisocial behavior, including substance abuse. Withdrawal from the family and school difficulties are common. Elderly adults with depression may be misdiagnosed as having dementia. In fact, a number of symptoms of Alzheimer-type dementia are also symptoms of depression, such as decreased interest, poor concentration, fatigue, and changes in psychomotor activity (35). Careful diagnosis is important, because depression is usually reversible with appropriate treatment. When physical symptoms of depression predominate, the person may undergo many unnecessary diagnostic procedures if depression is not considered.

Course and Prognosis

Depression may be acute or chronic, but even in acute cases, there is a typical duration of 6 months. At a minimum, 2 weeks of symptoms are required to diagnose a major depressive episode (1). For people with a chronic depression, some symptoms may persist, even when the major symptoms have lifted. A person may have a single episode of depression or recurring episodes over a lifetime.

Depression may, in time, lift without treatment, but there is no reason for a person to go through the pain and disruption of a major depression, waiting for it to go away by itself. This is a very treatable disorder, at least in terms of alleviating symptoms. However, people often go without treatment because they, and others around them, do not recognize the depression, or they fail to seek help because of the stigma of having a mental illness. Knowledge of the biological causes of depression may make seeking treatment more acceptable. It has been my experience that people who are managing to function in their daily lives, even if symptoms of depression are making this difficult, often resist the notion of having a psychiatric disorder.

Until recently, few studies were done of the long-term prognosis for depression. It was assumed that people returned to normal functioning once the symptoms of depression had subsided. Studies now show that this is not universally true. About 20% of persons who have major depression may develop chronic depression (22), and about the same proportion may have a recurrence during the first year. It is not yet clear how patients function over time in their daily occupational performance after major depression.

The major complication of depression is the high risk of suicide. It is estimated that more than half the suicides in the United States are related to depression. Ten to 15% of people who are hospitalized with depression will eventually commit suicide (3, 19). The risk of suicide is high for those who are in the hospital for medical conditions and who suffer from depression and for people in the months after discharge from a psychiatric unit.

Potential suicide should always be a consideration when working with an individual who is depressed. Clinicians must observe closely for signs that someone might be thinking of hurting himself or herself, or might have a suicide plan. All such suggestions must be taken very seriously. In an inpatient setting, patients considered to be acutely suicidal are usually placed on a one-to-one staffing ratio or are given ward restrictions with 15-minute checks. In occupational therapy, careful counts are kept of any potentially dangerous implements, and toxic materials are kept locked up when not in use. Use of any dangerous tools or substances is closely monitored. Suicide may be a risk with other conditions, and similar precautions should be followed as standard practice.

Another common complication of depression is substance abuse. Depressed people may turn to alcohol or drugs as means of "self-medication," or the depression may be secondary to the substance abuse problem.

Diagnosis

As stated earlier, depression is diagnosed on the basis of symptoms. In addition to meeting criteria for symptoms, the person must have had the symptoms for at least 2 weeks and must not be going through a normal reaction to a bereavement. The clinician must be sure that there is no organic cause for the symptoms and must rule out other disorders with similar characteristics, such as schizophrenia, delusional disorder, and anxiety disorder.

Some scales and inventories are used to help diagnose depression, such as the Beck depression inventory (23), the Hamilton rating scale (24),

the schedule of affective disorders and schizophrenia (SADS) (25), and the research and diagnostic criteria (21). These seem most useful in classifying subtypes of depression or in ensuring homogeneity of subjects for research purposes. They have demonstrated concurrent validity with each other and with other diagnostic criteria. These instruments may not be useful for cross-cultural studies of depression. No laboratory or other medical tests are able to diagnose depression reliably at this time.

Medical/Surgical Management

Medications

Antidepressant medications fall into four categories: the heterocyclics (*tricyclics* until fairly recently), the monoamine oxidase inhibitors (MAOI) (7), the selective serotonin reuptake inhibitors (SSRIs), and those chemically unrelated to any of those categories. Antidepressant medications are summarized in the Medications Appendix at the end of this book. The various types of antidepressant medications are equally effective in treating depression, but individuals respond to them differently.

Until recently, the most commonly used drugs were the tricyclics. These take several weeks to reach full therapeutic benefits, as do all of the antidepressant medications. No particular type is more effective than another, but they vary in their side effects. Physicians often choose a particular drug because of such factors as side effects and patient preference. For example, a person with a cardiac problem would be given a medication with no known cardiovascular side effects, and a person with an agitated depression might be given a drug that had sedative side effects. If a patient had good results with a particular medication in the past, it will usually be the first one tried.

Monoamine oxidase inhibitors are used less frequently than heterocyclics in the treatment of depression because they require more careful management and are somewhat less effective. They work by inhibiting the production of monoamine oxidase, a normally occurring enzyme that breaks down certain amines in the body, including serotonin and norepinephrine. When the levels of monoamine oxidase are reduced, the levels of serotonin and norepinephrine rise, effecting a remission of the depression. Unfortunately, the effects of monoamine oxidase are general, and some of the amines it breaks down become toxic. These substances that break down into dangerous products come from a wide variety of food, much of it aged or fermented, including aged cheese, pickled herring, red wine, beer, and cured meats, as well as some over-the-counter and prescribed medications. Patients must be well educated in what foods to avoid and motivated to follow the dietary restrictions. (Therapists should check with the dietician or nurse before any use of food in occupational therapy treatment groups.) If dietary restrictions are not followed, the person taking MAOIs may develop increased blood pressure, headaches, and intracranial bleeding resulting in death. In spite of the care that must be followed when taking MAOIs, they are the only effective medication for some people.

Selective serotonin reuptake inhibitors were developed recently but have rapidly become the most prescribed antidepressants because they have fewer side effects than earlier drugs. Most side effects, if they do occur, are transient. Sexual dysfunction is a common and persistent side effect (7). Fluoxetine hydrochloride (Prozac), the most widely used SSRI, is controversial. Whereas this medication appears to be very effective for many people, there was early concern that it might increase the risk of suicide or violence. The belief that it is being overprescribed is common in the popular press—a perception based on Prozac's becoming the most widely prescribed antidepressant in the United States within 2 years of its introduction (26). Newspaper columns, periodicals, and books raise issues about people taking medication to improve their mood, linking this to drug abuse directly or by implication. The belief that people ought to be able to pull themselves out of their depressed moods, identifying depression as a problem of moral weakness, is basic to these concerns.

Antidepressant medications are toxic, with lethal doses being only a few times greater than the normal daily dose. Thus suicidal patients must be carefully monitored to be sure that they are taking medication as prescribed (not saving pills), and outpatients should not be given large supplies of medication until the risk of suicide has declined. The SSRIs are less toxic than other antidepressants, but they should be monitored.

Antidepressants usually take 3 to 4 weeks to alleviate depression, and even after the obvious symptoms of depression begin to lift, the individual may still *feel* very depressed. The period after treatment begins and before effects are felt can be very difficult for depressed patients, the lack of immediate relief adding to their feelings of hopelessness. Much reassurance and education are needed during this time, and caregivers and family should watch for signs of potential suicide. A person may not do well while taking a particular medication, experiencing unacceptable side effects or not achieving therapeutic benefits. Changes in medication will prolong the time before a person feels improvement.

Electroconvulsive Therapy

Electroconvulsive therapy (ECT) is "the brief application of an electrical stimulus to the brain to produce a generalized seizure" (27). Electroconvulsive therapy can be very effective in short-term treatment for some people who have depression, notably when the depression includes delusions, when it has no known antecedents, or when the person is at extremely high risk for suicide (7, 27). Effects of treatment are seen more rapidly than with antidepressant medication.

Unfortunately, ECT has received "bad press" because it was massively misused in treatment of psychiatric patients in the past. Public reaction to this abuse continues to limit access to this treatment. It is also frightening, and the reason it works is not understood. Thus, it is probably not used as much as it could be, and often it is considered only as a last resort, when medications have not been effective or the patient's depression is considered life threatening.

When ECT is used, strict protocols are followed, including consultation with other physicians and careful attention to informed consent of the patient and family. A thorough medical screening is completed before use of ECT.

A physician gives ECT on an inpatient or outpatient basis, with a professional anesthetist and nursing personnel in attendance. Treatment is usually given in the morning after 8 to 12 hours of fasting. Before treatment, the patient is given an anticholinergic agent, a brief anesthetic, and a muscle relaxant. Oxygen is administered throughout the procedure, and the electrocardiogram (EKG), blood pressure, and pulse rate are continuously monitored. A brief electrical stimulus is given to the brain through one or two electrodes, using the lowest amount of electrical energy needed to produce a seizure (as evidenced by electroencephalogram monitoring or physical evidence of a seizure). Usually a patient has 6 to 12 of these treatments at the rate of 2 to 3 per week (7).

After treatment, patients are monitored in the recovery room and then returned to the patient ward or home to rest. Often they can engage in activity in the afternoon after early morning treatment, although they may still feel tired.

The major adverse effect of ECT is memory loss, which is seen in almost all cases. The severity of the memory deficit varies according to the individual and the degree of treatment. For many patients, memory problems relate to the time around the treatment and persist for as long as 3 years. During the time patients are receiving treatment and for a few weeks after its comple-

tion, they may have transient difficulty learning and retaining new information (27). The treatment does carry some risk of complications such as cardiorespiratory problems, severe confusion, and falls (28). It is, however, viewed as a safe and effective treatment choice.

In addition to medication or ECT, psychotherapy is often helpful for people with depression. Although such therapy might not alleviate symptoms or prevent relapse, it can enhance social functioning (29). Psychotherapy may be either focused and short term, or more psychodynamically oriented and long term.

Impact on Occupational Performance

All occupational performance areas may be affected by this condition, a fact reflected in the number of symptoms that relate directly to functioning. In a very large study of functioning and well-being of depressed patients, Wells et al. demonstrated that depression is associated with limitations in functioning (physical, social, and role) and well-being. They also concluded that depressed people have comparable or worse functioning than patients with chronic medical conditions, with the exception of current heart conditions (30). Table 6.5 highlights the performance areas and components where dysfunction is most likely to be seen.

Any of the occupational performance areas may be affected. The typical symptoms of major depressive disorder affect occupational performance according to each individual's characteristics (e.g., age, sex, life situation, roles) and environmental expectations (e.g., family responsibilities, support systems, roles). The individual's social and cultural contexts have substantial impact on how he or she experiences depression. Thus, there is no single, "typical" depressed person. The following case study shows how occupational performance is affected for one person with major depressive disorder (Table 6.5).

TABLE 6.5   Occupational Performance Profile

I. PERFORMANCE AREAS	II. PERFORMANCE COMPONENTS	III. PERFORMANCE CONTEXTS

I. PERFORMANCE AREAS

A. Activities of Daily Living*
  1. Grooming
  2. Oral Hygiene
  3. Bathing/Showering
  4. Toilet Hygiene
  5. Personal Device Care
  6. Dressing
  7. Feeding and Eating
  8. Medication Routine
  9. Health Maintenance
  10. Socialization
  11. Functional Communication
  12. Functional Mobility
  13. Community Mobility
  14. Emergency Response
  15. Sexual Expression
B. Work and Productive Activities*
  1. Home Management
    a. Clothing Care
    b. Cleaning
    c. Meal Preparation/Cleanup
    d. Shopping
    e. Money Management
    f. Household Maintenance
    g. Safety Procedures
  2. Care of Others
  3. Educational Activities
  4. Vocational Activities
    a. Vocational Exploration
    b. Job Acquisition
    c. Work or Job Performance
    d. Retirement Planning
    e. Volunteer Participation
C. Play or Leisure Activities
  1. Play or Leisure Exploration
  2. Play or Leisure Performance

II. PERFORMANCE COMPONENTS

A. Sensorimotor Component
  1. Sensory
    a. Sensory Awareness
    b. Sensory Processing
      (1) Tactile
      (2) Proprioceptive
      (3) Vestibular
      (4) Visual
      (5) Auditory
      (6) Gustatory
      (7) Olfactory
    c. Perceptual Processing
      (1) Stereognosis
      (2) Kinesthesia
      (3) Pain Response
      (4) Body Scheme
      (5) Right–Left Discrimination
      (6) Form Constancy
      (7) Position in Space
      (8) Visual–Closure
      (9) Figure Ground
      (10) Depth Perception
      (11) Spatial Relations
      (12) Topographical Orientation
  2. Neuromusculoskeletal
    a. Reflex
    b. Range of Motion
    c. Muscle Tone
    d. Strength
    e. Endurance
    f. Postural Control
    g. Postural Alignment
    h. Soft Tissue Integrity
  3. Motor
    a. Gross Coordination
    b. Crossing the Midline
    c. Laterality
    d. Bilateral Integration
    e. Motor Control
    f. Praxis
    g. Fine Coordination/Dexterity
    h. Visual–Motor Control
    i. Oral–Motor Control

III. PERFORMANCE CONTEXTS

A. Temporal Aspects
  1. Chronological
  2. Developmental
  3. Lifecycle
  4. Disability Status
B. Environment
  1. Physical
  2. Social
  3. Cultural

(continued)

		III. PERFORMANCE

TABLE 6.5 Occupational Performance Profile (Continued)

I. PERFORMANCE AREAS	II. PERFORMANCE COMPONENTS	III. PERFORMANCE CONTEXTS

B. Cognitive Integration and Cognitive
   Components
   1. Level of Arousal
   2. Orientation
   3. Recognition
   4. Attention Span
   5. Initiation of Activity
   6. Termination of Activity
   7. Memory
   8. Sequencing
   9. Categorization
   10. Concept Formation
   11. Spatial Operations
   12. Problem Solving
   13. Learning
   14. Generalization
C. Psychosocial Skills and
   Psychological Components
   1. Psychological
      a. Values
      b. Interests
      c. Self-Concept
   2. Social
      a. Role Performance
      b. Social Conduct
      c. Interpersonal Skills
      d. Self-Expression
   3. Self-Management
      a. Coping Skills
      b. Time Management
      c. Self-Control

*All may be affected

CASE STUDIES

CASE 1

Major Depression

M. K. is a 38-year-old married woman with 2 children, aged 14 and 16. For 2 months prior to admission to an inpatient unit, M. K. complained of constant fatigue and being unable to sleep at night. She began to stay up late to avoid tossing and turning and to decrease the chance that her husband would want to have sex, something she no longer enjoyed. M. K. works part-time in the grade school library, a job she always said she loved. She now says that "the job hasn't been the same lately" and reports that she called in sick frequently over the past 2 months and knows her work performance has deteriorated. Lately she has been preoccupied with thoughts that she will be fired, although her supervisor has always been pleased with her work.

In the past M. K.'s interests were broad, including doing things with her husband and children such as attending church, going on picnics, and participating in school social events. She bowled in a neighborhood league with her husband and socialized with a group of friends on a regular basis. M. K. also enjoyed cooking and playing cards. When she started feeling tired all the time, she discontinued all of these interests except attending church, explaining to everyone that she was not feeling well and had to save her energy for work.

At home, M. K. started to pay less and less attention to her usually immaculate house and carried out only those chores necessary to keep the home functioning. When her husband or children offered help, she reacted with tears and accusations that they didn't think she was able to do anything. M. K. tells the occupational therapist that she feels terribly guilty about not taking care of her family.

M. K. used to dress stylishly and wear carefully applied makeup. Lately her clothes have not always matched, and she rarely applies makeup or bothers to style her hair. She says it doesn't matter anyway because nobody cares how she looks.

M. K.'s usual "sunny" relationships with her family and friends have also changed. She no longer participates in mutual activities, and her concerns with her own feelings override concern for others. Her children complain openly that she is not fun as she used to be. They no longer bring friends to the house and avoid spending time there. Her husband has gently tried to discuss the situation, but each time he does, M. K. starts crying and accuses him of not loving her anymore, of having an affair, and of not understanding her. He, too, is starting to stay away from home, often working late. M. K. has cut off all contact with friends, many of whom have stopped calling after repeated failed attempts to involve M. K. in some activity. M. K.'s job performance has suffered less than other occupational performance areas, but lately she has had difficulty handling unusual situations, has stopped taking time to talk with the children, and has difficulty managing the physical demands of the job because of fatigue.

For 2 weeks before coming to the hospital, M. K. often found herself crying for no apparent reason. She was unable to get out of bed for several mornings and only went to work twice. Her husband brought her to the hospital emergency room because she said she couldn't breathe and felt like she was dying.

M. K. was given a diagnosis of major depression and started on a treatment program that included antidepressant medication, group and individual therapy, and occupational therapy. It is anticipated that she will be discharged after 5 days of inpatient care, with 2 weeks of partial hospital treatment, and ongoing outpatient treatment with a psychiatrist.

To summarize her occupational performance, M. K.'s performance of activities of daily living is affected with respect to grooming, socialization, and sexual expression. In work activities, almost all areas of home management are affected, as is care for her family and job performance. Neither leisure exploration nor performance occurs.

With appropriate treatment (antidepressant medication and psychotherapy), it is highly likely that M. K. will return to her previous lifestyle. She may have a recurrence of the depression in the future, but her psychotherapist has educated her and her family to recognize the early symptoms and seek treatment as soon as she feels that she may be becoming depressed.

BIPOLAR DISORDER

Etiology

Bipolar disorders, often referred to as manic-depressive disease, have been clearly linked to heredity. About 50% of people with bipolar disorder have a parent with the disease (7). Evidence that this disorder is genetic has been found in studies of family incidence, twin studies, and adoption studies. The existence of any blood relative with a history of bipolar disorder, depression, or for that matter, mental illness, lends support to this diagnosis for persons meeting other diagnostic criteria. Where there is doubt about presenting symptoms, the family history often provides sufficient support for the physician to prescribe lithium, a medication known to treat the symptoms of bipolar disorder effectively. In a roundabout way, good response to lithium confirms the diagnosis.

Although the genetic component of bipolar disorders is well established, it is not clear what triggers individual episodes. In some cases there appears to be a correlation with levels of psychosocial stress in the individual's environment, but this is not universally true. Often there seems to be no relation between episodes and life circumstances.

Incidence and Prevalence

"The lifetime expectancy of developing bipolar disorder is about 1% in both men and women"

(7). Variations in rates between the United States and other countries suggest differences in patterns of diagnosis by physicians, rather than a difference in prevalence. The onset of manic episodes occurs in the early 20s on average, but people may develop a bipolar disorder at any age.

Signs and Symptoms

A person with bipolar I disorder will, at the least, experience manic or mixed episodes and may also have one or more major depressive episodes (Tables 6.1–6.3.) The symptoms of the depression are the same as those described earlier. A person with bipolar II disorder will have a history of one or more major depressive episodes and at least one hypomanic episode (Table 6.4). If a person has had a manic or mixed episode, they meet the criteria for bipolar I disorder. An occupational therapist is most likely to work with persons with bipolar II disorder during the depressive episodes. On the other hand, people with bipolar I disorder are often seen during manic episodes.

Persons in the manic phase of a bipolar disorder are often easy to spot, especially if their illness is severe enough to require hospital treatment. There is an "excessive" quality about everything they do. They may start sleeping very little without experiencing fatigue; become unusually euphoric, expansive, "high," or irritable; and become more active in work or school. The unusually elevated mood is recognized by those close to the individual. However, the euphoric outlook may explode into rage with little provocation. During a manic episode, the individual may speak rapidly and loudly, expressing intense enthusiasm for everything planned or accomplished. Sometimes people with this disorder believe they are very powerful or special. People with mania may take risks in their activities because they feel invincible. For example, a businessman may start a number of new ventures with very little capital, or a student may party the night before an examination because she "knows" that she will "ace" the test. If the individual is delusional, the content of the delusions is usually grandiose: a patient may tell you that he owns the hospital and will see to it that you receive a big bonus. John repeatedly told me that all the women in the world were his wives, including me!

Many of the symptoms may be enjoyed by the individuals and those around them, as long as they do not get out of hand. Some symptoms, at controlled levels, may be an asset in certain jobs. For example, not needing much sleep may benefit the long-distance truck driver, or increased goal-directed activity might help the employee in an advertising firm when a new campaign is being developed. Individuals who experience their symptoms as pleasurable may reject treatment. Hypomanic episodes may not trouble the individual.

The occupational therapy clinic is often very exciting for the patient in a manic episode. Plans are stated enthusiastically to make every available project bigger and more complex than ever before. A simple project is described as a "masterpiece," and accepted rules and standards of performance are rejected as "not creative" or "too restrictive." On the hospital unit, the patient in a manic episode will keep things stirred up, and more than one person with this diagnosis may create chaos. Mental health professionals often describe manic patients as being extremely intrusive.

Until symptoms are partially controlled by medication and by the natural course of the illness, management of the patient with mania is focused on avoiding stimulation (thus you might not see this patient in the occupational therapy clinic during the early stages of hospitalization) and providing a firm and consistent structure.

Course and Prognosis

Manic episodes usually develop rapidly over a few days and may last for a few days to a few months (1). Symptoms often respond well to pharmacological intervention, and people who receive prophylactic medication may function well for years. As with depression, few studies of functioning over time have been completed for people with this diagnosis. Harrow et al. completed a prospective follow-up study of patients with bipolar disorder and found that many had moderately impaired or poor functioning in the period following hospitalization. Very poor outcomes were found in 30% (31). People with bipolar disease should be carefully monitored as outpatients, to ensure that medication levels are sufficiently high and to identify stressful life circumstances that might lead to relapse or recurrence.

Some people with bipolar I disorder experience rapid cycling of moods from manic to depressed. Others never experience a clear depression. For some, the intervals between episodes are brief; for others relatively long, stretching into years without clinically significant symptoms.

Common "complications" for persons with bipolar disorders result from behaviors during manic episodes. The incidence of "risky" behaviors, such as substance abuse, excessive spending, gambling, sexual promiscuity, and reckless driving, is high. People may experience effects on their physical and mental well-being, work performance, and social relationships as sequelae to such behaviors. Even with remission of symptoms, occupational performance may not improve (32), perhaps because the social structures that support this performance were destroyed by the person's behavior while manic. Potential complications during depressive episodes are the same as for major depressive disorder.

Diagnosis

Persons who experience symptoms of mania without marked impairment in occupational performance or risk of harming themselves or others are said to have a *hypomanic* episode. When occupational performance is significantly impaired, the symptoms are called a "manic episode".

Bipolar disorders are diagnosed according to the symptoms of mood episodes using the *DSM-IV* criteria (Tables 6.1–6.4). In addition, presence of mood disorders or any history of mental illness in blood relations indicates the possibility of this diagnosis. Diagnosis includes ruling out other possible causes, such as use of psychoactive substances or brain disorders. Sometimes it is difficult to distinguish between psychotic disorders and manic episodes, especially when onset occurs in young males and involves irritability and delusions of grandeur and persecution. Again, family history supports a bipolar diagnosis.

Medical/Surgical Management

Bipolar disorders usually respond well in both manic and depressive episodes to treatment with a compound of lithium (a carbonate or citrate) or an anticonvulsant (carbamazepine, valproate), and people may be maintained on medication for many years with few side effects. Lithium is metabolized differently by different individuals and over time by the same person. Because it is highly toxic, patients receive a careful medical screening before administration, and monitoring of blood levels is essential for safe and effective use. Initially, blood is drawn for analysis several times a week, then tapered over time. With maintenance doses, blood levels are determined as infrequently as once a year. A level between 0.6 and 1.2 mEq/liter is considered therapeutic (7, 33). Anything lower is ineffective, and higher levels are dangerous and potentially fatal.

Side effects of lithium treatment include a fine tremor of the hands, nausea, and vomiting. These usually occur in the first few days of treatment. Signs of possible toxicity include drowsiness, blurred vision, fatigue, thirst, dizziness, gait problems, coarse tremor, and muscle twitching. Moderate toxicity may be indicated with more severe neuromuscular symptoms, seizures, and confusion. Severe toxicity can result in coma and death.

At this time, lithium is believed to be an extremely effective method of treating bipolar disorders and preventing recurrences. It is not, however, a panacea. Some people discontinue taking it because of weight gain, polyuria, and fine hand tremor. It is also known to be teratogenic, so use in women of childbearing age must be considered cautiously (34). Furthermore, only about 20% of those taking it have no further recurrences, although it probably moderates the rate of occurrence and severity of manic or depressed episodes (34). A number of individuals respond well to anticonvulsants for treatment of bipolar I disorder. Effective drug treatment for bipolar II disorder is still being investigated (7).

Impact on Occupational Performance

The sensorimotor components of occupational performance are not likely to be affected by this disorder, except as side effects of medications. Any cognitive or psychological component may be disturbed, according to the individual, the severity of the episode, and the manner in which symptoms are manifested (Table 6.5).

The following case shows how a person's occupational performance may be affected by this illness.

CASE STUDIES

CASE 1

Bipolar Disorder

P. J. is a 32-year-old college graduate who owns a small business. He is married and has two children. His wife describes him as usually fun to be around, well liked, and good with the children. Once in college, and again just prior to his marriage 7 years ago, P. J. went through periods of several weeks when he hardly slept at all. The first time he was planning a fraternity party, which he was determined would be the best ever held, and was working extra hours to have money for a summer vacation. He says he felt as if he was invincible and on a "natural high." At first all of his friends were eager to be with him, but as the episode went on he became irritable and friends dropped away. One night he began to shout that he was the leader of the universe and no one could tell him what to do. He fought off those who tried to quiet him down. He was taken by police to the campus clinic and was hospitalized for 2 weeks in a psychiatric unit. His psychiatrist was unsure of a diagnosis, and when symptoms cleared spontaneously, P. J. was discharged with the recommendation that he receive counseling.

P. J. successfully completed college and took a job in business. He used a small inheritance to make some investments and made enough money to buy a small retail business. Usually P. J. put in a 12-hour day at work. He spent a great deal of time contacting new customers, putting together new product lines, developing displays, and supervising a small staff. After 2 years, he and his live-in girlfriend from college decided to get married. Two months before the wedding, P. J. started talking constantly about how great it was to be single, how much women liked him, plans he had to develop a retail chain, plans to return to school for a degree in law, and other diffuse and generally grandiose ideas he had for his immediate and future life. He started staying up late and often left home for hours in the evening. One night his fianceé received a call from the jail where P. J. had been taken after a fight over a woman at a bar. When she went to the jail to bail him out, P. J. told her not to bother, he knew the judge and would be out the next day. He yelled at her loudly, telling her he was the best thing that had ever happened to her and she ought to appreciate him more.

P. J. was taken to a psychiatric hospital and given the diagnosis of acute intoxication and bipolar I disorder. After he became sober, he continued to exhibit a state of euphoria for several days until the medication (lithium carbonate) took effect. After P. J. returned home, he continued to take the lithium, returned to work, and got married as planned. At work he noticed that some of his old customers had not returned and that his financial records were in disarray. Bills had not been paid for many months, and his stock inventory was at an unusually high level, reflecting excessive ordering he had done during his manic episode.

From then until the present episode, P. J. worked hard and put his business back in order. He and his wife enjoyed an active social life together that included bowling, softball, and card playing with friends. Such activities often included heavy drinking and occasional use of marijuana. Sometimes P. J. would become loud and "obnoxious," but often he was the life of the party, and the couple was sought out by others.

Six weeks ago, P. J. started to talk about adding new lines to his stock and took out several bank loans to buy large orders. He began to stay late at work and sometimes would go home with one or another of the female employees. He contacted local business leaders to propose partnerships, bought himself a luxury car, and planned to take his wife on a trip to the Riviera to gamble. His wife, however, was more concerned about his not coming home at night, and when she objected, P. J. became verbally abusive toward her. Two weeks ago she told him she'd had enough, and she and the children went to her parents to stay. P. J. called her frequently, telling her that he had changed, reminding her of the fun they had together, and then becoming angry again when she refused to move back.

One week ago, P. J. started to feel very tired and overwhelmed. He says it was like a black cloud, a weight, descending on his head. He could hardly bring himself to go to work in the morning, and when he got there would often find himself crying for no apparent reason. He decided that there was no reason to go on—his marriage was in trouble, he was heavily in debt, and one of his female employees was threatening to sue him for harassment if he didn't give her a raise. P. J. purchased a gun and wrote a suicide note, but decided to give his wife a last call. The tone of his voice was so different that she became worried and called the police to go to the house. They found P. J. with the gun in his hand, easily disarmed him, and took him to the psychiatric emergency room. Even though P. J. was having a major depressive episode, his diagnosis was bipolar I disorder because of previous manic episodes.

P. J. again responded well to medication, but the effects of his illness on his life were not so easy to mend. After individual and couple counseling, his wife agreed to return to the home on a trial basis. The business was in such a bad state that P. J. had to declare bankruptcy and sell it at a loss. In addition, he discovered that one of the employees with whom he'd had sexual relations is an I.V. drug user, and he worries about the possibility that he might have contracted AIDS. Because P. J. has very little work experience in anything but his own business he has not been able to find work, and his wife has returned to work to make ends meet. Still, P. J. talks of the big plans he has to succeed, and he continues to be enjoyable company most of the time.

P. J.'s occupational performance areas have all been affected by his bipolar disorder. These effects have varied over time. In summary, P. J. shows dysfunction in the area of activities of daily living of health maintenance and socialization. In the occupational performance area of work activities, he does not manage money well and has failed to take appropriate safety precautions in his sexual activity. His ability to care for others is questionable. P. J.'s work performance in the past has been both excellent and horrible. At this time he is not managing vocational exploration and job acquisition, both necessary to rebuilding his life. In leisure performance there does not seem to be any pres-

ent problem, but in the past P. J. has engaged in leisure activities that were dangerous or destructive to his family life. The temporal aspects of P. J.'s occupational performance are affected by the disabling nature of his illness and by his failure to participate effectively in the roles expected of him at this stage of his life. In a cultural environment that rewards his hard work, and a social environment that reinforces his expansive affect and activities that may be part of his manic episodes, P. J.'s symptoms may be encouraged.

P. J.'s prognosis is unclear. He is now taking lithium, which controls the symptoms of his bipolar disorder, but his behavior during past manic episodes has severely eroded his support systems. P. J. is a good candidate for psychotherapy, which should focus on setting and working toward realistic goals to get his life back in order. P. J. and his wife might also benefit from marital counseling.

POINTS FOR REVIEW

1. Give a brief and concise definition of mood disorder.

2. What are the two major categories of mood disorders?

3. Describe the major theories that try to explain the cause of depression.

4. What are the most common symptoms of depression?

5. What are the four categories of medications used for depression? What are their major side effects?

6. What is the distinction between bipolar I disorder and bipolar II disorder?

REFERENCES

1. American Psychiatric Association. Diagnostic and Statistical Manual of Mental Disorders. 4th ed. Washington, DC: American Psychiatric Association, 1994.

2. Styron W. Why Primo Levi died. New York Times, Dec 19, 1988.

3. Doherty K. The good news about depression. Business Week 1989; (Mar):39–42.

4. Sinaikin PM. A clinically relevant guide to the differential diagnosis of depression. J Nerv Ment Dis 1985;173:199–211.

5. National Depressive and Manic Depressive Association. Consensus statement on the under treatment of depression. JAMA 1997;277(4):333–340.

6. Andreasen NC. Concepts, diagnosis and classification. In: Paykel ES, ed. Handbook of Affective Disorders. New York: Guilford Press, 1982:24–44.

7. Kaplan HI, Sadock BJ. Synopsis of psychiatry. 8th ed. Baltimore: Williams & Wilkins, 1998.

8. Akiskal HS, Tashjian R. Affective disorders: II. Recent advances in laboratory and pathogenetic approaches. Hosp Community Psychiatry 1983;34: 822–830.

9. Wehr TA, Rosenthal NE. Seasonality and affective illness. Am J Psychiatry 1989;146:829–839.

10. Karasu TB. Toward a clinical model of psychotherapy for depression, I: Systematic comparison of three psychotherapies. Am J Psychiatry 1990;147: 133–147.

11. Beck AT. Depression: Causes and Treatment. Philadelphia: University of Pennsylvania Press, 1967.

12. Sackeim HA, Wegner AZ. Attributional patterns in depression and euthymia. Arch Gen Psychiatry 1986;43:553–560.

13. Silverman JS, Silverman JA, Eardley DA. Do maladaptive attitudes cause depression? Arch Gen Psychiatry 1984;41:28–30.

14. Ellis A, Harper, RA. A guide to rational living. Hollywood, CA: Wilshire, 1973.

15. Seligman MEP. Helplessness: on depression, development, and death. San Francisco: WH Freeman, 1975.

16. Lewinsohn PM, Libet J. Pleasant events, activity schedules and depression. J Abnorm Psychol 1972;79:291–295.

17. Lewinsohn PM, Youngren MA, Grosscup SJ. Reinforcement and depression. In: Depue RA, ed. The Psychobiology of the Depressive Disorders: Implications for the Effects of Stress. New York: Academic Press, 1979.

18. Lewinsohn PM, Munoz RF, Youngren MA, et al. Control Your Depression. Englewood Cliffs, NJ: Prentice-Hall, 1978.

19. Regier DA, Hirshfeld RMA, Goodwin FK, et al. The NIMH depression awareness, recognition, and treatment program: structure, aims and scientific basis. Am J Psychiatry 1988;145:1351–1357.

20. Kleinman A, Good B, eds. Culture and Depression: Studies in the Anthropology and Cross-Cultural Psychiatry of Affect and Disorder. Berkeley: University of California Press, 1985.

21. Spitzer RL, Endicott J, Robins E. Research diagnostic criteria: rationale and reliability. Arch Gen Psychiatry 1978;35:773–783.

22. Sargeant JK, Bruce ML, Florio LP, et al. Factors associated with 1-year outcome of major depression in the community. Arch Gen Psychiatry 1990;47:519–526.

23. Beck AT, Ward CH, Mendelson M, et al. An inventory for measuring depression. Arch Gen Psychiatry 1961;4:561–571.

24. Hamilton MA. A rating scale for depression. J Neurol Neurosurg Psychiatry 1960;23:56–62.

25. Endicott J., Skpitzer RL. A diagnostic interview: the schedule for affective disorders and schizophrenia. Arch Gen Psychiatry 1978;35:837–844.

26. Yudofsky S, Hales RE, Ferguson T. What You Need to Know about Psychiatric Drugs. Washington, DC: American Psychiatric Press, 1991.

27. National Institutes of Health. Electroconvulsive therapy. Consensus Development Conference statement. U.S. Department of Health and Human Services 1985;5(11).

28. Zorumski CF, Rubin EH, Burke WJ. Electroconvulsive therapy for the elderly: a review. Hosp Community Psychiatry 1988;39:643–647.

29. Weissman MM, Klerman GL, Paykel ES, et al. Treatment effects on the social adjustment of depressed patients. Arch Gen Psychiatry 1974;30:771–778.

30. Wells KB, Stewart A, Hays RD, et al. The functioning and well-being of depressed patients. JAMA 1989; 262:914–919.

31. Harrow M, Goldberg JF, Grossman LS, et al. Outcome in manic disorders. Arch Gen Psychiatry 1990;47:665–671.

32. Dion GL, Tohen N, Anthony WB, et al. Symptoms and functioning of patients with bipolar disorder six months after hospitalization. Hosp Community Psychiatry 1988;39:652–657.

33. O'Connell RA. Lithium update. In: Flach F, ed. Affective Disorders. New York: WW Norton, 1988.

34. Prien RF, Gelenberg AJ. Alternatives to lithium for preventive treatment of bipolar disorder. Am J Psychiatry 1989;146:840–848.

35. Rubin EH, Zorumski CF, Burke WJ. Overlapping symptoms of geriatric depression and Alzheimer-type dementia. Hosp Community Psychiatry 1988; 39:1074–1079.

CHAPTER 7

DEMENTIA

Joyce Fraker and Jacqueline McKillop

CRITICAL TERMS

Agnosia
Alzheimer's disease
Aphasia
Apraxia

Delirium
Dementia
Dysarthria
Lability

Neurofibrillary tangles
Plaques
Psychotropic

Mr. G. enters the hospital day room and approaches a staff nurse. "I don't know what to do." The nurse points to the chair and suggests that he have a seat. Mr. G. apparently does not recognize the purpose of the chair and responds, "What are these?"

Mr. G. was diagnosed as having dementia 5 years ago. For the past 2 years, his condition was severe enough to warrant his being placed in a nursing home. Ten days prior to this hospital admission, Mrs. G. took her husband home from the nursing home, needing his pension check to supplement their diminished savings. Within a week, she realized she could not manage his wandering, confusion, striking out at her, and need for total self-care assistance. The nursing home bed was no longer available, so she brought him to the hospital. The nurse reports that Mr. G. cannot hold a conversation but continually asks, with mild anxiety, what he should do or where he should go. Nursing care activities are focused on two basic needs: nutritional intake and toileting. He defecates or urinates wherever he may be, without searching for a bathroom or alerting staff to his need. The nurses escort him to the bathroom regularly to prevent accidents as much as possible.

Oral intake is also a management problem. He holds pills in his mouth until they dissolve, then spits them out. He doesn't seem to understand the concept of swallowing those hard little objects, or perhaps he cannot master the oral–motor task itself. At meal times, he needs verbal and physical prompts for every bite of food. One nurse confided his method for getting Mr. G. to take fluids: "I get us both a cup of water and say, 'Cheers, let's drink up.' He'll tell me, 'I really shouldn't have any more,' but I wink at him and say, 'One more won't hurt.'"

Mr. G. will leave the hospital as soon as another nursing home placement can be found.

COGNITIVE DISORDERS

Dementia, as defined by the *Diagnostic and Statistical Manual of Mental Disorders* (DSM-IV), is a condition characterized by multiple cognitive deficits, with the main deficit being impairment of memory. Former president Ronald Reagan brought national attention to the disorder when, in 1994, he announced that he had been diagnosed with Alzheimer's disease. In fact, Alzheimer's disease is the most prevalent form of dementia. Dementia, an often misunderstood disorder, has been variously identified in the past as organic brain syndrome, organic mental disorder, or senile dementia. The American Psychiatric Association no longer classifies dementia as an organic disorder, because "organic" implies that only dementia, and not other mental disorders, has a biological basis (1). Senile dementia is a term that was used when the medical community believed that memory loss was a normal part of the aging process. "Senile" literally means age 65 or older, but the term conjures up negative images of one who is weak and incompetent. Some memory loss may occur as a normal part of aging; this varies from person to person and should not interfere with occupational performance. In fact, well into late old age, individuals can learn new things. Memory loss that impairs function is a serious concern that calls for medical investigation (2).

Serious and persistent memory loss is the hallmark, or most significant symptom, of dementia. However, because memory loss is a symptom seen in other disorders, it is useful to review cognitive disorders in general.

The *DSM-IV* includes dementia in the chapter "Delirium, Dementia, and Amnestic and Other Cognitive Disorders." These disorders are grouped together because they share the symptom of a significant deficit in cognition or memory that represents a decline from a previous level of occupational performance.

Delirium and dementia are the cognitive disorders most commonly seen by health care practitioners. Although they differ greatly in the course and prognosis, they easily can be mistaken for each other. Therefore, the occupational therapist must be able to differentiate between them.

Delirium

The diagnostic criteria for delirium are as follows: 1) disturbed consciousness (reduced level of arousal) with decreased ability to focus, sustain, or shift attention; 2) change in cognition (such as memory loss, disorientation, language disturbance) or the development of a perceptual disturbance (hallucinations, paranoid thoughts) that cannot be explained by a preexisting, established, or evolving dementia; 3) disturbance quickly develops, usually within hours or days, and symptoms fluctuate throughout the course of a day; 4) medical evidence that the disturbance is either caused by a medical condition or developed during intoxification or withdrawal from a substance, including alcohol, illegal substances such as cocaine or hallucinogens, or prescription medications (1).

It is not unusual for delirium to occur when a person is being treated, or is in need of treatment, for an acute physical condition. A high fever can bring on delirium, causing the person to be confused, to misinterpret shadows, to be disoriented (especially in a hospital environment, which is unfamiliar and possibly frightening), and to be unable to express thoughts or needs clearly. These symptoms might fluctuate, just as the degree of a fever might fluctuate during the course of a day. The delirium ends as the acute medical condition clears.

For a person who is normally alert with intact memory, the symptoms of delirium are a significant cause for concern. If the person is recovering from a medical condition that resulted in delirium, care should be taken that long-term decisions, such as guardianship and nursing home placement, be avoided until the delirium has cleared. Consider the possibility of an individual who has a delirium caused by a prescribed medication, *f* the delirium is not accurately *...e* medication routine changed, *...d* be assessed as being unable to *...tly.* Delirium is a temporary condi- *...ourse* usually ends as the person *bo...* *...dically* stable.

Dementia

Memory impairment is the first and most prominent symptom to emerge. Recent memory is affected first, often manifested as the person uncharacteristically misplaces things. In addition to memory impairment, multiple cognitive deficits develop, including at least one of the following: aphasia, apraxia, agnosia, or a disturbance in executive functioning. For an individual to be diagnosed as having dementia, these deficits must be severe enough to impair occupational performance and represent a decline from a previous functional level (1).

A person who has dementia may experience other cognitive and personality disturbances as well. Topographical orientation may be affected, which, compounded by memory loss, can result in the person easily becoming lost. A disturbance in spatial relations creates difficulty with spatial tasks. The person with little or no awareness of memory loss, and who has other impairments, often displays poor judgement or poor insight. One who has awareness of cognitive deficits may become anxious or defensive. Dementia may be associated with gait disturbances that lead to falls, disinhibited behavior such as making inappropriate jokes, and psychotic symptoms such as delusional thinking or hallucinating (1).

The *DSM-IV* differentiates between the types of dementia based on their etiologies. Dementia of the Alzheimer's type is more commonly known as Alzheimer's disease (AD). The cause of AD is the subject of much debate and medical research and will be discussed in the section on etiology. Vascular dementia was formerly referred to as multiinfarct dementia. Dementias that result from other general medical conditions may be diagnosed when one of the following medical conditions is present: HIV disease, head trauma, Parkinson's disease, Huntington's disease, Pick's disease, Creutzfeldt-Jakob disease, normal-pressure hydrocephalus, hyperthyroidism, brain tumor, vitamin B_{12} deficiency, and intracranial radiation. Substance-induced, persisting dementia may be diagnosed when there is evidence that cognitive deficits are related to the effects of substance use, such as a drug of abuse or a medication. The *DSM-IV* lists alcohol, inhalants, sedatives, hypnotics, and anxiolytics as substances that may induce dementia.

ETIOLOGY
Alzheimer's Disease

There is no known cause for AD. The clinical diagnosis can be made only after ruling out the etiologies, such as cardiovascular disease or Parkinson's disease, for other dementias. However, much research has focused on associated features and laboratory findings relevant to AD in an attempt to discover its origin(s). We will review some of the major findings now being studied.

Neuropathology

The definitive diagnosis of AD is made at autopsy. The gross neuroanatomical findings include diffuse atrophy with flattened cortical sulci and enlarged cerebral ventricles. Microscopic findings include senile plaques, neurofibrillary tangles, neuronal loss, synaptic loss, and granulovascular degeneration of the neurons. Senile plaques, or amyloid plaques, are most indicative of AD but may be present in Down's syndrome and, to a lesser degree, in normal aging. The amount of senile plaques found in autopsy has been correlated to the severity of the dementia that affected the person with AD (3).

Amyloid Precursor Protein

There are four forms of amyloid precursor protein, one of which, the beta/A4 protein, is the major constituent of senile plaques. Current research suggests that beta amyloid deposits play a central role in the development of AD (4).

Genetic Predisposition

The genetic risk factors for AD have been linked to three chromosomal abnormalities. Research has found that each of these abnormalities results in an accumulation of insoluble beta amyloid within cortical and subcortical neurons (5).

Abnormal chromosome 21 has been linked to an altered amyloid precursor protein (6). Mutations in the amyloid precursor protein gene on chromosome 1 are known to cause early-onset (before age 65) AD (7).

Abnormal chromosome 19 has been associated with late-onset AD. Variable genes on this chromosome cause production of apolipoprotein E. Apolipoprotein E-4 causes diffuse depositions of insoluble beta amyloid (8).

Abnormal chromosome 14, associated with onset of AD before the age of 50, leads to a mutated form of the amyloid precursor protein (9, 10).

Neurotransmitter Abnormalities

The neurotransmitters most studied are acetylcholine and norepinephrine. Both are hypothesized to be hypoactive in AD. Several studies have found specific degeneration of cholinergic neurons in the nucleus basalis of Meynert in persons with AD. Other studies found decreases in acetylcholine and cholinergic acetyltransferase concentrations in the brains of individuals with AD, which suggests a decrease in the number of cholinergic neurons. Because it is known that cholinergic antagonists, such as scopolamine and atropine, impair cognitive abilities, and that cholinergic agonists, such as physostigmine and arecoline, enhance cognitive abilities, the cholinergic deficit hypothesis is further supported (3).

Some pathological examinations of brains from individuals with AD have found a decrease in the norepinephrine-containing neurons in the locus ceruleus. Two other neurotransmitters—the neuroactive peptides somatostatin and corticotropin—have also been reported to be decreased in AD (3).

Other Potential Causes

Some researchers are exploring the theory that abnormality in the regulation of membrane phospholipid metabolism results in membranes that are more rigid in AD (3). Others are looking for a possible viral connection or a combination of aforementioned factors as causing AD (11).

Vascular Dementia

Cerebral vascular disease is the primary cause of vascular dementia. Multiple infarcts of small and medium-size cerebral vessels produce lesions over wide areas of the brain. Men, especially those with preexisting hypertension or other cardiovascular conditions, have an increased risk for vascular dementia (3).

Other Disorders Related to Dementia

As seen in Table 7.1, a multitude of diseases and neurological disorders may be accompanied by a dementia. Some of the more common of these include alcoholism, head trauma, intracranial masses, and normal-pressure hydrocephalus. Parkinson's disease is a neurodegenerative condition in which an estimated 20 to 30% of those affected also have dementia. Two other of the more common neurodegenerative disorders, Huntington's disease and Pick's disease, are associated with the development of dementia (3).

INCIDENCE AND PREVALENCE

It is estimated that 4 million Americans have severely disabling dementia, and that 1 to 5 million may have mild to moderate dementia (11). The United States Congress Office of Technology Assessment has projected that, as the population

TABLE 7.1   Disorders That May Produce Dementia

Alzheimer's disease*
Vascular dementia†
   Varieties: Multiple infarcts (called multi-infarct
         dementia)
         Lacunae
         Binswanger's disease
         Cortical microinfarction
Drugs and toxins (including chronic alcoholic
   dementia)‡
Intracranial masses: tumors, subdural masses,
   brain abscesses‡
Anoxia
Trauma
   Head injury‡
   Dementia pugilistica (punch-drunk syndrome)
Normal-pressure hydrocephalus‡
Neurodegenerative disorders
   Parkinson's disease§
   Huntington's disease§
   Progressive supranuclear palsy§
   Pick's disease§
   Amyotrophic lateral sclerosis
   Spinocerebellar degenerations
   Olivopontocerebellar degeneration
   Ophthalmoplegia plus
   Metachromatic leukodystrophy (adult form)
   Hallervorden-Spatz disease
   Wilson's disease
Infections
   Creutzfeldt-Jakob disease
   AIDS§

Viral encephalitis
Progressive multifocal leukoencephalopathy
Behçet's syndrome
Neurosyphilis
Chronic bacterial meningitis
Cryptococcal meningitis
Other fungal meningitides
Nutritional disorders
   Wernicke-Korsakoff syndrome (thiamine
   deficiency)‡
   Vitamin B_{12} deficiency
   Folate deficiency
   Pellagra
   Marchiafava-Bignami disease
   Zinc deficiency
Metabolic disorders
   Metachromatic leukodystrophy
   Adrenal leukodystrophy
   Dialysis dementia
   Hypothyroidism and hyperthyroidism
   Renal insufficiency, severe
   Cushing's syndrome
   Hepatic insufficiency
   Parathyroid disease
Chronic inflammatory disorders‡
   Lupus and other collagen-vascular§ disorders
   with intracerebral vasculitis
   Multiple sclerosis
   Whipple's disease

*Accounts for 50 to 60% of cases.
†Accounts for 10 to 20% of cases.
‡Accounts for 1 to 5% of cases.
§Accounts for about 1% of cases.
No symbol: less than 1% of cases.
(Reprinted with permission from Rosser M: Dementia. In: Asbury AK, McKhann GM, McDonald WI, eds. Diseases of the
Nervous System: Clinical Neurobiology, 2nd ed. Philadelphia: Saunders, 1992:789.)

ages, the numbers of older Americans with severe dementia may increase dramatically, up to 8 million by the year 2020 (11).

Estimates of the prevalence of dementia vary among epidemiological studies, but it is clear that the prevalence of dementia increases dramatically with age. The American Psychiatric Association (12) reports that dementia affects approximately 5 to 8% of individuals older than age 65, 15 to 20% of those older than age 75, and 25 to 50% of individuals older than age 85. Alzheimer's disease accounts for 50 to 75% of all diagnosed dementias. Vascular dementia is the next most common dementia, but the prevalence is unknown (12). Table 7.1 gives some estimates of the occurrence of dementia related to various disorders.

SIGNS AND SYMPTOMS

The term "dementia" encompasses a group of disorders that may derive from differing etiologies but share the primary characteristic of the development of multiple cognitive deficits (1). The individual experiencing a dementing disease will exhibit cognitive deficits of memory impairment and at least one of the following: aphasia, agnosia, apraxia, and disturbance in executive functioning (1, 13). To represent a true dementia, the disturbances in cognitive function must be severe enough to interfere with occupational or social function and must signify a decline from previous levels of cognition. The earliest sign of dementia is memory loss manifested in either the inability to retrieve previously known information or to learn new material (1).

During the course of a dementia, an individual's ability to function and perform basic activities of daily living deteriorates. This decline in self-care is often the presenting symptom when medical advice is sought (14). Individuals may seek assistance in an early stage of dementia. The symptoms or subjective feelings about which they complain focus on memory loss. They have trouble remembering where objects have been placed and recalling names of familiar objects and places. Despite these complaints, the individuals and those close to them do not feel a sense of helplessness. At this point in the course of a dementia, the affected individual may be able to maintain psychosocial skills and satisfactory job performance. The person may have slight feelings of shame. At this point, no signs of the disease are observable.

As the disease progresses, the individual experiences growing problems with memory and difficulty with cognition. Others observe a greater inability to remember names, recover "lost" objects, recall past events, and manage finances. Incidences are reported of the individual becoming hopelessly lost while traveling to a location that should have been easy to find. The individual with dementia becomes less sociable and can-

not function as well on the job (15). He or she may experience some changes in personality, becoming more passive or more hostile toward others. Those who remain employed increasingly depend on others as memory loss and cognitive deficits become more pronounced (16).

Clinical signs become evident as the disease progresses. The affected person has sleep disturbances. Deficits in concentration and attention span are elicited by attempts to perform serial subtractions. Deficits also appear in long-term memory. The person cannot recall the current president, a personal address, the current year, or the present location (15). Short-term memory is affected. When given the names of three objects, the person cannot recall them after 5 minutes (16). Disorders of executive function become apparent. The individual has difficulty when directed to name as many animals as possible in 1 minute or to draw a continuous line of alternating m's and n's (1). The individual may have aphasia, apraxia, or agnosia. Constructional difficulty also develops: when given a specific design to replicate, the person cannot assemble blocks or sticks correctly.

Severe dementia is heralded by the inability to survive without constant supervision and support (15). A person with dementia may wander without regard for his or her whereabouts or personal safety. He or she may become increasingly agitated and combative or excessively passive and socially withdrawn.

The ability to maintain nourishment by feeding and eating and to maintain cleanliness deteriorates and ultimately disappears. The affected person cannot manipulate utensils and makes no attempt to eat. He or she becomes unaware of the urge to urinate or defecate and is incontinent of bladder and bowel. Gait becomes unsteady. The individual loses the desire and ability to bathe and may resist a caregiver's attempts to assist with the bath. A fear of water may develop, complicating baths. The person with dementia may refuse to get into bath water or may become combative when bathed.

All memories and cognition are lost. The individual does not know his or her own name, nor the name of a spouse. He or she does not recall any personal life history. The ability to count from 1 to 5 disappears. Eventually the ability to speak is lost and communication is reduced to a grunt in response to stimuli. During the last phase of a dementia, the affected person may develop psychiatric symptoms of overt paranoia, delusions, and visual or other hallucinatory experiences. Such symptoms make caring for the individual extremely difficult, forcing families to consider institutionalization (15).

Barry Reisberg, M.D. and colleagues have developed The Functional Assessment Staging (FAST) scale. The FAST identifies cognitive decline in Alzheimer's disease based on the appearance of deficits in the performance of activities of daily living (15). This highly detailed scale defines seven primary stages and nine substages of functional decline. Stage 1 corresponds to normal adult cognition. Stage 2 corresponds to the cognitive function of a normal, older adult in which there is personal awareness of functional decline. In stage 3, or early AD, deficits begin to emerge in situations or jobs requiring higher executive functioning. Needing assistance with complicated tasks, such as handling finances or planning a dinner party, is the hallmark of stage 4, or mild AD. Stage 5, moderate AD, is characterized by the need for assistance in choosing appropriate clothing. Stage 6, or moderately severe AD, is broken down into five substages, which identify the following declining functions: requiring assistance with dressing, requiring assistance in bathing properly, requiring assistance with the mechanics of toileting, urinary incontinence, and, finally, incontinence of bowel. Stage 7, or severe AD, is divided into six substages marking advancing decline: spoken vocabulary is limited to about six intelligible words; intelligible vocabulary is limited to a single word; ability to ambulate is lost; ability to sit up is lost; ability to smile is lost; and the ability to hold one's head up is lost. The decline in function appears in the reverse order in which children acquire developmental milestones (17).

COURSE AND PROGNOSIS

Although generally perceived as progressive or irreversible, the progression and prognosis of a dementia depends on the etiology of the disease process. The capacity for a dementia to be arrested or reversed depends on the underlying pathology, along with timely diagnosis and treatment intervention (1). Vascular dementia is usually abrupt in onset with stepwise loss of cognition as multiple strokes occur. Deficits in vascular dementia are limited to the areas of the brain destroyed by vascular accident. The course of vascular dementia may be halted by the treatment of hypertension and vascular disease (1).

Dementia caused by a single injury usually is not progressive. Repeated injuries, however, such as those sustained by boxers, may result in progressive dementia. In fact, the dementia that is seen in boxers is known as "pugilistic dementia."

Dementia may be the result of brain tumors, subdural hematoma, endocrine conditions (hypothyroidism, hypercalcemia, or hypoglycemia), vitamin deficiencies, infectious diseases, abnormal liver and kidney function, or other neurological conditions, such as multiple sclerosis. The course of dementia in the presence of other medical conditions depends on the accurate diagnosis and proper management of the underlying medical condition (1). Neurological disorders, such as Parkinson's disease, Huntington's disease, Pick's disease, and Creutzfeldt-Jakob disease, may cause dementias that are progressive (16).

Alzheimer's disease is insidious in onset and slowly progressive, with gradual worsening of memory and other cognitive functions (16). There is a loss of 3 to 4 points per year on standard assessment tests such as the Mini-Mental State Exam (MMSE). Alzheimer's disease may have plateaus of up to 1 year during which the individual does not decline. In general, the length of the course of disease process varies from 7 to 12 years (18), with progression from onset of symptoms until death being as brief as 2 years to as long as 20 years (19). How well the individual copes with and compensates for cognitive losses is influenced by premorbid personality, intelligence, and level of education (3). The greater the individual's fund of knowledge, resources, and coping strategies, the greater the ability to compensate for cognitive losses. The disease process is irreversible. At this time, only two approved medications have shown modest effect in slowing cognitive decline (19, 20).

DIAGNOSIS

According to the *DSM-IV* (1), the essential feature of dementia is the development of multiple cognitive deficits that include memory impairment and at least one of the following cognitive disturbances: aphasia, apraxia, agnosia, or a disturbance in executive functioning (1). These deficits must be severe enough to affect occupational or social functioning, causing a decline from a previously higher level of function (1).

An algorithm-based approach to diagnosis is used by the Veterans' Health Administration (13). Table 7.2 shows a diagram of this diagnostic approach. The recommended sequence in diagnosis begins with the presenting complaint of disturbance in memory or cognitive function as identified by the affected individual, a family member, or significant other.

In the first step of the diagnostic sequence, a complete history is taken. A functional evaluation, psychiatric evaluation, mental status examination, neurological/physical examination, and caregiver assessment are conducted. Structured tests may be given including the MMSE, the Six-Item Blessed Orientation-Memory-Concentration (BOMC) test, the 26-Item Blessed Information-Memory-Concentration (BIMC) test, and the Functional Activities Questionnaire (1, 13, 18). Neuropsychological evaluation is a more comprehensive assessment of cognitive function, general intelligence, sensorimotor function, and mood; it is particularly able to detect cerebral dysfunction (13, 21). If the findings from this process do not meet the criteria for dementia, other factors that may cause memory disturbances, such as delirium, amnesia, or depression, are investigated (13).

After determining that the findings are consistent with dementia, an apparent cause is sought.

The various disorders known to cause dementia are ruled out through a process of elimination. No further diagnostic assessment is required if the person relates a history of trauma, anoxic insult, or other definite cause of dementia (e.g., Huntington's disease) and if cognitive deficits are considered stable. If no cause for the dementia is apparent, the presence of medical illness is evaluated and laboratory tests are checked for abnormalities. Required laboratory tests include complete blood count, serum electrolytes, glucose, BUN and creatinine, liver function test, thyroid function tests, and vitamin B_{12} and syphilis serology (13). When the history or examination indicates the need, an HIV screen, heavy metal screen, and blood or urine tests for illicit drugs or prescribed medications may be done. If found, other medical conditions that may cause dementia are diagnosed; appropriate treatment is then initiated.

Should no other medical condition or abnormal laboratory findings be found, neuroimaging is indicated. A computerized tomography (CT) or a magnetic resonance imaging (MRI) scan may be done, particularly when the dementia is of recent onset, is concomitant with focal neurological signs, is atypical, or presents with history of headache. Pathologies that may be detected are tumors, abscess, hydrocephalus, subdural hematoma, multiple sclerosis, or evidence of cerebrovascular accident. Differential diagnoses of frontotemporal dementias and Huntington's disease may also be made, based on patterns of atrophy (13).

Motor system evaluation for the presence of disorders is conducted as part of the neurological examination. Those findings are integrated with the findings of neuroimaging. In AD, the neurological examination is normal until the very late stages of the disease. Diagnoses of extrapyramidal syndromes and Creutzfeldt-Jakob disease may be confirmed or eliminated at this time (13).

The individual is next evaluated for evidence of a depression syndrome. The history is checked for depression with short duration since onset, past history of depression, or family history of depression. If symptoms of depression are present, a diagnosis of dementia syndrome of depression is made. In the event that treatment for depression

TABLE 7.2 Algorithm Guiding the Differential Diagnosis of Dementia

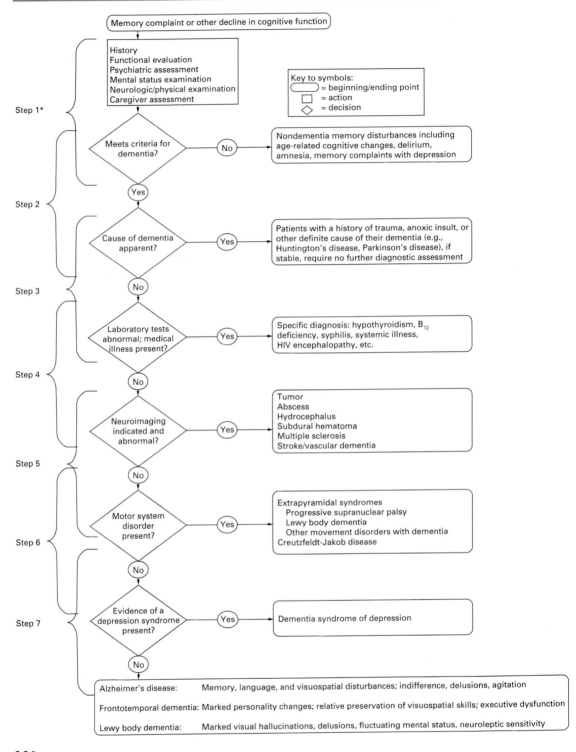

Memory complaint or other decline in cognitive function

Step 1*
History
Functional evaluation
Psychiatric assessment
Mental status examination
Neurologic/physical examination
Caregiver assessment

Key to symbols:
⬭ = beginning/ending point
▢ = action
◇ = decision

Meets criteria for dementia? — No → Nondementia memory disturbances including age-related cognitive changes, delirium, amnesia, memory complaints with depression

Yes

Step 2
Cause of dementia apparent? — Yes → Patients with a history of trauma, anoxic insult, or other definite cause of their dementia (e.g., Huntington's disease, Parkinson's disease), if stable, require no further diagnostic assessment

No

Step 3
Laboratory tests abnormal; medical illness present? — Yes → Specific diagnosis: hypothyroidism, B_{12} deficiency, syphilis, systemic illness, HIV encephalopathy, etc.

No

Step 4
Neuroimaging indicated and abnormal? — Yes → Tumor
Abscess
Hydrocephalus
Subdural hematoma
Multiple sclerosis
Stroke/vascular dementia

No

Step 5
Motor system disorder present? — Yes → Extrapyramidal syndromes
  Progressive supranuclear palsy
  Lewy body dementia
  Other movement disorders with dementia
Creutzfeldt-Jakob disease

No

Step 6

Step 7
Evidence of a depression syndrome present? — Yes → Dementia syndrome of depression

No

Alzheimer's disease: Memory, language, and visuospatial disturbances; indifference, delusions, agitation

Frontotemporal dementia: Marked personality changes; relative preservation of visuospatial skills; executive dysfunction

Lewy body dementia: Marked visual hallucinations, delusions, fluctuating mental status, neuroleptic sensitivity fails to alleviate cognitive deficits, alternate dementia diagnoses should be considered (13).

When all other disorders have been eliminated, AD, frontotemporal dementias, and Lewy body dementia must be considered. Alzheimer's disease is the most common diagnosis in this group. Typically, persons with AD present with a triad of cognitive deficits, including memory impairment, language changes, and visual–spatial deficits (13). The probable diagnosis of AD is given when an individual has dementia that cannot be attributed to systemic disorders or other brain diseases. A definite diagnosis of Alzheimer's disease can be made only when the individual has demonstrated signs and symptoms of dementia while living and histopathological evidence is found during autopsy.

MEDICAL/SURGICAL MANAGEMENT

Successful interventions in the management of dementia, regardless of whether the dementia is reversible, static, or progressive, depend on early detection and diagnosis. Screening may be done with the elderly during routine physicals or when they seek management of illnesses other than cognitive impairment (21–23).

In a dementia for which there are identifiable and treatable pathologies, medical or surgical interventions are directed at ameliorating underlying pathology. If an individual has dementia attributable to low thyroid function or vitamin B_{12} deficiency, providing appropriate replacement therapies may reduce or eliminate symptoms. Follow-up care over time is warranted to ensure that interventions have been successful. Neurosurgical consultation and surgical intervention are indicated when intracranial pathologies (tumors, abscess, subdural hematoma, hydrocephaly) are present. Control of hypertension and vascular disease may prevent progression of vascular dementia (1).

Depressive pseudodementia is a depression accompanied by cognitive changes similar to dementia. Treatment relies on the use of antidepressant medications, assessment of underlying medical conditions, and counseling once atten-

tion span and insight are improved (18). It is important to note that depression may accompany a true dementia. Careful diagnosis of the clinical presentation is crucial in planning the appropriate intervention.

For progressive, irreversible AD, early intervention focuses on educating the patient and his or her family about community resources, advocacy, and safety, including when to stop driving (23). Early intervention may delay the occurrence of medical and behavioral problems associated with dementia. Early and appropriate intervention can have a significant impact on the affected individual, the caregiver, the family, and society. Individuals in the earliest stages of the disease should be made aware of the diagnosis immediately, so that they may express their wishes regarding life-prolonging measures and extended care options (24, 25). Drug therapies may be needed to slow the progression of the disease, manage AD-related depression, normalize sleep/wake cycles, and minimize aggressive behaviors. Although the absence of effective drug therapy that will cure the disease can be a problem for families, the health care provider can help by providing emotional support, symptom management, and informed counseling (19). Physical exercise and social activity are important, as is proper nutrition. A calm, well-structured environment may help the affected person to continue functioning (26).

It is also important to attend to the needs of the caregiver, making sure that he or she addresses and maintains personal and health care needs. Caregiver depression and insomnia are common. Because they have neglected their own medical problems, caregivers often predecease a spouse who has dementia (18). Caregivers should be encouraged to attend support groups to get information on strategies for dealing with their loved one and emotional support (18).

Medications

Tacrine (Cognex) and donepezil hydrochloride (Aricept) are two drugs currently approved by the Food and Drug Administration (FDA) specifically for use by persons with AD. These medications have been shown to slow the progression of cognitive loss. Tacrine was first approved by the FDA in 1993. Patients with mild to moderate symptoms may be candidates for tacrine (24). It inhibits the action of acetylcholinesterase, an enzyme that breaks down the neurotransmitter acetylcholine (20). Acetylcholine is used by neurons in the hippocampus and other regions of the brain affected by AD. Loss of cholinergic neurons is highly correlated with the severity of dementia symptoms (20). Tacrine also blocks the function of enzymes that normally break down excess acetylcholine, thereby making more of the neurotransmitter available to brain cells (19).

Early trials of the use of tacrine showed only mild symptomatic improvement (20, 27). In subsequent trials, the doses of tacrine were increased. In patients taking 80 mg of tacrine daily, 27% showed improvement equivalent to the reversal of normal decline from AD in 1 year (20). Cognitive improvement using tacrine usually occurs within the first 2 weeks of administration and reaches a maximum benefit at 1 month (28). Unfortunately, many patients are unable to tolerate tacrine, with 28% developing abnormally high levels of liver enzymes and 17% being withdrawn from the medication because of liver problems (20, 29). The usual effective dose is 120 to 160 mg daily, divided into 4 doses. The patient begins taking the medication at 40 mg a day and increases the dose by 40 mg per day every 6 weeks to reduce the likelihood of adverse effects (18).

Approved by the FDA in 1996, donepezil hydrochloride, also an acetylcholinesterase inhibitor, is recommended for patients with mild to moderately severe AD (13, 18). Donepezil appears to be better tolerated by patients than tacrine. Side effects are primarily gastrointestinal disturbances (nausea, vomiting, and diarrhea) and are usually transient (18). Published data regarding the effectiveness of donepezil are limited. Improvements of 3 to 4.2 points on the Alzheimer's Disease Assessment Scale-Cognitive Subtests correspond roughly to decrements typically occurring over 6 to 8

months in patients with moderate AD (30, 31). Donepezil is administered in 5-mg or 10-mg doses, given once a day. It is often the drug of choice. Once-a-day dosing is more convenient for the patient and caregiver. Donepezil may be more effective than tacrine; early studies show no liver toxicity with donepezil (18).

Other medications being investigated for their potential to stall the rate at which cognitive function is lost are antioxidants. Two common medications, vitamin E in high doses and selegiline (an anti-parkinsonism drug), have shown dramatic effects when given to patients with moderately severe AD (32).

Behavioral problems inevitably arise during the course of the disease. Common behavioral abnormalities are agitation, aggression, incontinence, and wandering (18). Aggression may become a distressing, potentially harmful, and challenging behavior for caregivers and health care providers. Understanding, acceptance, and management skills are required of those looking after aggressive individuals (33). The individual with AD, by nature of his or her illness and loss of judgment, is often unaware of safety issues or dangerous behaviors (1). He or she may become anxious, fearful, and unwilling to cooperate with necessary care. Managing difficult behaviors becomes a challenge in promoting quality of life for the individual with AD. It is important for the clinician to investigate and treat behavior changes in the affected individual that may be the result of pain, hypoxia, infection, drug toxicity, electrolyte imbalances, dehydration, delirium, anxiety, depression, or environmental changes (18, 34).

A systematic approach in behavior management may be useful. This begins by identifying the exact nature of the behavior, reviewing possible physical and emotional stressors, and evaluating the individual for coexistent depression or psychosis. The degree of environmental stimulation may be reduced and the individual's tasks simplified (35). Other interventions may include leaving lights or music on if reduced sensory input triggers problem behaviors; distracting the individual by changing the topic of conversation or the person's location; providing familiar, reassuring objects such as a wallet or purse; and comforting the individual through touch or tone of voice (18).

Environmental management of agitation and aggression consists of avoiding events that precipitate the behavior, removing precipitating or perpetuating stimuli, distracting the agitated individual, and providing emotional support (18).

Day care centers for individuals with moderate to severe AD may aid in improving behaviors by providing structured physical and social activities, stimulation, and a sensitive environment. Day care centers also offer respite for overtaxed caregivers, which can in turn improve the quality of time the caregiver and the individual with AD spend together (18, 26).

Medications remain the standard in controlling agitated behaviors that do not respond to environmental controls. Medications that increase serotonin levels, such as trazadone, carbamazepine, buspirone, or propranolol, are the first treatment choice (13, 18). The use of antipsychotic or antianxiety medications is reserved for those behaviors that a) do not respond to behavioral interventions, b) present a clear danger to the individual or others, or c) interfere with the provision of necessary care (35). Antipsychotic medications, or dopamine antagonists, are effective medications; however, they often have unacceptable side effects or cause a worsening of the dementia symptoms (18). Drugs must be introduced at low dosages, and the dose must be increased gradually. Individuals with AD must be monitored closely for side effects, especially as they may be unable to report or describe adverse reactions (13).

Eventually, persons with AD become totally incapable of caring for themselves. When they can no longer be maintained by a family caregiver, placement in a long-term care facility may be necessary. Special units have been designed to respond to the needs of residents with AD (36). Management of the individual on a special unit has been shown to result in less patient discomfort (37). For residents in special care units, there are fewer chemical and physical restraints, a decreased number of problem behaviors, and

environmental adaptations that provide a sense of personal freedom and dignity (36).

Medical management in advanced AD consists of ensuring proper nourishment and hydration, maintaining skin integrity with regular bathing and perineal care after bowel and bladder incontinence, providing a safe environment, and reducing discomfort (36). Death usually occurs as a result of aspiration pneumonia, urinary tract infection, asphyxiation from placing an object into the mouth, or separate disorders such as myocardial infarction or cancer (13).

IMPACT ON OCCUPATIONAL PERFORMANCE

Cognitive integration and cognitive components are most seriously affected by AD. As the disease progresses, the number of performance areas affected increases, as does the severity of the dysfunction. We will address the impact of the condition on occupational performance for each of the three identified phases of Alzheimer's disease.

Early or Forgetful Phase (Table 7.3)

Early in the disease process, the individual develops difficulty in short-term and recent memory. In the orientation component, there is intermittent or consistent confusion about time and place. Concept formation tends to be concrete and problem solving begins to be difficult (16). Integration and synthesis of learning are also affected.

These cognitive losses begin to affect several occupational performance areas. The individual who cannot adapt to the memory loss and other cognitive deficits has difficulty with job performance. The inability to recall names and faces, the tendency to forget where objects have been placed, poor orientation to time and place, the inability to learn new procedures and to resolve problems in a timely manner may result in a change of work assignment or the loss of a job.

In the performance area of home management, affected individuals begin to need assistance with

TABLE 7.3 Occupational Performance Profile: Early or Forgetful Phase

I. PERFORMANCE AREAS

A. Activities of Daily Living*
1. Grooming
2. Oral Hygiene
3. Bathing/Showering
4. Toilet Hygiene
5. Personal Device Care
6. Dressing
7. Feeding and Eating
8. Medication Routine
9. Health Maintenance
10. **Socialization**
11. **Functional Communication**
12. Functional Mobility
13. **Community Mobility**
14. **Emergency Response**
15. **Sexual Expression**
B. Work and Productive Activities
1. Home Management
a. Clothing Care
b. Cleaning
c. Meal Preparation/Cleanup
d. **Shopping**
e. **Money Management**
f. **Household Maintenance**
g. **Safety Procedures**
2. **Care of Others**
3. **Educational Activities**
4. **Vocational Activities**
a. **Vocational Exploration**
b. **Job Acquisition**
c. **Work or Job Performance**
d. Retirement Planning
e. Volunteer Participation
C. **Play or Leisure Activities**
1. **Play or Leisure Exploration**
2. **Play or Leisure Performance**

II. PERFORMANCE COMPONENTS

A. Sensorimotor Component
1. Sensory
a. Sensory Awareness
b. Sensory Processing
(1) Tactile
(2) Proprioceptive
(3) Vestibular
(4) Visual
(5) Auditory
(6) Gustatory
(7) Olfactory
c. Perceptual Processing
(1) Stereognosis
(2) Kinesthesia
(3) Pain Response
(4) Body Scheme
(5) Right–Left Discrimination
(6) Form Constancy
(7) Position in Space
(8) Visual–Closure
(9) Figure Ground
(10) Depth Perception
(11) Spatial Relations
(12) Topographical Orientation
2. Neuromusculoskeletal
a. Reflex
b. Range of Motion
c. Muscle Tone
d. Strength
e. Endurance
f. Postural Control
g. Postural Alignment
h. Soft Tissue Integrity
3. Motor
a. Gross Coordination
b. Crossing the Midline
c. Laterality
d. Bilateral Integration
e. Motor Control
f. Praxis
g. Fine Coordination/Dexterity
h. Visual–Motor Control
i. Oral–Motor Control

III. PERFORMANCE CONTEXTS

A. Temporal Aspects
1. Chronological
2. Developmental
3. Lifecycle
4. Disability Status
B. Environment
1. Physical
2. Social
3. Cultural

(continued)

TABLE 7.3 Occupational Performance Profile: Early or Forgetful Phase (Continued)		
I. PERFORMANCE AREAS	**II. PERFORMANCE COMPONENTS**	**III. PERFORMANCE CONTEXTS**
	B. Cognitive Integration and Cognitive Components	
	1. Level of Arousal	
	2. Orientation	
	3. Recognition	
	4. Attention Span	
	5. Initiation of Activity	
	6. Termination of Activity	
	7. Memory	
	8. Sequencing	
	9. Categorization	
	10. Concept Formation	
	11. Spatial Operations	
	12. Problem Solving	
	13. Learning	
	14. Generalization	
	C. Psychosocial Skills and Psychological Components	
	1. Psychological	
	a. Values	
	b. Interests	
	c. Self-Concept	
	2. Social	
	a. Role Performance	
	b. Social Conduct	
	c. Interpersonal Skills	
	d. Self-Expression	
	3. Self-Management	
	a. Coping Skills	
	b. Time Management	
	c. Self-Control	

*All may be affected.

shopping and money management. Functional communication is also affected. Patients may experience anomia (the inability to find a name for something) or expressive aphasia (the inability to say what one wants to say) (37). There also may be perseveration (the uncontrollable repetition of a word or phrase) and some inability to speak in a coherent manner (16).

The awareness of increasing cognitive loss often leads to problems in psychosocial skills and components. Depression may manifest early in the disease process, along with irritability and hostile behavior (18). An altered self-concept results in feelings of shame. Coping skills and time management begin to disintegrate, and socialization may be affected. Family relationships are strained, and the affected individual may begin to curtail social and leisure activities. Feelings of inadequacy may impair the fulfillment of sexual expression (38).

Confusional Phase (Table 7.4)

The confusional phase is marked by increasing deficits in recent memory, as well as short-term,

TABLE 7.4 Occupational Performance Profile: Confusion Phase

I. PERFORMANCE AREAS	II. PERFORMANCE COMPONENTS	III. PERFORMANCE CONTEXTS
A. Activities of Daily Living*	A. Sensorimotor Component	A. Temporal Aspects
1. Grooming	1. Sensory	1. Chronological
2. Oral Hygiene	a. Sensory Awareness	2. Developmental
3. Bathing/Showering	**b. Sensory Processing**	3. Lifecycle
4. Toilet Hygiene	**(1) Tactile**	4. Disability Status
5. Personal Device Care	**(2) Proprioceptive**	B. Environment
6. Dressing	**(3) Vestibular**	1. Physical
7. Feeding and Eating	**(4) Visual**	2. Social
8. Medication Routine	**(5) Auditory**	3. Cultural
9. Health Maintenance	**(6) Gustatory**	
10. Socialization	**(7) Olfactory**	
11. Functional Communication	**c. Perceptual Processing**	
12. Functional Mobility	**(1) Stereognosis**	
13. Community Mobility	**(2) Kinesthesia**	
14. Emergency Response	**(3) Pain Response**	
15. Sexual Expression	**(4) Body Scheme**	
B. Work and Productive Activities	**(5) Right–Left Discrimination**	
1. Home Management	**(6) Form Constancy**	
a. Clothing Care	**(7) Position in Space**	
b. Cleaning	**(8) Visual–Closure**	
c. Meal Preparation/ Cleanup	**(9) Figure Ground**	
d. Shopping	**(10) Depth Perception**	
e. Money Management	**(11) Spatial Relations**	
f. Household Maintenance	**(12) Topographical Orientation**	
g. Safety Procedures	2. Neuromusculoskeletal	
2. Care of Others	a. Reflex	
3. Educational Activities	b. Range of Motion	
4. Vocational Activities	c. Muscle Tone	
a. Vocational Exploration	d. Strength	
b. Job Acquisition	e. Endurance	
c. Work or Job Performance	f. Postural Control	
d. Retirement Planning	g. Postural Alignment	
e. Volunteer Participation	h. Soft Tissue Integrity	
C. Play or Leisure Activities	3. Motor	
1. Play or Leisure Exploration	a. Gross Coordination	
2. Play or Leisure Performance	b. Crossing the Midline	
	c. Laterality	
	d. Bilateral Integration	
	e. Motor Control	
	f. Praxis	
	g. Fine Coordination/Dexterity	
	h. Visual–Motor Control	
	i. Oral–Motor Control	

(continued)

TABLE 7.4 Occupational Performance Profile: Confusion Phase (Continued)		
I. PERFORMANCE AREAS	**II. PERFORMANCE COMPONENTS**	**III. PERFORMANCE CONTEXTS**

	B. Cognitive Integration and Cognitive Components
	  1. Level of Arousal
	  2. Orientation
	  3. Recognition
	  4. Attention Span
	  5. Initiation of Activity
	  6. Termination of Activity
	  7. Memory
	  8. Sequencing
	  9. Categorization
	  10. Concept Formation
	  11. Spatial Operations
	  12. Problem Solving
	  13. Learning
	  14. Generalization
	C. **Psychosocial Skills and Psychological Components**
	  1. Psychological
	    a. Values
	    b. Interests
	    c. Self-Concept
	  2. Social
	    a. Role Performance
	    b. Social Conduct
	    c. Interpersonal Skills
	    d. Self-Expression
	  3. Self-Management
	    a. Coping Skills
	    b. Time Management
	    c. Self-Control	

*All may be affected.

long-term, and remote memory. Individuals cannot recall their address, familiar telephone numbers, or the names of close family members. Orientation to person, place, and time is impaired, with concepts of time most seriously affected (16). Concentrating is difficult and ability to make sense of incoming stimuli is lessened (39).

At this phase, occupational performance becomes so dysfunctional that these individuals require the help of a caregiver. They no longer can perform on the job, and home management skills are seriously impaired. They may lose valuables and cannot manage finances, as number concepts are very poor or nonexistent (16, 39). They may create hazards, such as turning on a stove and forgetting to turn it off. Habits become rigid, and a self-care routine, if interrupted, may be difficult or impossible to complete. Dressing problems include difficulty selecting proper clothing and dressing in a sequential fashion.

Bathing problems include fear of bathing, refusal to bathe, or inadequate performance (16).

Functional communication continues to deteriorate. Speech content may be confused or irrelevant, with increased difficulty choosing words and the addition of irrelevant words at the end of a sentence. Circumlocution appears, in which the individual avoids the issue by speaking in a roundabout way and never getting to the point. There is increased anomia and paraphasia (substituting inappropriate words in a sentence). Agnosia, which is difficulty seeing or reading, also affects communication (16). Functional mobility becomes impaired, and the individual begins to wander and habitually gets lost.

In the second phase of Alzheimer's disease, psychosocial skills and components continue to decline. Self-concept further deteriorates, and there is a sense of helplessness and feelings of impotence (39). Social conduct is affected. There may be excessive passivity or impulsive verbalizations. Time management is seriously affected, and disturbances of the sleep-wake cycle create difficulties for the caregiver. Individuals may display frequent repetitive behaviors, making termination of activity difficult. In addition, hallucinations, paranoia, and emotional lability may be present (16).

Dysfunction in psychosocial skills and components also affect occupational performance. Depression can cause loss of appetite, and intimacy becomes increasingly impaired (38). Personality changes found in AD include overtly antisocial behavior and sexual excesses and indiscretions (40). Problems related to these behaviors may surface during the second phase and may worsen as the disease progresses.

Dementia Phase (Table 7.5)

In the dementia phase, AD begins to take its toll on the cognitive and psychosocial components, as well as the sensorimotor components of functioning. At this point, affected individuals need complete supervision and, eventually, total care.

The cognitive components of memory and orientation are severely impaired. These individuals cannot identify close relatives, although they may be able to distinguish between strangers and those who are familiar. Eventually they may lose this awareness along with the ability to recall their own name. Familiar surroundings are confusing, and there is no awareness of season or year. The ability to process information is severely limited; they may not be able to follow through with an action such as picking up a spoon and putting it into the mouth (16).

These cognitive losses cause an inability to perform work activities and severe limitations in leisure and daily living activities. These individuals cannot bathe alone, may be incontinent, and may need assistance with feeding. Functional communication continues to deteriorate. Language comprehension is impaired, and affected individuals tend to lapse into unintelligible mumbling. At the very end of this stage, speech is either limited to a few words or there is no intelligible vocabulary (16).

Sensory integration is impaired. Distortions in sensory perceptions may lead to paranoia and aggression. Patients with AD may experience wandering pain, being unable to locate internal cues of physiologic distress (38). Motor skills are affected; individuals become unsteady and eventually lose ambulation and voluntary movement. Speech becomes slurred because of motor dysfunction (dysarthria). Visual agnosia occurs (difficulty interpreting visual stimuli in the absence of significant visual impairment) (16). Eating problems become a primary concern. Whereas early in the dementia phase patients may have an overeating problem, at the end of this phase they cannot swallow food. The end stage of AD involves physical complications, as noted in the section on medical management.

TABLE 7.5   Occupational Performance Profile: Dementia Phase

I. PERFORMANCE AREAS	II. PERFORMANCE COMPONENTS	III. PERFORMANCE CONTEXTS
A. Activities of Daily Living*	A. Sensorimotor Component	A. Temporal Aspects
1. Grooming	1. Sensory	1. Chronological
2. Oral Hygiene	a. Sensory Awareness	2. Developmental
3. Bathing/Showering	b. Sensory Processing	3. Lifecycle
4. Toilet Hygiene	(1) Tactile	4. Disability Status
5. Personal Device Care	(2) Proprioceptive	B. Environment
6. Dressing	(3) Vestibular	1. Physical
7. Feeding and Eating	(4) Visual	2. Social
8. Medication Routine	(5) Auditory	3. Cultural
9. Health Maintenance	(6) Gustatory	
10. Socialization	(7) Olfactory	
11. Functional Communication	c. Perceptual Processing	
12. Functional Mobility	(1) Stereognosis	
13. Community Mobility	(2) Kinesthesia	
14. Emergency Response	(3) Pain Response	
15. Sexual Expression	(4) Body Scheme	
B. Work and Productive Activities	(5) Right–Left Discrimination	
1. Home Management	(6) Form Constancy	
a. Clothing Care	(7) Position in Space	
b. Cleaning	(8) Visual–Closure	
c. Meal Preparation/	(9) Figure Ground	
Cleanup	(10) Depth Perception	
d. Shopping	(11) Spatial Relations	
e. Money Management	(12) Topographical Orientation	
f. Household Maintenance	2. Neuromusculoskeletal	
g. Safety Procedures	a. Reflex	
2. Care of Others	b. Range of Motion	
3. Educational Activities	c. Muscle Tone	
4. Vocational Activities	d. Strength	
a. Vocational Exploration	e. Endurance	
b. Job Acquisition	f. Postural Control	
c. Work or Job Performance	g. Postural Alignment	
d. Retirement Planning	h. Soft Tissue Integrity	
e. Volunteer Participation	3. Motor	
C. Play or Leisure Activities	a. Gross Coordination	
1. Play or Leisure Exploration	b. Crossing the Midline	
2. Play or Leisure Performance	c. Laterality	
	d. Bilateral Integration	
	e. Motor Control	
	f. Praxis	
	g. Fine Coordination/Dexterity	
	h. Visual–Motor Control	
	i. Oral–Motor Control	

(continued)

TABLE 7.5	Occupational Performance Profile: Dementia Phase (Continued)	
I. PERFORMANCE AREAS	**II. PERFORMANCE COMPONENTS**	**III. PERFORMANCE CONTEXTS**

	B. Cognitive Integration and Cognitive Components
	   1. Level of Arousal
	   2. Orientation
	   3. Recognition
	   4. Attention Span
	   5. Initiation of Activity
	   6. Termination of Activity
	   7. Memory
	   8. Sequencing
	   9. Categorization
	   10. Concept Formation
	   11. Spatial Operations
	   12. Problem Solving
	   13. Learning
	   14. Generalization
	 C. Psychosocial Skills and Psychological Components
	   1. Psychological
	     a. Values
	     b. Interests
	     c. Self-Concept
	   2. Social
	     a. Role Performance
	     b. Social Conduct
	     c. Interpersonal Skills
	     d. Self-Expression
	   3. Self-Management
	     a. Coping Skills
	     b. Time Management
	     c. Self-Control	

*All may be affected.

CASE STUDIES

CASE 1

Alzheimer's Disease

Mrs. L. was born in South America. She was bilingual, speaking her native Spanish as well as faultless English. In her early years, she had the luxury of maids and a cook. She was a widow before her two children were grown. When Mrs. L. was about age 60, her adult daughter died, leaving Mrs. L. as the primary caregiver for her two young grandchildren. Soon after her daughter's death, Mrs. L. fled her native land for political reasons, bringing her orphaned grandchildren to live in New York. After raising them, she continued to live with her adult granddaughter, G.

Early Phase

When Mrs. L. was 82, G. married and her new husband moved into their home. Mrs. L. had always told G. that "when you marry and no longer need me, it will be my time to die." She seemed angry at G. and showed her irritation by complaining. Nevertheless, she continued to prepare the family meals, make beds, and do some laundry. In spite of failing vision, she was aware of the need to dust. She continued to take impeccable care of her appearance, always setting her hair at night and never going out without wearing hose and high heels. Her social life was full, with friends and neighbors frequently visiting. She took pride in serving tea and dessert to her weekly women's support group who met at her apartment.

There were times when Mrs. L. misplaced her dentures (in odd places such as in a plant pot) or forgot to use detergent when washing the dishes. She was often anxious and needy when G. came home from work, and she became defensive and easily upset when questioned about mistakes. Her granddaughter attributed these aberrations to Mrs. L.'s increased stress as a result of the marriage.

Forgetful Phase

At age 86, Mrs. L. broke her hip, her granddaughter had a new, colicky baby, and the family moved to a larger apartment in the same complex. As a result of these crises, Mrs. L. seemed to have slowed down and became more dependent on G. She began making more obvious mistakes, such as using the toilet brush to scrub the floor and neglecting to wash the dishes before putting them away. G. took over the housekeeping and cooking duties.

Mrs. L.'s hearing and sight continued to decline, and she complained about "nothing ever being right." G. got her books on tape, but Mrs. L. could not learn to operate the tape player. She continued to entertain her weekly women's group, basking in the compliments from her friends for the tasty desserts that they knew were now being made by G.

Mrs. L. became a picky eater, putting catsup on everything, including salads and fruit. She was still very particular about her appearance, but she began to need help doing her hair and became neglectful of her denture care. She could still fold laundry, make beds, and take her bath independently.

There were times when Mrs. L. became fearful of G.'s husband, accusing him of wanting to hurt her granddaughter.

At age 91, the family moved out of the apartment complex, where they had lived for many years, to a new home. Mrs. L. was no longer able to make impromptu visits to her neighbors, and her circle of friends now rarely visited. Mrs. L. was afraid to use anything in the new kitchen, especially the unfamiliar gas stove. Her appetite continued to be poor, and she was losing weight.

Strategies to enable her to make her own tea and toast were unsuccessful, and she would forget to eat food left for her in the refrigerator when G. went to work.

Mrs. L. began to have incontinence of bowel and bladder, yet she would resist her granddaughter's suggestions that she needed to shower or bathe. Ironically, when Mrs. L. fell and broke her wrist, she became amenable to assistance. Insurance covered about 6 weeks of home health care, and Mrs. L. seemed to enjoy the attention.

Dementia Phase

At age 92, it was clear that Mrs. L. could not be left alone. She continued to be incontinent; she couldn't lift herself from the toilet and seemed afraid to use a bedside commode. When her granddaughter came home from work, she would follow her about, repeating the same question over and over. She was not eating lunch or dinner. Her granddaughter, pregnant with her second child, was having difficulty bathing Mrs. L. On one occasion they both ended up falling on the bathroom floor during a bathing session. In-home care proved unaffordable, and G. made the difficult decision to place Mrs. L. in a nursing home.

The nursing home, known for its excellence, proved to be a positive move for Mrs. L. She regained some of her weight and seemed much less anxious. Mrs. L.'s deep-rooted social personality and gift for charming those around her made a reappearance. This served to ensure that a constant stream of staff and residents dropped by her room for brief chats. When G. and her family visited, Mrs. L. remained cool, as if to reprimand G. for sending her away.

Within a year, Mrs. L. was not always able to recognize G. when she came to visit. Sometimes she mistook G. for her daughter. Eventually she completely lost the ability to recognize G. Her granddaughter continued to visit with her own children, who delighted in playing word games with Mrs. L. The youngest child, himself learning to speak, would say a few words or phrases to Mrs. L., which she would mimic. This would set both children to giggling, in turn pleasing Mrs. L. to have had such an amusing effect on the children.

At age 94, Mrs. L. seemed no longer able to speak English. Her verbalizations in Spanish were limited to a few words, which were sometimes unintelligible. She was no longer able to ambulate and needed total care for feeding. Shortly after her 95th birthday, Mrs. L. died peacefully of heart failure.

CASE 2

Vascular Dementia

Mr. B. is a 71-year-old African American who is cared for at home by his wife. Mrs. B. describes him as having been a quietly dignified person before the onset of his illness. He enjoyed spending time with his family, including his four children and other members of his extended family.

As a young college graduate, Mr. B. was unable to find work in his field of engineering but did get an unskilled job with the phone company. His supervisors recognized his talents and abilities, and over time, he had a series of promotions that eventually took him to the position of personnel manager.

When Mr. B. was 60, his company was bought out and he was given an early retirement. Soon after this, he started taking classes in cabinet making, and began working for an architect who was building a local church.

At age 64, Mr. B. began making errors in measurement in his work. He was aware of, and troubled by, this difficulty He decided to cut back his hours at work. Mrs. B. noted at this time that he sometimes appeared confused. During family gatherings he was not only quieter than his usual self, but he would actually distance himself by sitting in another room. Although he was still driving, he began misplacing things. Mrs. B. had some concerns about these behaviors but attributed them to the stress of life changes.

It was when Mr. B. was no longer able to read a ruler that Mrs. B. began to realize something was seriously wrong. At about this time, Mr. B. had an episode in which he got lost on the way to the dentist. Mrs. B. turned to her family physician for help, and an 18-month period of medical and neurological testing ensued.

At age 66, Mr. B. had a stroke. During hospitalization, the diagnosis of vascular dementia was finally made. When Mr. B. left the hospital, he was able to walk and perform his self-care activities independently.

At first, things went well at home. Both Mr. and Mrs. B. adjusted to a routine in which she would make sure that he was up, dressed, and had breakfast before she left the house for work. His lunch was prepared and left for him to retrieve from the refrigerator. One day Mrs. B. came home from work and found that the stove had been left on. At this point, she realized that Mr. B. was no longer safe when left alone, and she enrolled him in a day care program.

About 8 months later, Mrs. B. made the decision to stop working. The day program cost almost as much as her pay. It was becoming more and more difficult to help Mr. B. get dressed and out of the house every morning. In fact, Mr. B. started choosing to undress himself several times a day. He began having problems speaking and understanding what others said to him. Mrs. B. felt he was losing his personality; he wasn't able to focus on conversation or show interest, even when his grandchildren visited. He was still ambulating with help. He began to have difficulty swallowing, was losing weight, and was having bladder infections. He was no longer continent of bowel or bladder.

At age 69, Mr. B. had another stroke. Despite the efforts of the rehabilitation service, he could no longer ambulate. He returned home in a wheelchair. His home did not have a ground-floor bedroom, so Mrs. B. converted the living room to his bedroom. For about 1 month, his insurance provided a home health aide who would give Mr. B. a weekly bed bath. Eventually Mrs. B. took over this responsibility, along with complete care for dressing and feeding him. Mr. B. often did not recognize Mrs. B. and no longer recognized his children.

During a recent visit to the outpatient clinic, Mrs. B. talked about the difficulty of getting through each day. "I rarely get out unless one of the family members can stay with my husband, and even then I'm just too tired. I think about the reality that someday I may need to put him in a nursing home. I'll do it when it gets to the point where I'm no longer able to take care of him or if my health gets bad. But if that happens, I'll lose our life savings—it's not much, but enough to help pay bills with my social security check." She also related an incident that illustrated the small daily frustrations of caring for her husband: "I was feeding him lunch, and he reached for the glass of milk with his left hand. I helped place the glass in his outstretched hand, but he began raising his right hand to his mouth as if to drink. Obviously that wasn't working, so I took the glass out of his left hand and put it in his right hand. This must have totally confused him, and he just stopped, giving me a wounded look as if to say 'what did you do that for?' I felt so helpless, and so bad that I couldn't even help him."

Mr. B., who at 71 is still handsome, sits straight and tall in his wheelchair, appearing to emanate dignity and calm, faintly smiling and nodding as his wife tells their story.

1. List the diagnostic criteria for delirium.
2. Describe the course of delirium.
3. What is the hallmark symptom of dementia? In addition to this symptom, what other cognitive deficits must be present, and to what degree, to establish a diagnosis?
4. How are the different types of dementia differentiated in the *DSM-IV*?
5. Describe the neuropathology of AD.
6. List the various diseases and neurological disorders that may be accompanied by a dementia.
7. The FAST defines seven primary stages and nine substages of functional decline. Describe behaviors that would be observed in each of the stages.
8. Can treatment with medications alter and reverse the course of dementia?
9. Profile the effect of early-stage dementia on occupational performance.
10. Describe the behaviors you will likely observe in persons with dementia who have progressed to the confusional phase.
11. What behavioral changes occur that mark the transition to the dementia phase of dementia?

REFERENCES

1. Diagnostic and Statistical Manual of Mental Disorders. 4th ed. Washington, DC: American Psychiatric Association, 1994.
2. Geldmacher DS, Whitehouse PJ. Evaluation of dementia. New Engl J Med 1996;335(5):330–336.
3. Kaplan HI, Sadock BS, Grebb JA. Kaplan and Sadock's Synopsis of Psychiatry. 7th ed. Baltimore: Williams & Wilkins, 1994.
4. Hardy J, Allsop D. Amyloid depositions as the central event in the aetiology of Alzheimer's disease. Trends Pharmacol Sci 1991;12:383–388.
5. Shua-Haim J, Gross J. Alzheimer's syndrome, not Alzheimer's disease. J Am Geriatr Soc 1996;44:96–97.
6. Goate A, Chartier-Harlin M, Mullan M, et al. Segregation of a missense mutation in the amyloid precursor protein gene with familial Alzheimer's disease. Nature 1991;349:704–706.
7. Levy-Lahad E, Wijsman E, Nemens E, et al. A familial Alzheimer's disease locus on chromosome 1. Science 1995;269:970–977.
8. Saunders A, Strittmatter W, Schmechel D, et al. Association of apolipoprotein E allele 4 with late-onset familial and sporadic Alzheimer's disease. Neurology 1993;43:1467–1471.
9. Kennedy AM, Newman SK, Frackowiak RS, et al. Chromosome 14 linked familial Alzheimer's disease. Brain 1995;118:185–205.
10. Lampe TH, Bird TD, Nochlin D, et al. Phenotype of chromosome 14-linked familial Alzheimer's disease in a large kindred. Ann Neurol 1994;36(3):368–378.
11. Hales D, Hales R. Caring for the Mind: the Comprehensive Guide to Mental Health. New York: Bantam Books, 1995.
12. American Psychiatric Association. Practice guidelines for the treatment of patients with Alzheimer's disease and other dementias of late life. Am J Psychiatry 1997;154(5):1–38.
13. Veterans Health Administration. Dementia identification and assessment. Oak Brook, IL: University Health System Consortium, 1997.
14. Pfeffer TI, Kurosaki TT, Harrah CH. Measurement of functional activities in older adults in the community. J Gerontol 1982;37:323–329.
15. Reisberg B, Sclan SG. Functional assessment staging (FAST) in Alzheimer's disease: reliability, validity and ordinality. Int Psychogeriatr 1992;4(suppl 1):55–69.
16. Glickstein J. Therapeutic Interventions in Alzheimer's Disease. Rockville: Aspen Publishers, 1988.
17. Reisberg B, Ferris SH, Anand R, et al. Initial description of the characteristic functional progression of Alzheimer's disease. Ann N Y Acad Sci 1984;435:481–483.
18. Shankle WR. Dr. Dementia's medical student lecture on Alzheimer's disease and other dementias. University of California Institute for Brain Aging and Dementia; March 15, 1996.
19. Cimons M. FDA approves first Alzheimer's disease treatment medications. Los Angeles Times, Sept. 10, 1993: Vol.113, No. 40.

20. The Harvard Mental Health Letter. Dementia of the Alzheimer type: is tacrine worth it? November, 1994.

21. Pinholt EM, Kroenke K, Hanley JF, et al. Functional assessment of the elderly: a comparison of standard instruments with clinical judgment. Arch Intern Med 1987;147:484–488.

22. Roca RP, Klein LE, Kirby SM, et al. Recognition of dementia among medical patients. Arch Intern Med 1984;144:73–75.

23. Bennett DA, Knopman DS. Alzheimer's disease: a comprehensive approach to patient management. Geriatrics 1994;49(8):20–26.

24. Bennett DA, Evans DA. Alzheimer's disease. Dis Mon 1992; 38(1):1–64.

25. Ham RI. After the diagnosis. Postgrad Med 1997;10(6):57–66.

26. Alzheimer's Association, Inc. Alzheimer's disease: fact sheet, 1997.

27. Meador KJ. Alzheimer's disease and dementia. J Med Assoc Ga 1993;82(9):495–499.

28. Eagger S, Morant N, Levy R, et al. Tacrine in Alzheimer's disease: time course of changes in cognitive function and practice effects. Br J Psychiatry 1992;160:36–40.

29. van Reekum R, Black SE, Conn D, et al. Cognition-enhancing drugs in dementia: a guide to the near future. Can J Psychiatry 1997;42(suppl):35S–50S.

30. Stern RG, Mohrs RC, et al. A longitudinal study of Alzheimer's disease measurement: rate and predictors of cognitive deterioration. Am J Psychiatry 1994;161:390–396.

31. Aricept package insert. Roerig Division of Pfizer, Inc., New York.

32. Thompson D. Buying time: the onset of Alzheimer's delayed by vitamin E. Time 1997;149:18.

33. Page S. Aggression in Alzheimer's disease. Nurs Stand 1992;6(24):37–39.

34. Sky AJ, Grossberg GT. The use of psychotropic medication in the management of problem behaviors in the patient with Alzheimer's disease. Med Clin North Am 1994;78(4):811–822.

35. Banazak DA. Difficult dementia: six steps to control problem behaviors. Geriatrics 1996;51(2):36–42.

36. Sand BJ, Yeaworth RC, McCabe BW. Alzheimer's disease: special care units in long-term care facilities. J Gerontol Nurs 1992;18:328–334.

37. Constantinidis J. Heredity and dementia. Gerontology 1986;32(suppl 1):73–79.

38. Ninos M, Makohon R. Functional assessment of the patient. Geriatric Nurs 1985;6:139–142.

39. Reisberg B, ed. Alzheimer's Disease. New York: Free Press, 1983.

40. Mancall E. Essentials of the Neurological Examination. 2nd ed. Philadelphia: FA Davis, 1982.

SUGGESTED READINGS

Bennett G, Vourakis C, Woolf D, eds. Substance Abuse: Pharmacological, Developmental, and Clinical Perspectives. New York: John Wiley, 1983. *This book offers easy-to-read information on the autonomic and central nervous system as well as central nervous system depressants and stimulants. It includes information on substance abuse problems throughout the life span and clinical practice in substance abuse treatment.*

Gold M. The Facts about Drugs and Alcohol. 3rd ed. New York: Bantam Books, 1988. *This book discusses addiction, adolescent drug abuse, cocaine, marijuana, alcohol, prescription drugs, drug testing, and assessing treatment programs.*

Milkman H, Shaffer H, eds. The Addictions: Multidisciplinary Perspectives and Treatments. Lexington, MA: Lexington Books, 1985. *This book discusses several theories of addiction and reviews various treatment perspectives.*

Nicholi AM Jr, ed. The New Harvard Guide to Psychiatry. Cambridge, Mass: Belknap Press of Harvard University Press, 1988. *The chapter on substance use disorders gives a description of the disorders as well as adverse effects, tolerance, and withdrawal.*

CHAPTER 8

CEREBROVASCULAR ACCIDENT

Susan Nassar Bierman and Ben Atchison

CRITICAL TERMS

Aneurysm
Apoplexy
Apraxia
Arteriovenous
Associated reactions
Ataxia
Atheroma
Atherosclerosis
Cerebrovascular accident

Collateral circulation
Decussation
Deep vein thrombosis
Dysarthria
Dysphagia
Embolism
Endarterectomy
Flaccidity

Hematoma
Hemianopsia (hemianopia)
Hemorrhagic stroke
Ischemia
Spasticity
Thrombus
Transient ischemic attack
Unilateral spatial neglect

J. S., a 50-year-old black man, was born and raised in a small farming community in Alabama. His father worked long, hard hours on the family farm and died of a stroke at the age of 52. J. S. decided at a young age that farming was not for him, and he went to college to earn a degree in management. His current position as director of hourly employees in a large industrial firm is a highly stressful one, and he often puts in long hours. He smokes about a pack of cigarettes every day, is moderately overweight, and does not have time for exercise. His blood pressure, when last checked by his family physician 2 years ago, was at the upper limit of normal. Yesterday, J. S. went to work earlier than usual to catch up on some desk work. He noticed difficulty seeing out of his right eye and he was unable to control his pen when writing. However, after resting his head on his desk for a few minutes, these symptoms disappeared. J. S. attributed them to lack of sleep and forgot about them quickly. Unfortunately, his symptoms are indicative of an impending stroke.

INTRODUCTION

Strokes have afflicted mankind since earliest times. Studies of the remains of ancient Egyptian mummies have shown that people in that era suffered strokes (1). In the past, strokes were referred to as apoplexy, meaning a sudden shock to the senses. Hippocrates, the father of Western medicine, wrote, "It is impossible to remove a strong attack of apoplexy and not easy to remove a weak attack" (2). This bleak statement demonstrates the pessimistic view once held about strokes; however, much has changed since Hippocrates' time. Having a stroke does not mean one must give up all hope and be resigned to a life of disability. Modern medical and surgical techniques, state-of-the-art rehabilitation programs, and knowledge of risk factor control now offer more hope than ever before (3).

The effect a stroke has on a person's life depends on many factors, each of which will be discussed in this chapter. It is possible to survive, recover, and resume daily activities after a stroke, as demonstrated by the lives of many famous people. Louis Pasteur, one of our greatest medical and scientific geniuses, experienced a stroke at the age of 46. While still bedridden, he dictated a brilliant bacteriological technique. Later he went on to prove that germs cause disease, founded the science of immunology, and created the basis for all modern aseptic surgery (2). Sir Winston Churchill, despite his stroke at age 79, went on to regain the prime ministry of Great Britain (1). He also subsequently published his four-volume book, *A History of the English Speaking Peoples* (2). George Frederick Handel experienced a stroke at the age of 52 but still produced some of his greatest works, including the *Messiah*. Presidents Dwight Eisenhower and Franklin Delano Roosevelt, dancer and choreographer Agnes de Mille, actress Patricia Neal, and Chairman Mao Tse-tung all suffered strokes, and they too went on to lead active lives (2).

ETIOLOGY

A stroke may be defined as an interruption in the blood flow that causes an inadequate supply of oxygen and nutrients to reach portions of the brain. Medical practitioners use the term "cerebrovascular accident," often abbreviated as CVA, for stroke. A stroke can occur in any part of the brain, the cerebral hemispheres, the cerebellum, or the brainstem.

Strokes are divided into two main types: hemorrhagic, including intracerebral and subarachnoid hemorrhages, and ischemic, including atherothrombotic, lacunar, and embolic infarctions, in that order of frequency (4). Lack of blood supply (ischemia) and leakage of blood outside the normal vessels (hemorrhage) can cause acute neuronal death. These two groups of strokes can be differentiated further by the location of the insult and the precise causes of the hemorrhage or ischemia (5). In most cases, a loss of blood supply is the result of long-standing degeneration of the body's blood vessels. Less commonly, a CVA occurs because of an inborn abnormality or weakness of the brain's vascular supply (6). These two types of strokes are described in detail after the review of cerebral circulation.

The Brain's Blood Vessels

The blood supply of the brain is extremely important because of the metabolic demands of nervous tissue. The brain is one of the most metabolically active organs of the body. Although it comprises only 2% of the body's weight, the brain receives approximately 17% of the cardiac output and consumes about 20% of the oxygen used by the entire body (7).

In the brain, the arteries of the anterior circulation supply the front, top, and side portions of the cerebral hemispheres. The brainstem,

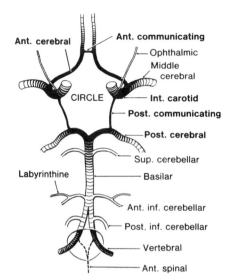

FIGURE 8.1. Circle of Willis. (Reprinted with permission from Moore KL, ed. Clinically Oriented Anatomy. 2nd ed. Baltimore: Williams & Wilkins, 1985:880.)

cerebellum, and back and undersurface of the cerebral hemispheres are supplied by the posterior circulation. These two parts of circulation are further categorized into the extracranial portions (arising from outside the skull and traveling toward the brain) and the intracranial portions (arising from within the skull) (5) (Fig. 8.1).

Extracranial Vessels

The extracranial anterior circulation consists of the two carotid arteries that travel in the front of the neck on each side of the trachea and esophagus (6). The word "carotid" is derived from the Greek word "karos" meaning "deep sleep," indicating the significance of this main artery in maintaining consciousness and brain function (8). The right common carotid artery arises from the innominate artery. The left com-

mon carotid artery originates directly from the aortic arch. Around the fifth or sixth vertebrae, these common carotid arteries divide into external carotid arteries, whose branches supply the face and its structures, and the internal carotid arteries, which supply the eyes and the cerebral hemispheres.

The vertebral arteries arise from the subclavian arteries and make up the extracranial posterior circulation. They remain within the vertebral column for part of their course from about C6 to C2. The vertebral arteries enter the cranium through the foramen magnum (6).

Intracranial Vessels

The internal carotid arteries enter the skull through the carotid canal and form an S-shaped curve called the carotid siphon (6). The artery then enters the subarachnoid space by piercing the dura mater. It gives rise to the ophthalmic arteries, which supply the eyes, the posterior communicating arteries, which join with the posterior circulation, and the anterior cerebral arteries, which supply the orbital and medial surfaces of the frontal lobes and part of the basal frontal lobe white matter and caudate nucleus. It also gives off the middle cerebral arteries, which supply almost the entire lateral surface of the frontal, parietal, and temporal lobes, as well as the underlying white matter and basal ganglia (6). The middle cerebral artery is the largest of the terminal branches of the internal carotid artery and is the direct continuation of this vessel.

The vertebral arteries enter the cranium within the posterior fossa and travel along the side of the medulla, where they give off their longest branch, the posterior inferior cerebellar artery, which supplies the lateral medulla and the back of the undersurface of the cerebellum (6). The two vertebral arteries then join at the junction between the medulla and pons to form the single midline basilar artery (9). The basilar artery gives off penetrating arteries to the base of the pons and two vessels (the anterior inferior and superior cerebellar arteries) that supply the upper and anterior undersurfaces of the cerebellum (6). At the level of the midbrain, the basilar artery bifurcates into the two posterior cerebral arteries (9). As they circle the brainstem, these two arteries give off penetrating branches to the midbrain and thalamus and then divide into branches that supply the occipital lobes as well as the medial and undersurfaces of the temporal lobes (6). One of the branches of the posterior cerebral artery, the calcarine artery, is of special significance because it is the main supplier of the blood for the visual area of cortex (7).

Communicating Arteries

The right and left carotid vessels connect with each other when they enter the brain, each sending out a small lateral branch that meets in the space between them. These are the anterior communicating arteries. They also branch backward to join with the right and left posterior cerebral arteries, called the posterior communicating arteries. This communicating vascular interchange, the circle of Willis, protects the brain should one of the four major supplying arteries coming up through the neck be blocked (2). The circle of Willis, named for Dr. Thomas Willis, was first described in the mid-17th century. The original diagram of this structure was first drawn for Dr. Willis by Sir Christopher Wren, the architect of St. Paul's Cathedral. Although known primarily for his architectural genius, he was also deeply involved in biology and medicine (2).

Thus we have an arterial circle to provide backup supplies for the essential functions and tissues of the brain. Starting from the midline anteriorly, the circle consists of the anterior communicating, anterior cerebral, internal carotid, posterior communicating, and posterior cerebral arteries, from which it continues to the starting point in reverse order (7). When one major vessel supplying the brain is slowly occluded, either within the circle of Willis or proximal to it, the normally small communicating arteries may enlarge slowly to compensate for the occlusion (9). This system is imperfect, however, and it often fails to prevent strokes for several reasons. In many individuals, the same atherosclerotic processes that caused a stroke also may damage communicating arteries. In addition, only about one-fourth of strokes are caused by a blockage of the major neck vessels (2). Also, approximately half the population have anomalies or deviations in the circle of Willis. The most common defect is the absence of the posterior communicating arteries, so that the two blood supply systems, anterior and posterior, cannot interchange. It is interesting that such anomalies are more common in those who have strokes than in the general population. Experts feel that such anomalies increase the chances of stroke in persons who also have atherosclerosis (2).

TYPES OF STROKES
Ischemic Stroke

Cerebral infarction or brain tissue death results from obstruction of circulation to an area of the brain (ischemia) as in thrombotic, embolic, or lacunar strokes. The infarcted area has two components: the tissues that have died as a result of blood supply loss and the peripheral area in which there may be temporary dysfunction as a result of edema. Edematous brain tissue sometimes recovers slowly and gradually, resulting in a reappearance of function after a period of 4 to 5 months (10).

The actual physiological events that follow an ischemic stroke occur in characteristic steps.

First, the membrane surrounding each affected neuron leaks potassium (a mineral necessary for producing electrical impulses) and adenosine triphosphate (ATP, an energy-producing biochemical found in the body). Fluid quickly accumulates between the blood vessel and neuron, making it difficult for oxygen and nutrients to pass from the bloodstream into the damaged neuron. The initial injury produces a vicious circle in which more cellular injury results. Irreversible cell death will occur in 5 to 10 minutes if oxygen and nutrients are unable to pass to them from the bloodstream or in a slightly longer period if blood flow is only partially interrupted. These dead cells form a zone of infarction that is dead tissue that will not regenerate.

Downstream from the infarcted zone is a zone of injury (penumbra). This area may be served by collateral blood vessels and is capable of returning to normal functioning. A third area that reacts differently to the stroke process may also exist. In this area of hyperemia, the blood vessels are congested and swollen and also may have the potential for recovery.

The presence of these two zones, the regions of penumbra and hyperemia, may serve to minimize the total area of infarction. However, they do present problems for treatment, because interventions may benefit one region and not the other (1).

Thrombosis

Cerebral thrombosis occurs when a blood clot forms in one of the arteries supplying the brain, causing vascular obstruction at the point of its formation. The size and location of the infarct depends on which vessel is occluded and the amount of collateral circulation. Thrombosis occurs most frequently in blood vessels that have already been damaged by atherosclerosis (1).

Atherosclerosis is a gradual degenerative vessel-wall disease that is pathological and not a normal aspect of human aging (1). It appears as rough, irregular fatty deposits formed within the intima and inner media of the arteries. Large-vessel atherosclerosis accounts for 60% of ischemic stroke. In nearly all cases, this atherosclerosis leads to the occurrence of stroke through the generation of a thrombus. Only rarely does stenosis alone cause stroke (11). The body's blood vessels have a significant reserve capacity, so atherosclerosis does not usually occur until the vessel is two-thirds blocked (1).

To understand the process that produces a mass of degenerated, thickened material (plaque) called atheromas, imagine a glue bottle that has been allowed to collect the residuals of dried glue. The more clogged the cap of the bottle becomes, the more difficult it is for the glue to flow through. Squeezing the glue through the opening can push already dried glue more firmly against the opening. The opening will become smaller and smaller until it closes completely or bursts from the increased pressure.

In the cerebral circulation, atherosclerosis and thrombus formation are most likely to occur in areas where blood vessels turn or divide, such as the origins of the internal carotid artery and the middle cerebral artery and the junction of the vertebral and basilar arteries (1, 12).

Cerebral thrombosis often causes stuttering or progressive symptoms that occur over several hours or days. Onset during sleep is common. Often a patient notices mild arm numbness at night and then awakens the next morning with paralysis. Transient ischemic attacks precede actual infarction about half the time (4).

Lacunar Strokes

Lacunar strokes were first described by the French physician, Pierre Marie, at the beginning of the 20th century (1). These are small infarcts usually lying in the deep noncortical parts of the cerebrum and brainstem including the basal ganglia, thalamus, pons, internal capsule, and deep white matter (12, 13). Within a few months of onset of a lacunar stroke, a small cavity ("lacune" in French) is left (1).

Lacunar strokes result from an occlusion of small branches of larger cerebral arteries—middle cerebral, posterior cerebral, basilar, and, to a lesser extent, anterior cerebral and vertebral arteries (13). Lacunar infarcts range in size from 2 to 15 mm (12). Because of their small size, only minimal neurological symptoms usually result, and many go undetected.

Commonly, lacunar strokes produce purely motor deficits (weakness or ataxia), purely sensory deficits, or a combination of motor and sensory deficits. Symptoms usually do not include aphasia, changes in mental activity or personality, loss of consciousness, homonymous hemianopsia, or seizures (13).

Causes of vascular occlusion in lacunar infarcts include atheroma in a small vessel, an embolic particle of a thrombus lodging in a small vessel, or lipohyalinosis, in which hypertension reduces the wall of the artery to connective tissue shreds (13). Hypertension is the most consistently identified risk factor for lacunar infarction, so treatment is aimed at controlling it (12). Prognosis for recovery after a lacunar stroke is excellent (13).

Embolism

Embolism occurs when a clot that has formed elsewhere (thrombus) breaks off (embolus), travels up the bloodstream until it reaches an artery too small to pass through, and blocks the artery (5). At this point, the effects of the embolus are similar to those produced by thrombosis. Approximately 5 to 14% of strokes are the result of this process (1).

Embolic materials that travel to the arteries of the brain can originate from many sources, including the aortic arch and arteries arising from it, the extracranial carotid and vertebral arteries, and thrombi in the heart. Cardiac-source emboli are common and are referred to as cardiogenic. Many cardiac abnormalities can give rise to a cerebral embolism, including atrial fibrillation, coronary artery disease, valvular heart disease, and arrhythmias. The middle cerebral artery is by far the most common destination of cardiac emboli, followed by the posterior cerebral artery (6).

In contrast to thrombotic strokes, embolic strokes typically occur during daytime activity. The embolism can be precipitated by a sudden movement, or even a sneeze. Clinical symptoms are usually maximal at onset, but in some cases the neurological symptoms improve or stabilize somewhat, then worsen as the embolus moves and blocks a more distal artery. A history of transient ischemic attacks is rare. Seizures are often associated with embolic strokes (6).

Hemorrhagic Stroke

Hemorrhagic strokes are caused by a rupture in a blood vessel or an aneurysm with resultant bleeding into or around cerebral tissue. These types of strokes have a much higher fatality rate than those caused by clots. An aneurysm is a bulging or out-pouching of a wall of an artery owing to weakness in the vessel wall; it is prone to rupture at any time. Aneurysms often are seen in young persons, and hemorrhagic strokes are more common than infarcts in young people. The vessel wall anomaly is often congenital. There are two types of hemorrhagic strokes. An intracerebral hemorrhage refers to bleeding directly into brain substance, whereas a subarachnoid hemorrhage is bleeding occurring within the brain's surrounding membranes and cerebrospinal fluid (11). These two types of hemorrhage differ in incidence, etiology, clinical signs, and treatment.

Subarachnoid Hemorrhages

Subarachnoid hemorrhages account for about 7% of all strokes (5). Their most common cause is leakage of blood from aneurysms. A combination of congenital and degenerative factors, usually at the points of origin or bifurcations of arteries, can precipitate formation of an aneurysm. Blood may break through the weak point of the aneurysm at any time and, because of the force of arterial pressure, spread quickly into the cerebrospinal fluid surrounding the brain. A subarachnoid hemorrhage also may be caused by bleeding from an arteriovenous malformation, which is an abnormal collection of vessels near the surface of the brain. Other less common causes of subarachnoid hemorrhages are hemophilia, excessive anticoagulation therapy, and trauma to the skull and brain (6).

Extravasated blood irritates the meninges, and intracranial pressure is increased owing to extra fluid in the closed cranial cavity. This can lead to headache, vomiting, and an altered state of consciousness. Sleepiness, stupor, agitation, restlessness, and actual coma are various manifestations of reduced consciousness. Headaches are usually severe and are described as the worst in the patient's life. Because the bleeding takes place around the brain and not in the actual brain substance, motor, sensory, or visual abnormalities on one side of the body usually are not seen. Lumbar puncture with analysis of the cerebrospinal fluid is the most reliable method of diagnosing subarachnoid hemorrhage (6).

Intracerebral Hemorrhages

Intracerebral hemorrhage usually begins with bleeding from small, deep penetrating vessels under arteriolar or capillary pressure as opposed to arterial pressure as with a subarachnoid hemorrhage. Therefore, symptoms from intracerebral hemorrhages develop gradually over minutes, hours, or even days. Release of blood into brain tissue and surrounding edema will then disrupt the function of that particular brain region (6). Hypertension is the most common cause of bleeding into the brain. Less common causes are arteriovenous malformations, aneurysms, drugs (especially methamphetamines and cocaine), use of anticoagulants, and trauma (14).

Clinical signs of intracerebral hemorrhage are usually focal at first and depend on the location of the bleeding. There are also some general symptoms regardless of the location, and extremely small hemorrhages may go undetected. A large hematoma causes headache, vomiting, convulsions, and decreased levels of alertness (14).

Stupor and coma are common signs of very large hemorrhages and carry a poor prognosis. Nevertheless, recovery is possible. Agnes de Mille's book *Reprieve: A Memoir* is a story of cerebral hemorrhage and subsequent recovery (1).

Cerebral injury caused by intracerebral bleeding results from the damaging effect that the abnormal presence of blood has on the neurons. Abnormal pressure on neurons distorts their normal architecture. It also prevents oxygen and nutrients from passing to the cells from the bloodstream. Eventually, bleeding will stop and a hard clot will form. During a period of months, the clot slowly recedes, breaks down, and is absorbed by the body's white blood cells (1).

INCIDENCE AND PREVALENCE

Stroke is the third leading cause of death in the United States, surpassed only by heart disease and cancer (3). It is the most common diagnosis among clients seen by occupational therapists for the treatment of physically disabled adults. At least 500,000 people suffer an episode each year. Of the 2 million individuals in this country who have experienced a stroke and who are alive at any one time, 10% will fully recover, 40% will be left with a mild disability, and 50% will be severely disabled and may require institutional care (3). Of the two main types, hemorrhagic strokes occur much less frequently (20% of all strokes) than ischemic strokes, which account for about 80% of all strokes (6). Approximately 10% of all strokes result from intracerebral hemorrhage (5) and approximately 18% are lacunar (15).

Despite these grim statistics, there is some good news. With the exception of subarachnoid hemorrhage, all types of strokes have shown a significantly decreased incidence in the last 4 to 5 decades. This may be partly the result of increased control of risk factors such as hypertension, diabetes mellitus, and heart disease and the fact that individuals are trying to lead healthier lives (16). Individuals who have had a stroke now live almost twice as long (4). Fewer people now die of stroke, notwithstanding the continuing debate as to whether this decline is the result of the occurrence of fewer strokes occurring or to better medical treatment (5).

Stroke in young children occurs in about 2.5 cases per 100,000 children per year as compared to 100 cases per 100,000 in the adult population. It is more frequent in children under 2 years of age than in older children. The effects of stroke among children are similar to those described in adults. Whereas the cause of stroke in children is often unknown, the most common known cause is a developmental defect of the heart that affects the structure of the heart. Sickle cell disease, which affects blood clotting mechanisms, and genetic disorders are the next most common known causes. Fortunately, the outcome of stroke is better for children than adults, as the extent of permanent disability is less than it is for adults. Children often have minor delays in the development of sensorimotor and cognitive functioning (17).

SIGNS AND SYMPTOMS
Stroke Warning Signs

To educate the public, the American Heart Association has published several pamphlets listing signs that are considered preliminary warnings of an impending serious stroke. These include sudden weakness or numbness of the face, arm, and leg on one side of the body; loss of speech or trouble talking or understanding speech; dimness or loss of vision, particularly in one eye only; and unexplained dizziness, unsteadiness, or sudden falls (1).

Some general medical symptoms related to *type* of stroke were discussed under Etiology, above. The outward signs and symptoms also depend on the size and location of the injury, and neurologists can often predict location by the symptoms the individual demonstrates. However, it is important to remember that a stroke is complex and visible symptoms are as different as each individual. Relying on stereotypical models of stroke leads to generalized, and often inappropriate, therapy.

Symptoms that result from a partial reduction or temporary change in the blood flow to the brain are extremely important warning signs for stroke (16). Several of these conditions are discussed below.

Transient Ischemic Attacks

Transient ischemic attacks, or TIAs, result from a temporary interference of the blood supply to the brain. The symptoms occur rapidly and last for about 1 minute up to but not exceeding 24 hours. The specific signs and symptoms depend on the portion of the brain affected, but they may include fleeting blindness in one eye, hemiparesis, hemiplegia, aphasia, dizziness, double vision, and staggering. Carotid artery disease and vertebral basilar artery disease may lead to TIAs (1). The main distinction between TIAs and stroke is the short duration of the symptoms and the lack of permanent neurological damage. People who have had TIAs are 9 1/2 times more likely to have a stroke than those of the same age and sex who have never had a TIA (16).

Small Strokes

In some cases, the symptoms of a TIA may last longer than 24 hours. If they last a day or more and then completely resolve, or if they leave only minor neurological deficits, they are called "small strokes." Often, the remaining neurological deficits are barely noticeable. Like TIAs, however, these small strokes are important warning signs that a more serious CVA may occur (1). A small stroke that completely resolves is called a reversible ischemic neurological deficit (RIND). An episode that lasts more than 72 hours and leaves some minor neurological impairments is called a partially reversible ischemic neurological deficit (PRIND). The mechanism of injury in RIND and PRIND is the same as that for a stroke or TIA. Blood flow to the brain is reduced below the critical level needed for normal neurological activity (1).

Many small strokes are not reported to a medical practitioner, which makes the exact frequency of occurrence of these strokes difficult to determine. However, the occurrence of a small stroke increases the risk of a serious stroke by as much as tenfold (1). It is important to recognize the symptoms of a small stroke so that it can be treated early, reducing the risk of more permanent injury.

Subclavian Steal Syndrome

This is a rare condition in which there is a narrowing of the subclavian artery that runs under the clavicle. Symptoms occur when the arm on the side of the narrowed vessel is exercised. Usually, movement of the arm produces light-headedness, numbness, and weakness. Other neurological symptoms also may be present. In this syndrome, blood is "stolen" from the brain and instead is delivered to the exercised arm. It is a warning sign that advanced atherosclerosis may be present in the arteries throughout the body, including the cerebral arteries (1).

Neurological Effects of Stroke

An occlusion that causes a serious stroke can occur anywhere in the extracranial or intracranial system, but the most common site is in the distribution of the middle cerebral artery and its branches in the cerebrum. The majority of cerebral strokes occur in one or the other cerebral hemisphere, but not both (1). It is important to note that even in individuals with the same neurological deficit, the impact of disability is different, depending on the individual's life situation.

Left-Sided Cerebral Injuries: Middle Cerebral Artery

The left cerebral hemisphere controls most functions on the right side of the body because of the decussation of motor fibers (decussation of the pyramids) in the medulla. These fibers that cross, or decussate to the opposite side, form the lateral corticospinal tract. The rest of the fibers descend ipsilaterally, forming the anterior corticospinal tract (18). The proportion of crossing fibers varies from person to person, with an average of about 85% (7).

A CVA in the region of the middle cerebral artery in the left cerebral hemisphere may produce the following symptoms:

1. Loss of voluntary movement and coordination on the right side of the face, trunk, and extremities.
2. Impaired sensation, including temperature discrimination, pain, and proprioception on the right side (hemianesthesia).

3. Language deficits, called aphasia, in which the patient may be unable to speak or understand speech, writing, or gestures. The breakdown of language function is complex; the many types of aphasia will be discussed later in this chapter.
4. Produce problems with articulation of speech because of disturbances in muscle control of the lips, mouth, tongue, and vocal cords (dysarthria).
5. Create blind spots in the visual field, usually on the right side.
6. Produce a slow and cautious personality.
7. Produce memory deficits for recent or past events (1).

Right-Sided Cerebral Injuries: Middle Cerebral Artery

The right cerebral hemisphere controls most of the functions on the left side of the body. The right cerebral hemisphere also is responsible for spatial sensation, perception, and judgement.

Injury to the middle cerebral artery of the right cerebral hemisphere may produce a combination of the following deficits:

1. Weakness (hemiparesis) or paralysis (hemiplegia) on the left side of the body (face, arm, trunk, and leg).
2. Impairment of sensation (touch, pain, temperature, and proprioception) on the left side of the body.
3. Spatial and perceptual deficits.
4. Unilateral neglect, in which the patient neglects the left side of the body or the left side of the environment.
5. Dressing apraxia, in which the patient is unable to relate the articles of clothes to the body (19).
6. Defective vision in the left halves of visual fields or left homonymous hemianopsia in which there is defective vision in each eye (the temporal half of the left eye and the nasal half of the right eye).

7. Impulsive behavior, quick and imprecise movements, and errors of judgment (1).

Anterior Cerebral Artery Stroke

The territory of the anterior cerebral artery is rarely infarcted because of the side-to-side communication provided by the anterior communicating artery in the circle of Willis (15). Symptoms of an anterior cerebral artery stroke include:

1. Paralysis of the lower extremity, usually more severe than the upper extremity, contralateral to the occluded vessel.
2. Loss of sensation in the contralateral toes, foot, and leg.
3. Loss of conscious control of bowel or bladder
4. Balance problems in sitting, standing, and walking.
5. Lack of spontaneity of emotion, whispered speech, or loss of all communication.
6. Memory impairment or loss (1).

Vertebrobasilar Stroke

The vertebrobasilar system of arteries supplies blood primarily to the posterior portions of the brain, including the brainstem, cerebellum, thalamus, and parts of the occipital and temporal lobes. This posterior circulation is not divided into right and left halves, as in the anterior circulation. An occlusion here might produce:

1. A variety of visual disturbances, including impaired coordination of the eyes.
2. Impaired temperature sensation.
3. Impaired ability to read and/or name objects.
4. Vertigo, dizziness.
5. Disturbances in balance when standing or walking (ataxia).
6. Paralysis of the face, limbs, or tongue.
7. Clumsy movements of the hands.
8. Difficulty judging distance when trying to coordinate limb movements (dysmetria).

9. Drooling and difficulty swallowing (dysphagia).
10. Localized numbness.
11. Loss of memory.
12. Drop attacks in which there is a sudden loss of motor and postural control resulting in collapse, but the individual remains conscious (1). Transient ischemic attacks in this area are common in the elderly. The vertebral arteries travel up to the brainstem through a bony channel in the cervical vertebrae. In older individuals, osteoarthritis may develop in cervical bones, causing narrowing of the cervical canal, especially when the head is extended or rotated.

Wallenberg's Syndrome

Wallenberg's syndrome is a classic brainstem stroke that also is referred to as the lateral medullary syndrome (15). It occurs as the result of an occlusion of the posterior inferior cerebellar artery or one of its branches supplying the lower portion of the brainstem (1). It is located in an area of the brainstem that both relays nerve fibers from the spinal cord and regulates many vital senses (1). Strokes in this area may produce contralateral pain and temperature loss, ipsilateral Horner's syndrome (sinking of the eyeball, ptosis of the upper eyelid, and a dry cool face on the affected side), ataxia, and facial sensory loss. Ischemia to ipsilateral cranial nerve fibers 8, 9, and 10 results in palatal paralysis, hoarseness, dysphagia, and vertigo. There is no significant weakness in this syndrome (15).

Brainstem strokes often result in coma because of damage to the centers involved with alertness and wakefulness (reticular system) (15). A hemorrhage into the brainstem area is rare, quickly accompanied by loss of consciousness, and usually fatal. Among patients who survive brainstem stroke, however, recovery is often good.

Other Complications of Stroke

Secondary conditions may occur in addition to these deficits. These are important manifestations that are important to the patient's recovery and rehabilitation and may actually be more disabling than the stroke itself (10). It is necessary to be aware of these complications so that they may be prevented.

Seizures

Brain scars that result from stroke may irritate the cortex and cause a spontaneous discharge of nerve impulses that may generalize to a full grand mal convulsion (10). Seizures develop in up to 10% of stroke patients and are more common with embolic than thrombotic infarcts (10). Anticonvulsant drugs are sometimes used in patients with early seizures, but their use is controversial. Some studies have shown that seizures usually resolve spontaneously (10).

Infection

Alteration of swallowing function, aspiration, hypoventilation, and immobility in the stroke patient often lead to pneumonia. Changes in bladder function may lead to bladder distention and urinary tract infection (6). Impaired sensation and inadequate position changes may result in pressure sores (decubitus) and consequent infection of these areas.

Thromboembolism

Immobility of the legs and bed rest often lead to thrombosis of dependent leg veins. In deep vein thrombosis (DVT), local pain and tenderness may develop in the calf, with some swelling and a slight increase in temperature. The risk of venous thrombosis occurring in a paralyzed leg approaches 60% (10). If the thrombosis is confined to the calf, it may not be serious. However, if the thrombosis spreads up toward the groin to involve the veins in the pelvis, then there is a very real possibility of a clot breaking off into the bloodstream. The clot will then travel through the right side of the heart and enter the lungs through the pulmonary arteries, resulting in sudden collapse and death owing to obstruction of the pulmonary arteries (10). Early mobilization of the patient is of utmost importance in preventing deep vein thrombosis and subsequent pulmonary embolism.

RISK FACTORS

The best way to prevent a stroke from occurring is to control the risk factors that can cause it. Regular visits to a family physician are important, and modifications in lifestyle and diet are best made early in life. Risk factors for stroke are similar to those for heart attack, because atherosclerosis is a common underlying cause for both.

1. Race—African Americans are 50% more likely to have hypertension than white Americans, and they suffer strokes more often and at a younger age. According to one study, African-American men aged 35 to 74 were 2 to 3 times more likely than whites to die of stroke (20).
2. Age—In the Framingham Heart Study, it was reported that 45- to 64-year-old men had a 25.4% incidence rate of first stroke, compared with only 5.5% in the 30- to 44-year-old age range. Approximately 29% of people who suffer a stroke in a given year are younger than age 65 (5).
3. Heredity—A family history of stroke increases one's risk (5).
4. Obesity—Being overweight is a known risk factor for hypertension and diabetes mellitus and also is associated with stroke. Many overweight individuals have hyperlipidemia (raised levels of cholesterol and

triglycerides in the blood) (1). The Framingham Study found that in men between the ages of 30 and 62, cholesterol levels of 250 carried about 3 times the risk of heart attack and stroke as did cholesterol levels that were under 194 (2).

5. Hypertension—It has long been known that hypertension is the major risk factor for stroke. It is, however, a risk that can be controlled through antihypertensive drug therapy, stress reduction, dietary control, and regular exercise. Chronically elevated blood pressure exerts pressure on intracranial and extracranial cerebral vessels, often resulting in lacunar infarctions or intracerebral hemorrhage. It also has been implicated in the atherosclerotic process by driving fatty substances into the walls of arteries making them brittle, narrowed, and hardened (1). Hypertension has been called "the silent disease" because often there are no symptoms (1). An occasional headache, dizziness, or light-headedness, which are all symptoms of hypertension, can easily be attributed to other factors. High blood pressure that continues for several years also can damage the heart. If a person has a stroke, the already damaged heart will be less capable of delivering needed blood to the brain tissues. This may influence the severity of the episode (1). It is important to have regular blood pressure checks and to follow the drug treatment and recommendations prescribed by a physician to control this major risk factor.
6. Smoking—There is strong evidence for a relationship between smoking and increased risk of stroke (8). Quitting smoking reduces the likelihood of stroke, even in a long-term smoker.
7. Transient ischemic attacks—Most medical professionals consider a TIA to be an important risk factor for an impending

stroke. Approximately 30% of all patients who have had a TIA are at risk of having a stroke within 2 years. This risk is greatest in the first month, so it is important to seek medical intervention quickly (1).

8. Geographic location—The number of deaths from strokes in the United States is greatest in North and South Carolina, Georgia, northern Florida, Alabama, Mississippi, and Tennessee. Specific pockets of high death rates in Texas, Oklahoma, and all of the Hawaiian islands have been noted. This geographical strip, often termed the "stroke belt," is the source of numerous studies on environmental, cultural, or other geographically determined risk factors. A person who grows up in a high-risk area and then moves to a lower-risk area as an adult continues to carry the greater likelihood of having a stroke. This has led to speculation that the causes may be diet related, cultural, or possibly even related to water supply or altitude (2).

9. Diabetes mellitus—This disease is more common in stroke patients than in a normal population of similar age. However, because diabetes is associated with hypertension, obesity, and hyperlipidemia, it is difficult to be certain of a relationship with stroke when these other conditions are also present (2). Individuals with diabetes mellitus are two to four times more likely to have a stroke, a fact that is even more true for women than men (5).

10. Oral contraceptives—Women who have taken birth control pills, especially those with a high estrogen content, have an increased risk for stroke as they become older. Smoking while taking the pill further increases the risk (1).

11. Polycythemia—Increased blood viscosity (polycythemia) causes blood to flow sluggishly. This increases the likelihood of thrombosis and embolism and, ultimately, heart attack and, to a lesser extent, stroke (1).

12. Asymptomatic carotid bruits—A bruit is an abnormal sound or murmur heard when a stethoscope is placed over the carotid artery. This slushing noise indicates turbulent blood, often caused by a significant degree of stenosis. Carotid bruit clearly indicates increased stroke risk. Complete occlusion of the carotid artery sometimes follows, resulting in stroke (16).

13. Prior stroke—The risk of stroke for a person who has already suffered a stroke is increased four to eight times (16).

14. Heart disease—A diseased heart (whether it be chronic disease, acute heart attacks, or prosthetic heart valves) increases the risk of stroke. Independent of hypertension, people with heart disease have more than twice the risk of stroke than people with normally functioning hearts (5).

15. Alcoholism—Consistently, the Stroke Council's Subcommittee on Risk Factors and Stroke has stated that alcohol is a "less well-documented" risk factor for stroke but nevertheless is felt to be a contributing factor in a majority of reports on risk behaviors (21).

Of these many risk factors, several can be controlled by changes in lifestyle, including elevated blood cholesterol and lipids, cigarette smoking, use of oral contraceptives, excessive drinking of alcohol, and obesity. Some, such as hypertension, heart disease, TIAs, carotid bruits, and polycythemia, can be controlled by medical intervention. Factors that cannot be changed are age, sex, race, family history, diabetes mellitus, and a prior stroke. The potential benefits of all medical and surgical interventions currently available for cerebrovascular disease pale in comparison to what can be achieved through risk factor control (22). Understanding and awareness of these risk factors for stroke is an important first step in reducing the likelihood of having stroke.

COURSE AND PROGNOSIS

Strokes result in anoxic damage to nervous tissue that causes various neurological deficits, depending on where the blood supply was lost. If neuronal cell death occurs, it is considered irreparable and permanent, as no way has yet been found to regenerate nerve cells (2). However, the nervous system has a high level of plasticity, especially during early development, and individual differences in neural connections and learned behaviors play a major role in functional recovery. No two brains can be expected to be structurally or functionally identical (23). Spontaneous recovery may occur as edema subsides or viable neurons reactivate. Recovery also may occur with physiological reorganization of neural connections or developmental strategies. Any injury brings different factors into play, affecting axonal and dendritic sprouting or collateral rearrangement, synaptic formation, the excitability of neurons, "substitution of parallel channels," and "mobilization of redundant capacity" (24).

Accuracy in the prediction of function or rate of return in a given stroke patient is difficult because of individual variability of anatomy and extent of brain damage, as well as differences in types of CVA, learning ability, premorbid personality and intelligence, and motivation (25). Generally, the prognosis for recovery of function is greater in young clients, possibly because the young brain is more plastic or because the young are generally in better physical condition.

Secondary complications are important to recovery and rehabilitation and may actually be more disabling than the stroke itself (10). These complications are discussed in detail in this chapter and include depression, seizures, infection, bowel/bladder incontinence, thromboembolism, shoulder subluxation, painful shoulder, shoulder–hand syndrome, abnormal muscle tone, and associated reactions and movements.

Individuals with good sensation, minimal spasticity, some selective motor control, and no fixed contractures seem to make the greatest improvements in functional abilities. If an individual has no concept of the affected side and cannot localize stimuli to the affected side, or if he or she has fecal or urinary incontinence, the outlook for independence is generally poor. Some individuals may continue to have strokes, complicating recovery (26).

Medications and surgery may make a difference in the prognosis of an individual at risk for, or having had, a CVA.

DIAGNOSIS

Preventive treatments, surgical interventions, and general lifestyle changes can reduce the likelihood or severity of stroke (1). The best way to prevent a stroke from occurring is to control risk factors and be aware of warning signs and symptoms. The diagnosis of stroke requires a knowledge of the incidence of the different types of stroke and awareness of the presence of these risk factors. Symptoms must be carefully obtained from either the patient or the family, if the patient is too ill, frightened, or confused (6). Neurologists, neurosurgeons, and some internists are the specialists usually involved in this acute diagnostic phase of treatment (10).

The physical examination of the patient with a suspected stroke or TIA includes a search for possible cardiac sources of emboli by listening to the heart and arteries of the neck. Also useful in the determination of cardiac-source emboli are electrocardiography (ECG), echocardiography, and monitoring for arrhythmias. A neurological examination assists in determining the neurological disability and usually includes evaluation of higher cortical function (memory and language), level of alertness, visual and oculomotor system, behavior, and gait (6).

Laboratory and other diagnostic procedures are carefully selected to test, confirm, and elaborate on the suggested hypothesis of the mechanism and location of the stroke (6). Blood studies are essential and very useful in the diagnosis. Other diagnostic methods include neuroimaging techniques, noninvasive studies of blood vessels, and invasive techniques.

Neuroimaging Techniques

Computed tomography (CT) and magnetic resonance imaging (MRI) are invaluable noninvasive tools that depict pathological changes in the brain in patients with stroke (6). One or the other of these is almost always used at some point for every patient with a suspected stroke.

Computed Tomography

Computed tomography is a type of radiographic examination that allows accurate analysis of cerebral injury (1). An important distinction that a CT scan can make is the difference between a hemorrhagic stroke and an ischemic stroke. It is useful in clarifying the location and the mechanism and severity of stroke. It also can determine associated changes such as edema, shift of brain contents, hematomas, and infarcts that result from ischemia. It is most useful in the diagnosis of stroke caused by hemorrhage; CT findings may even be normal in patients with recent infarction. It is often not diagnostic in patients with TIAs and is not useful for imaging brainstem infarcts (6).

Magnetic Resonance Imaging

Magnetic resonance imaging is more sensitive than a CT scan and does not expose the patient to radiation from radiographs. It provides detailed pictures of the brain by using a magnetic field. Magnetic resonance imaging is particularly helpful in revealing arteriovenous malformations (AVMs) (6). It is superior to CT in imaging the cerebellum, brainstem, thalamus, and spinal cord. It also provides better anatomical definition of the injury, but it does not distinguish hemorrhage, tumor, and infarction as well as CT.

Positron Emission Tomography

Positron emission tomography, or PET scan, is being used experimentally. This scan shows how the brain uses oxygen, glucose, and other nutrients. With PET scanning, weakened or damaged areas can be identified (1).

Noninvasive Study of Blood Vessels

Two noninvasive procedures used to evaluate both extracranial and intracranial blood flow are duplex scanning and transcranial Doppler ultrasound. These techniques can localize and determine the approximate size of the lesions within the arteries (6).

Duplex scanning is useful in detecting the presence and severity of disease in the common and internal carotid arteries and in the subclavian and vertebral arteries in the neck. This scan can reliably differentiate between minor plaque disease, stenosis, and occlusive lesions. It is an excellent method of monitoring the progression or regression of atherosclerotic disease in the neck (6).

Transcranial Doppler ultrasound gives information about pressure and flow in the intracranial arteries. A probe is placed on the head and is then attached to a computer. This procedure is useful in monitoring changes in arterial flow later in the course of the patient's disease (6).

Invasive Techniques

Cerebral angiography involves radiography of the vascular system of the brain after injection of a dye or other contrast medium into the arterial blood system. The entire visible length of cerebral arteries can be defined as well as the nature, location, and extent of pathological changes. This technique is now safer than before (less than 1% incidence of mortality and serious morbidity) (6).

Analysis of cerebrospinal fluid is helpful in diagnosing subarachnoid hemorrhage. In a lumbar puncture, the subarachnoid space (usually between the third and fourth lumbar vertebrae) is tapped and cerebrospinal fluid is withdrawn. Analysis of the pigments in the spinal fluid also can help in estimating the age of the hemorrhage and detecting rebleeding (6).

Other Techniques

Other diagnostic techniques used for stroke include electroencephalography (EEG), single photon emission tomography (SPET), and special cardiac and coagulation tests that are useful in detecting unusual heart and blood disorders that can bring on a stroke (6). After this diagnostic phase of evaluation, a physiatrist will evaluate the brain-damaged person's ability to function. Rehabilitation often will begin at that point to return the patient to the highest possible level of independent functioning.

MEDICAL/SURGICAL MANAGEMENT

At present, the treatment of acute stroke is limited to management of the results of the primary event and preventive measures against further injury or occurrence (27). Much controversy

remains about the routine use of agents to reverse the cause or decrease the effects of stroke. The value of secondary preventative measures is far from clear (27); however, many treatments have been tried with acute stroke. Before the stroke can be treated, it must be accurately identified as either cerebral infarction or cerebral hemorrhage (27). Medications that are beneficial with one of these types of stroke may be potentially dangerous to the other. Therefore, careful and exact diagnosis must be made first.

Some common categories of drugs used for cerebral infarction are:

Anticoagulants

These drugs inhibit clotting by interfering with the activity of chemicals in the liquid portion of blood that are essential for the coagulation process (1). Heparin is one of the most commonly used drugs, although recent studies fail to support its use in completed cerebral infarct unless a cardiac source of emboli is likely (28). Nevertheless, 70% of neurologists questioned in one survey felt that prevention of stroke progression was a potential indication for the use of heparin (28). Subcutaneous heparin also has been found to dramatically reduce DVT formation, a serious complication of stroke.

Antiplatelet Therapy

Aspirin and ticlopidine are two antiplatelet agents that can reduce the risk of stroke recurrence. The use of aspirin in TIAs can result in a 30% reduction in the development of full stroke (28). It also benefits patients who have had a mild stroke but is not as effective in those with moderate or severe strokes (28). Two major studies, each with about 20,000 patients, have examined the effects of aspirin in the treatment of ischemic strokes (28, 29). The first, the International Stroke Trial, tested two methods of treatment: aspirin (in a dose of 300 mg a day) and heparin, a blood thinner that must be given by injection. A control group of subjects did not receive either drug. Treatment was started as soon as possible after stroke, given to patients whose CT scan indicated an ischemic, not hemorrhagic, stroke. Treatment proceeded for 2 weeks. The results suggested that 6 months after the stroke, heparin therapy produced no results and aspirin produced only a marginal improvement. The second study, the Chinese Acute Stroke Trial, included 20,000 Chinese patients who had recently experienced an ischemic stroke. In this study, aspirin in a smaller dose (160 mg a day) was compared to placebo treatment. The aspirin resulted in a small, but definite reduction in mortality after stroke.

It has been suggested that patients who have elevated blood levels of cholesterol and other lipids may need to take higher doses of aspirin to prevent a second stroke. Aspirin is clearly not suitable for patients with cerebral hemorrhage or those at risk of bleeding. It is less successful when used by women as compared with men. Aspirin is relatively safe and inexpensive. Recently published studies have recommended a lower dose of aspirin to reduce harmful side effects (28).

Ticlopidine is a new drug being tested that may be better than aspirin in preventing the formation of clots. Based on early studies, ticlopidine has been just as effective for women as men (1).

Thrombolysis

Thrombolysis, the dissolution of an occluding thrombus, is used frequently in the acute treatment of myocardial infarction. When it is used within the first few hours after cerebral infarction, substantial tissue recovery results. This benefit must be weighed against reperfusion damage, a bleeding tendency, and the possibility of reocclusion. Some common thrombolytics are strep-

tokinase, urokinase, and acetylated plasminogen-streptokinase complex (APSAC).

Cerebral Hemorrhage

Very little work has been done on the specific treatment of cerebral hemorrhage with medication. Some promising studies have been done on the use of calcium antagonists for prevention or reduction of poor neurological outcome owing to vasospasm. Nimodipine, one of these calcium antagonists, has been tested in several clinical trials and shown to have some positive benefits in aneurysmal subarachnoid hemorrhage. It limits the flow of calcium into the cells. Nimodipine dilates the blood vessels, allowing more blood to flow to the brain. (Please see Medications Appendix for a detailed chart of medications.)

After cerebrovascular accident, there are specific pathophysiological sequelae. Important treatment is aimed at these secondary effects of stroke. Two of the cerebral effects of stroke are edema and ischemia. Oxygen therapy to reduce hypoxia, vasodilation to improve blood flow through ischemic areas, therapeutic hypertension, and hemodilution therapy are some of the treatments used for ischemia. Hemodilution results in a significant rise in cerebral blood flow and increased oxygen transfer (27).

Edema often complicates ischemic strokes and must be controlled, because most deaths during the first week after a massive stroke are caused by extensive cerebral edema and increased intracranial pressure. This pressure can displace the cerebrum downward and interfere with the functioning of the midbrain and lower brainstem, which control such basic vital functions as respiration and heart action (2).

Corticosteroid therapy can cause a significant reduction in interstitial cerebral edema. Osmotic agents, such as mannitol and glycerol, can reduce both intracellular and interstitial edema. It appears logical that elevation of the patient's head might reduce edema formation, but this upright posture could also reduce cerebral blood flow. Formal studies have not been performed (22).

In some cases, surgical treatment may be the best choice for the patient. The neurosurgeon must carefully consider many factors before surgery is performed. Carotid endarterectomy is among the most commonly performed vascular surgeries in the United States. During the procedure, the diseased vessel is opened, the clot is removed, and an artificial graft put in place (1). Carotid endarterectomy is a treatment option for patients with more than 50% stenosis of the carotid artery ipsilateral to the affected hemisphere (11).

Subarachnoid hemorrhages are often caused by ruptured aneurysms or arteriovenous malformations. Surgical clipping or lesion removal is the most effective treatment of these anomalies. If the patient survives the initial bleeding, the goal of surgery is to correct the problem before bleeding recurs. In intracerebral hemorrhage, small hematomas usually resolve spontaneously. Large hematomas, however, often produce death. Some lesions may expand, causing gradually increasing neurological signs. These expanding lesions can be drained surgically if they are near the surface of the brain, especially in the cerebral or cerebellar white matter. Generally, hemorrhages are evacuated only if they are large and life threatening or when surgery is necessary to treat an aneurysm, tumor, or arteriovenous malformation (6).

Superficial temporal artery bypass is a new, more delicate surgical therapy for preventing future strokes (1). The procedure begins with craniotomy to expose the brain; then a scalp artery is connected to an intracranial artery microsurgically. This operation is trickier and, therefore, performed less frequently than carotid endarterectomy. Surgeons who do the procedure, however, are enthusiastic about the results and claim that it revascularizes the brain better than endarterectomy (2).

IMPACT ON OCCUPATIONAL PERFORMANCE

Sensorimotor, cognitive, and psychosocial components are almost always affected by a CVA. Deficits in these areas and any secondary complications profoundly affect an individual's occupational performance areas across all categories of activities of daily living, work and productive activities, and play or leisure activities.

Sensorimotor: Sensory and Perceptual Processing

Sensory functions can be affected at the very basic level of awareness and at the point of processing and modulation of sensory input. Loss of protective tactile functions, such as diminished awareness of temperature and pain, are common concerns for those with a cerebrovascular accident. Individuals with proprioceptive dysfunction in this area may show asymmetrical posture, have difficulty maintaining balance, appear to forget affected body parts, be unable to describe position or movement of limbs, and be susceptible to joint damage. Individuals with a loss of tactile sensation may demonstrate a lack of awareness of body parts simply because they forget what they cannot feel. They are also susceptible to damage of affected body parts, particularly to skin breakdown. Depending on the location of the infarct, individuals may experience diminished vestibular processing, which will limit mobility efficiency and safety. Impaired balance may cause difficulties in assuming and maintaining a vertical posture and in automatic adjustments to changes of position and antigravity movement. As a result, individuals demonstrate an asymmetrical posture at rest, leaning or falling to the hemiplegic side during mobility, or fail to use normal protective reactions when falling.

Visual field defects may impair reading, even in the absence of language dysfunction. Reading may also be impaired by right cerebral lesions, because the visuospatial deficits result in poor tracking across the printed page. Patients with homonymous hemianopsia of either side demonstrate a lack of response to people, objects, or the environment on the affected side. They may bump into objects or be startled by their sudden appearance. With visual inattention, individuals have difficulty scanning and shifting their gaze, particularly toward the affected side. Visual agnosia and visuospatial agnosia—difficulty in understanding the relationship between objects and between self and objects—are also present. Individuals lose their way in a familiar environment; they cannot trace a route on a map, pick out objects from a cluttered environment, copy drawings or simple construction, and may have difficulty in functional (spatial) tasks, such as dressing and reading a newspaper. Agnosia for sounds may also occur, characterized by not understanding or confusing nonverbal sounds (19). Astereognosis affects functional use of the affected hand whenever vision is occluded, so that tasks such as finding keys or coins in a pocket or a glass on a bedside table when it is dark may be difficult.

Somatoagnosia, in which an individual has no awareness of his or her own body and its condition, is commonly seen in right parietal lobe lesions. Deficits that result from right cerebral injuries often cause unilateral perceptual problems of the left body side and space, such as unilateral neglect, whereas lesions in the left cerebral hemisphere cause bilateral problems, such as right/left discrimination (19). Impairment of the left parietal lobe results in apraxia, whereby individuals are unable to adjust movement of their own body parts; impairment of the right parietal lobe causes an inability to adjust the position of external objects. Lesions of frontal lobes result in apraxia, in which sequencing of movement is a major difficulty. Individuals may be unable to carry out a verbal request (for even a simple task such as combing the hair), although often they can perform such tasks automatically. They may perseverate in purposeless movement, be unable to complete a required sequence of acts or to copy gestures, drawings, or simple spatial constructional tasks.

Neuromusculoskeletal and Motor Components

Sensory loss seldom occurs in isolation; rather, it goes along with motor loss and compounds the loss of functional activity. Motor dysfunction after a stroke usually results in initial hypotonicity (flaccid hemiplegia), followed by increasing hypertonicity (spastic hemiplegia). The spasticity makes it difficult to dissociate gross motor movements and interferes with efficient completion of most tasks. Occasionally the person will progress into a final stage of normal movement patterns.

The person with an intact central nervous system has a wide range of muscle tone, which can be changed according to the activity that is to be performed. Normal muscle tone is high enough to stabilize and maintain a person through an activity, while at the same time low enough to allow ease of movement. The mix of tone allows mobility to be superimposed on stability (30).

When a stroke occurs, abnormal muscle tone often can be felt. Normal tone is felt as an appropriate amount of resistance, allowing the movement to proceed smoothly. Hypotonus, or flaccidity, is felt as too little resistance or floppiness. When released, the extremity will drop.

Hypertonus, or spasticity, is felt as too much resistance as a result of hyperactive reflexes and loss of moderating or inhibiting influences from higher brain centers (30). Spasticity may be enhanced by pain, emotional upset, or trying to hurry. Spasticity is never isolated to one muscle group but is always a part of extensor or flexor synergy or grouping of stereotypical movements. These usually involve a flexion pattern in the arm (scapular retraction and depression, shoulder adduction and internal rotation, elbow flexion, forearm pronation, wrist flexion, finger and thumb flexion and adduction) and an extension pattern in the leg (pelvis rotated back and internal rotation, knee extension, foot plantar flexion and inversion, toe flexion and adduction). In addition to the extremities, abnormal tone is manifested in the head and trunk. The head is usually flexed toward the hemiplegic side and rotated so that the face is toward the unaffected side. The trunk is rotated back on the hemiplegic side with side flexion of the hemiplegic side (30). These typical patterns of spasticity interfere with the normal, smooth, efficient, and coordinated movement necessary for locomotion in and manipulation of the environment. If untreated, this spasticity may lead to contractures.

A common concern related to motor function involves the shoulder. Typical problems include shoulder subluxation, pain, and immobility. The causative factors in shoulder subluxation after stroke are related to changes in muscle tone and movement, the position of the scapula, and joint capsule stability. Shoulder subluxation at the glenohumeral joint occurs when the weight of the arm and pull of gravity draws the head of the humerus out of the glenoid fossa of the scapula. Two-thirds of the humeral head is not covered by the glenoid fossa. This lack of stability is partly compensated for by a strong surrounding musculature. In the normal orientation of the scapula, there is an upward slope of the glenoid fossa, which plays an important role in preventing downward dislocation of the humerus. The humeral head would have to move laterally to move downward. When the arm is adducted, the superior part of the capsule and the coracohumeral ligament are taut, which prevents lateral movement of the humeral head and guards against downward displacement. The supraspinatus muscle reinforces the horizontal tension of the capsule. The infraspinatus and the posterior portion of the deltoid also play an important role in preventing subluxation, because of their horizontal fibers. When the humerus is abducted sideways or flexed forward, the superior capsule becomes lax, eliminating

support, and joint stability must then be provided by muscle contraction. The integrity of the joint then depends almost exclusively on the rotator cuff muscles.

In hemiplegia, patients have lost the voluntary movement in relative muscles. These include the supraspinatus, infraspinatus, and posterior fibers of the deltoid. In addition, the muscles that support the scapula in its normal alignment are affected, allowing a change in angulation of the glenoid fossa. Subluxation is, therefore, inevitable (30).

Another typical complication is "the painful shoulder." This condition may either develop quickly after a stroke or at a much later stage. It presents with flaccid or spastic muscle tone and with or without subluxation. In hemiplegia, the normal, coordinated, and timed movement of the scapula and humerus (scapulohumeral rhythm) has been disturbed by abnormal and unbalanced muscle tone. The typical hemiplegic postural components of depression and retraction of the scapula and internal rotation of the humerus are especially important to the mechanism of pain. Fear of pain during passive movement of the arm will further increase abnormal flexor tone, which can become a vicious circle (30).

A chronically painful shoulder can lead to shoulder–hand syndrome. This complex condition produces severe pain, edema of the hand, and limitations in range of motion on the involved side (10).

Associated reactions in hemiplegia are abnormal reflex movements of the affected side that duplicate the synergy patterns of the arm and leg. These movements are observed when the patient moves with effort, is trying to maintain balance, or is afraid of falling. A flexor pattern of involuntary movement in the arm is often seen with a yawn, cough, or sneeze. Associated reactions also are seen when new activities, such as running or putting on socks, are attempted after a stroke. They are stereotyped reactions and may occur even if no active movement is present in the limb.

The limb returns to its normal position only after cessation of the stimulus and usually does so gradually.

Associated movements accompany voluntary movements and are normal, automatic postural adjustments. They reinforce precise movements of other parts of the body or occur when a great amount of strength is required. They are not pathological and can be stopped at will, as opposed to associated reactions. Associated movements often can be observed in the unaffected extremities of stroke patients' who are trying new activities.

Orofacial weakness may cause difficulties in expression, speech (dysarthria), mastication, and swallowing (dysphagia).

Bladder or bowel incontinence may result from a communication disorder or from disruption of normal routine and diet, lack of awareness of body function, or emotional disorder (10).

Cognitive Integration

Cognitive disturbance often occurs with more severe strokes (31). However, cognitive deficits may be more subtle in milder strokes, and the person should be observed in a variety of occupations. Commonly used psychometrics are not always sensitive to the wide range of cognitive components, including initiation, recognition, attention, orientation, sequencing, categorization, concept formation, spatial operations, problem solving, and learning abilities (32). Because basic visual deficits may be present, these factors will have a greater impact on cognitive performance. For example, visual attending and scanning deficits lead to a decrease in the efficiency required for cognitive performance.

Psychosocial

Stroke patients may experience a number of psychological changes, including depression. These changes often are a major cause of concern to relatives and the individual (e.g., irritability due to loss of interest and depression of mood, an inability to withstand stressful situations, fear and anxiety, anger, frustration, swearing, emotional lability, and catastrophic reactions). Significant depression has been recorded in 30 to 50% of stroke survivors (22). This depression usually is viewed by family and medical practitioners as a natural and understandable consequence of reduced function caused by stroke. Appropriate attention to depression, however, can result in observable improvement. Depression is more frequent and severe with lesions in the left hemisphere, as compared with right hemisphere or brainstem strokes (33, 34). Both organic and psychological factors are probably involved in poststroke depression. Patients usually respond well to antidepressants, psychological support, and encouragement (6).

Emotional lability may appear mostly through a release of inhibition. The individual may switch from laughing to crying for no apparent reason. Excessive crying is the most common problem and is frequently the result of organic emotional lability rather than depression or sadness over perceived losses. Organic emotional lability is characterized by little or no obvious relation between the start of emotional expression and what is happening around the person.

Catastrophic reactions are outbursts in which frustration, anger, and depression are combined. When individuals cannot perform tasks that used to be very easy, they may be unable to inhibit emotional expression and may begin sobbing, expressing a sense of hopelessness.

Outbursts and emotional difficulties are "normal" after stroke. Relatives and families should be told that a tendency to cry easily or get upset will improve with time. Families and therapists need to develop a positive, understanding attitude if the individual is to overcome psychological sequelae.

CASE STUDIES

CASE 1

The following story written by a man who had a stroke is an example of a left cerebral injury and illustrates some of the deficits that may result.

Wednesday, January 31, began as a normal day. This consisted of getting up for work at 4:45 AM, having breakfast, and arriving at Buick Engine Plant to begin my work shift of 6:00 AM to 2:30 PM. After spending 8 hours made up of 50% desk work and 50% floor work, I arrived back home feeling exceptionally fatigued. After a usual greeting and reading the mail, I proceeded to the couch for a nap. My wife woke me for dinner around 5:00 PM. Within a couple of hours, I returned to the couch, still feeling the need for rest. Waking up in time for the 11:00 PM news, I felt more refreshed and rested.

Just prior to retiring to the bedroom about midnight, I felt a "tingling" in my head that lasted for no more than a couple of minutes. Fifteen to 20 minutes later, the "tingling" returned, accompanied by the inability to move the limbs on my right side. Movement returned and the "tingling" ceased after about 10 minutes. Within another 15 minutes the sensation returned, along with a slurring of speech.

After I told my wife of these happenings, she called 911 and within a short time both a local ambulance and a sheriffs' paramedic arrived at our home. Noting the pattern that with each return of the "tingling," loss of limb movement and slurred speech occurred, the paramedics decided I needed immediate medical attention.

During my 4 to 5 hours in the emergency room, the sensation returned several times. During this time, they performed x-rays, ECG, blood pressure, and other tests. Emergency personnel later told me that the CVA was "evolving" with each recurrence of the symptoms. At about 5:00 AM, I was admitted to the hospital.

After being settled in a room, I became aware that I was there for more than a long weekend with hopes of returning to work on Monday. The next 2 days consisted of a series of tests, accompanied by a "state of confusion," being scared, questioning why and what the future held.

By late Friday afternoon, February 2, they had determined what had happened and why. I had suffered a cerebral hemorrhage on the left side of my brain. I was then transferred to the rehabilitation floor. Saturday and Sunday consisted of evaluating my abilities, or lack of abilities, of speech and limb movement. On Monday, February 5, therapy consisting of physical, occupational, and speech treat-ments, began. Speech therapy ended after 1 week, but I was advised to practice fundamentals.

During my 4-week stay at the Regional Medical Center, I began the journey to good health. Along with scheduled therapies, a bonus of mental therapy came about from the camaraderie with fellow rehabilitation patients. I was not alone! All at once the usual routines of earning a wage and maintaining a home were ended. The roles my wife and I previously played were now changed. She now became financial secretary, part-time mechanic, snow shoveler, and chauffeur, in addition to spending several hours each day at the hospital.

As a result of my affliction, the value of certain things such as good health, relationships of family and friends, and a closeness to God are no longer taken for granted. Only with hope and a firm determination to improve will my full recovery come about.

CASE 2

D. B., a 52-year-old male, left work and went to his doctor's office complaining of slurred speech and weakness in his left arm and leg. He was admitted to a local hospital, where a CT scan revealed infarction of embolic origin in the territory of the right middle cerebral artery. After 5 days, D. B. was transferred to another hospital's rehabilitation unit, where he began an intensive inpatient therapy program. D. B.'s previous medical history included diabetes mellitus for 12 years, coronary spasm 10 years prior to this admission, hypertension, bursitis in the right shoulder (at present), and arthritis in both knees. D. B. is a smoker and is moderately overweight.

D. B. is married, with two grown children and two grandchildren. He had been employed as a pharmacist for 27 years at a local drugstore and he enjoyed his job. His hobbies before his stroke included yard work, general handyman jobs around the house, playing cards, traveling, and helping his wife babysit the grandchildren. D. B. is an easygoing, friendly person who appears to have a positive attitude about his stroke and expected recovery. However, he is unable to answer questions about the cause of his stroke and risk factor control and does not have a plan for the future if he is unable to return to his job.

Some of the general symptoms that D. B. now exhibits 4 months after his stroke are hemiparesis and abnormal muscle tone in the left extremities, mild left unilateral neglect, decreased sensation in the left extremities, and impulsive behavior. D. B. can walk independently with a straight cane. He is fitted with an ankle–foot orthosis to maintain his ankle in a neutral position and prevent "toe-drag" during ambulation. He is right-handed and is now using the left upper extremity as a gross assist in some activities. The abnormal flexor tone in his hand interferes with function, so at night D.B. wears an antispasticity ball splint issued by the occupational therapist to control this hypertonicity. D. B.'s left unilateral neglect is most apparent while he is moving. He sometimes bumps into the left side of the doorway and is unable to find road signs while riding in the car with his wife. He often tries to get up from a chair before checking to be sure that his left foot is flat on the floor. D. B. also occasionally quickly slides his chair back from a table, letting his

left arm fall to his side. D. B.'s CVA results in many occupational performance deficits (Table 8.1).

D. B. is currently able to perform all self-care activities independently. He has been very resourceful and creative in coming up with new strategies to maintain his independence. He uses a tub bench, grab bar, and a handheld shower for bathing. He is anxious to resume driving but has been advised by his doctor and therapists to refrain from doing so because of his impulsiveness and unilateral neglect. D. B. has had some difficulty adjusting to the amount of time he now spends at home. He has found that he is physically unable to

TABLE 8.1   Occupational Performance Profile

I. PERFORMANCE AREAS	II. PERFORMANCE COMPONENTS	III. PERFORMANCE CONTEXTS

A. Activities of Daily Living
  1. Grooming
  2. Oral Hygiene
  3. Bathing/Showering
  4. Toilet Hygiene
  5. Personal Device Care
  6. Dressing
  7. Feeding and Eating
  8. Medication Routine
  9. Health Maintenance
  10. Socialization
  11. Functional Communication
  12. Functional Mobility
  13. Community Mobility
  14. Emergency Response
  15. Sexual Expression
B. Work and Productive Activities
  1. Home Management
    a. Clothing Care
    b. Cleaning
    c. Meal Preparation/Cleanup
    d. Shopping
    e. Money Management
    f. Household Maintenance
    g. Safety Procedures
  2. Care of Others
  3. Educational Activities
  4. Vocational Activities
    a. Vocational Exploration
    b. Job Acquisition
    c. Work or Job Performance
    d. Retirement Planning
    e. Volunteer Participation
	A. Sensorimotor Component
	  1. Sensory
	    a. Sensory Awareness
	    b. Sensory Processing
	      (1) Tactile
	      (2) Proprioceptive
	      (3) Vestibular
	      (4) Visual
	      (5) Auditory
	      (6) Gustatory
	      (7) Olfactory
	    c. Perceptual Processing
	      (1) Stereognosis
	      (2) Kinesthesia
	      (3) Pain Response
	      (4) Body Scheme
	      (5) Right–Left Discrimination
	      (6) Form Constancy
	      (7) Position in Space
	      (8) Visual–Closure
	      (9) Figure Ground
	     (10) Depth Perception
	     (11) Spatial Relations
	     (12) Topographical Orientation
	  2. Neuromusculoskeletal
	    a. Reflex
	    b. Range of Motion
	    c. Muscle Tone
	    d. Strength
	    e. Endurance
	    f. Postural Control
	    g. Postural Alignment
	    h. Soft Tissue Integrity
		A. Temporal Aspects
		  1. Chronological
		  2. Developmental
		  3. Lifecycle
		  4. Disability Status
		B. Environment
		  1. Physical
		  2. Social
		  3. Cultural

(continued)

| TABLE 8.1 Occupational Performance Profile (Continued) |

I. PERFORMANCE AREAS	II. PERFORMANCE COMPONENTS	III. PERFORMANCE CONTEXTS

C. Play or Leisure Activities
  1. Play or Leisure Exploration
  2. Play or Leisure Performance
	3. Motor
	  a. Gross Coordination
	  b. Crossing the Midline
	  c. Laterality
	  d. Bilateral Integration
	  e. Motor Control
	  f. Praxis
	  g. Fine Coordination/Dexterity
	  h. Visual–Motor Control
	  i. Oral–Motor Control
	B. Cognitive Integration and Cognitive Components
	  1. Level of Arousal
	  2. Orientation
	  3. Recognition
	  4. Attention Span
	  5. Initiation of Activity
	  6. Termination of Activity
	  7. Memory
	  8. Sequencing
	  9. Categorization
	  10. Concept Formation
	  11. Spatial Operations
	  12. Problem Solving
	  13. Learning
	  14. Generalization
	C. Psychosocial Skills and Psychological Components
	  1. Psychological
	    a. Values
	    b. Interests
	    c. Self-Concept
	  2. Social
	    a. Role Performance
	    b. Social Conduct
	    c. Interpersonal Skills
	    d. Self-Expression
	  3. Self-Management
	    a. Coping Skills
	    b. Time Management
	    c. Self-Control	

The potential for involvement in each component depends on the location of the infarct. Best practice is to assess each area to rule out functional impairment.

perform many household repairs and maintenance activities, such as cutting the grass, sweeping the driveway, and painting the trim around windows. He now requires assistance from his wife for money management and paying bills.

D. B. and his family, or occasionally some friends, get together to play cards. D. B. uses a card-holding device that was recommended by occupational therapy and recreational therapy to hold his cards. He enjoys this activity and the socialization that goes with it. He and his family just returned from a 1-week vacation near a lake, which he thoroughly enjoyed. Considering the extent of his disability, D. B. appears to be making an excellent adjustment to his stroke and, in fact, appears to deny the illness. He believes that soon everything will return to normal, that he will regain his physical abilities, and will be able to return to work.

POINTS FOR REVIEW

1. Define cerebrovascular accident (CVA).

2. Trace the circulatory supply of the major blood vessels in the brain.

3. What are the two major types of CVA and their subtypes?

4. Describe the characteristics of these types of CVA.

5. What is the incidence and prevalence of CVA?

6. Describe conditions that indicate warning of an impending CVA.

7. Given the site of arterial occlusion, list the neurological effects of a CVA.

8. Describe secondary complications that may occur as a result of a CVA.

9. List the prominent risk factors associated with a CVA.

10. Describe the progression of a stroke and the factors that affect the prognosis of a CVA.

11. Describe noninvasive diagnostic procedures used in the identification of a CVA.

12. Describe invasive diagnostic procedures used in the identification of a CVA.

13. List the actions of the common medications used to treat the various types of CVA.

14. Describe surgical options for prevention and treatment of CVA. Are these surgical interventions effective?

15. Profile the effects of a CVA on occupational performance components and occupational performance areas.

REFERENCES

1. Foley C, Pizer HF. The Stroke Fact Book. Golden Valley: Courage Press, 1990.
2. Freese A. Stroke—The New Hope and the New Help. New York: Random House, 1980.
3. Doolittle ND. Stroke recovery: review of the literature and suggestions for future research. J Neurosci Nurs 1988;20:169–173.
4. Miller VT. Diagnosis and initial management of stroke. Neuropsychiatry 1988;14(7):57–65.
5. Anonymous. Stroke Facts. Dallas, TX: American Heart Association, 1988.
6. Caplan LR. Stroke. Clin Symp 1988;40(4):1–32.
7. Barr ML. The Human Nervous System. 2nd ed. Hagerstown: Harper & Row, 1974.
8. Sherman DG. The carotid artery and stroke. Am Fam Physician 1989;40(5):415–495.
9. Nolte J. The Human Brain. St. Louis: CV Mosby, 1981.
10. Anderson TP. Stroke and cerebral trauma: medical aspects. In: Stolov WC, Clowers MR, eds. Handbook of Severe Disability. Seattle: University of Washington, 1981:119–126.
11. Nadeau SE. Stroke. Med Clin North Am 1989;73(6):1351–1369.
12. Gorelick PB. Etiology and management of ischemic stroke. Compr Ther 1989;15(3):60–65.
13. Fisher CM. Lacunar strokes and infarcts: a review. Neurology 1982;32:871–876.
14. Caplan LR, Stein RW. Intracerebral hemorrhage. In: Stroke: A Clinical Approach. Austin: Butterworth, 1986:261–292.
15. Kawalick M, Lerer A. Stroke syndromes. In: Erickson RV, ed. Medical management of the elderly stroke patient. Philadelphia: Hanley & Belfus, 1989:469–477.
16. Anonymous. Facts About Strokes. Dallas: American Heart Association, 1991.

17. Nicolaides P, Appleton RE. Stroke in children. Dev Med Child Neurol 1996;38:2.

18. Afifi AK, Bergman RA. Basic neuroscience. Baltimore: Urban & Schwarzenberg, 1986.

19. Siev E, Freishtat B, Zoltan B. Perceptual and Cognitive Dysfunction in the Adult Stroke Patient. Thorofare, NJ: Slack, 1986.

20. Gillum RF. Strokes in blacks. Stroke 1988;19(1):19.

21. Gorelick PB. The status of alcohol as a risk factor for stroke. Stroke 1989;20(12):1607–1610.

22. American Heart Association. AHA 21st International Joint Conference on Stroke and Cerebral Circulation. NR 96-4369 Abstract #25, Jan 25, 1996.

23. Devor M. Plasticity in the adult nervous system. In: Illis LS, Sedgewick EM, Glanville HJ, eds. Rehabilitation of the Neurological Patient. Oxford: Blackwell Scientific, 1982:44–84.

24. Moore JC. Recovery potentials following CNS lesions: a brief historical perspective in relationship to modern research data on neuroplasticity. Am J Occup Ther 1986;40(7):459–463.

25. Trombly C. Occupational Therapy for Physical Dysfunction. Baltimore: Williams & Wilkins, 1989.

26. Dobkin BH. Management of geriatric TIA and stroke. Geriatrics 1988;43(11):27–34.

27. Harper GD, Castleden CM. Drug therapy in patients with recent stroke. Br Med Bull 1990;46(1):181–199.

28. International Stroke Trial Collaborative Group. The international stroke trial: a randomised trail of aspirin, subcutaneous heparin, both or neither among 19,435 patients with acute ischemic stroke. Lancet 1997;349:1641–49.

29. Chinese Acute Stroke Trial Collaborative Group. Randomised placebo controlled trial of early aspirin use in 20,000 patients with acute ischemic stroke. Lancet 1997; 439:1641–49.

30. Utley J. Adult Hemiplegia NDT Certification Course. Flint, MI: McLaren Regional Medical Center, 1989.

31. Davies PM. Steps to Follow. Berlin: Springer-Verlag, 1985.

32. Restak RM. The Brain: The Last Frontier. New York: Warner Books, 1979.

33. Kilpatrick CJ, Davis SM, Tress BM, et al. Epileptic seizures in acute stroke. Arch Neurol 1990;47: 157–160.

34. Rose FC, Capileo R. Stroke. Oxford: Oxford University Press, 1981.

CHAPTER 9

CORONARY ARTERY DISEASE

Ben Atchison

Anastomosis
Aneurysm
Angina pectoris
Arteriosclerosis
Atherosclerosis

Diastole
Dyspnea
Infarct
Ischemia
Necrosis

Percutaneous transluminal
  coronary angioplasty
Stent
Systole
Tachycardia

He awoke with distinct discomfort around his chest and hoped the pain would go away as it had before. This time, though, the pain persisted. He had difficulty breathing and was sweating as if he had just run a mile. He felt weak and nauseated. An alarm went off in his mind. He felt impending doom as he realized that he was having a heart attack.

Does this man have a chance of surviving his heart attack? If so, what complications might he expect? Will he be able to resume his usual life roles and activities if he does survive? How did he develop coronary artery disease (CAD) that resulted in the heart attack?

This chapter reviews cardiac anatomy and circulation, incidence and prevalence, etiology, pathophysiology and clinical manifestations of CAD, and medical-surgical management issues. At the end, two case studies illustrate the impact of CAD on occupational performance.

CARDIAC ANATOMY AND CIRCULATION

How do people develop CAD? What occurs in the cardiac anatomy and physiology to create pathological changes? Understanding what goes wrong requires a basic comprehension of normal anatomy and physiology.

The heart is a muscle that works as a pump to provide oxygen and nourishment to the tissues in the body. It is hollow and is located slightly to the left of center in the chest. The major portion of the heart is a muscular wall called *myocardium*. The inner surface of the myocardium is raised into ridgelike surfaces that make up the papillary muscles. The interior of the myocardium is lined with smooth endothelial tissue called the endocardium. This smooth tissue allows the blood to pass through the heart chambers without cellular damage (1).

The interior of the heart is divided into upper and lower chambers called atria and ventricles. The ventricles—the lower chambers—are considerably larger and thicker than the atria, because they are required to perform heavier pumping action. These chambers of the heart are separated by two valves, called atrioventricular (AV) valves. The left one is the mitral valve and the right is the tricuspid. These valves prevent blood from flowing back into the atria from the ventricles when the heart is resting between beats. A review of these structures and cardiac circulation is provided in Figure 9.1.

The heart has its own system of arteries, called coronary arteries, that supply the heart with oxygen and nourishment. These major coronary arteries branch off the aorta, cross over the outside of the heart wall, and penetrate the muscle itself. The left main coronary artery divides into the left anterior descending (LAD) artery and the circumflex artery. The LAD supplies the left ventricle, the interventricular septum, the right ventricle, the inferior areas of the apex, and both ventricles (1). The circumflex artery supplies blood to the inferior walls of the left ventricle and to the left atrium (2) (Fig. 9.2).

In the body, the smallest arteries empty into one end of a profuse network of tiny blood vessels called *capillaries* that deliver oxygen and other nutritional substances to individual cells. At the capillary level, oxygen and nourishment are exchanged for carbon dioxide. These capillaries supply the heart, head, arms, legs, and various organs, such as the liver and stomach.

Like skeletal muscle, cardiac muscle requires innervation to contract. A specialized nervous conduction network of cells creates systematic depolar-

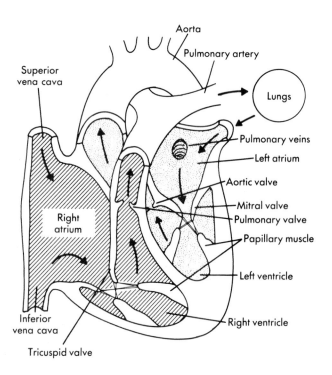

FIGURE 9.1. Anatomy of the heart. (Reprinted with permission from Andreoli KG, Fawkes VK, Zipes DR, et al, eds. Comprehensive Cardiac Care: A Text for Nurses, Physicians and Other Health Practitioners. St. Louis: CV Mosby, 1983.)

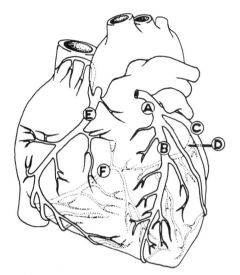

FIGURE 9.2. Coronary circulation. **A.** Left main coronary artery. **B.** LAD coronary artery. **C.** Left circumflex coronary artery. **D.** Posterior circumflex coronary artery. **E.** Right coronary artery. **F.** Posterior descending artery. (Reprinted with permission from O'Sullivan S, Schmitz TJ, eds. Coronary artery disease. In: Physical Rehabilitation: Assessment. 2nd ed. Philadelphia: FA Davis, 1988.)

ization that causes an action potential that elicits myocardial contraction (3). The origin of the electrical impulse is the sinoatrial node (SA), or the "pacemaker" of the heart, which is located in the right atrium. This impulse spreads through both atria, which then contract simultaneously and stimulate the AV node. The impulse travels next to the bundle branches, then to the Purkinje fibers (4). Because the Purkinje fibers merge with the walls of the ventricle, the impulse spreads through the Purkinje system to the cells of the ventricles, and the ventricles contract together. This sequence occurs, on average, 72 times per minute (1). Depolarization is the result of electrical cellular changes. Thus, it can be recorded graphically on an electrocardiogram (ECG) (5). To perform this test, surface electrodes are placed on the limbs and chest to monitor the sequence, timing, and magnitude of the impulse. Each graphic segment (P, QRS, and T waves) corresponds to the wave of depolarization as it travels through the heart chambers (6) (Fig. 9.3). The P wave indicates the electrical activity resulting

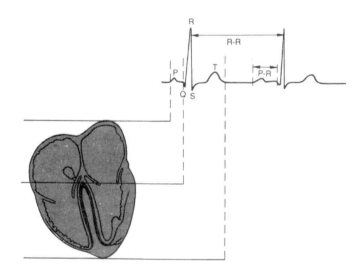

EKG COMPONENT	MYOCARDIAL EVENT
P wave	Atrial depolarization
QRS complex	Ventricular depolarization
T wave	Ventricular repolarization

FIGURE 9.3. Electrocardiographic recording of myocardial activity. (Reprinted with permission from Rothstein JM, Roy SH, Wolf SL. The Rehabilitation Specialists Handbook. Philadelphia: FA Davis, 1991.)

from depolarization in the atria, called atrial depolarization. The PR interval indicates the time that elapses from the beginning of the atrial contraction to the ventricular contraction. The QRS complex corresponds to the electrical activity known as ventricular depolarization, which occurs as electrical activity travels through the bundle branches and the ventricles. The T wave corresponds to ventricular repolarization, which is the reestablishment of an electrically polarized state in the ventricles. The timing of depolarization can be determined by counting the blocks on the ECG graph paper. For example, if the PR interval is too wide or the QRS is widened or longer than normal, a conduction abnormality would be suspected (7). See Figure 9.4 for examples of normal and abnormal ECG findings.

The American Heart Association recommends that therapists using ECG during treatment be familiar with the equipment and able to recognize a minimum of twelve ECG dysrhythmias (Table 9.1).

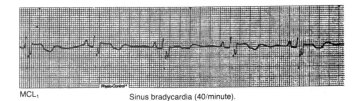

MCL₁   Sinus bradycardia (40/minute).

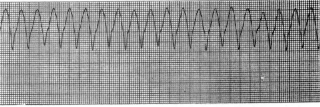

II   Regular or normal sinus rhythm (94/minute).

FIGURE 9.4. Examples of normal and abnormal ECGs. Strips illustrate normal heart rate, bradycardia, and tachycardia. (Reprinted with permission from Rothstein JM, Roy SH, Wolf SL. The Rehabilitation Specialists Handbook. Philadelphia: FA Davis, 1991.)

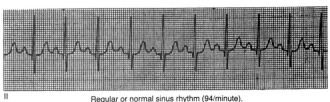

Ventricular tachycardia (180/minute).

TABLE 9.1 Dysrhythmias That Must Be Recognized by EKG

Sinus tachycardia	Junctional rhythms
Sinus bradycardia	Atrioventricular blocks of all degrees
Premature atrial complexes	Premature ventricular complexes
Atrial tachycardia	Ventricular tachycardia
Atrial flutter	Ventricular fibrillation
Atrial fibrillation	Cardiac standstill or asystole

Adapted from American Heart Association. Cardiopulmonary resuscitation: advanced life support. JAMA suppl Aug, 1980.

ETIOLOGY

Coronary artery disease is the result of an arteriosclerotic process created by a thickening in the intimal, or inner, layer of the vessel. This progressive thickening is caused by an accumulation of fatty tissue. (A detailed description of this process is given later in this chapter.)

The American Heart Association has identified several factors that increase the risk of a myocardial infarction (MI) (9). These risk factors are grouped into two classifications: a) major risk factors and b) contributing risk factors. Major risk factors are those shown by medical research to be definitely associated with a significant increase in risk. Contributing risk factors are those associated with increased risk of cardiovascular disease, but their significance and prevalence are not as certain. These risk factors are divided further into controllable and uncontrollable factors.

Three major, uncontrollable risk factors include increasing age, gender, and heredity (including race). About 4 of 5 people who die of CAD are age 65 or older. Interestingly, at older ages, women who have heart attacks are twice as likely than men to die of them within a few weeks. Overall, men have both a greater risk of MI than women and episodes that occur earlier in life. Even postmenopausal women—among whom the death rate increases—do not have as high an incidence as men. In terms of heredity, children whose parents have CAD are more likely to have the disease develop.

Risks identified as controllable factors include the use of cigarettes and tobacco, high blood cholesterol levels, high blood pressure, physical inactivity, and obesity and being overweight. Smokers' risk of CAD is more than twice that of nonsmokers. Evidence shows that chronic exposure to environmental tobacco smoke may increase the risk of CAD. Those with high blood cholesterol levels, combined with other risk factors, have even higher risks of CAD. In addition to these factors, diabetes seriously increases the risk of CAD. More than 80% of individuals with diabetes die of heart disease and stroke.

An epidemiological study initiated in 1949 in Framingham, Massachusetts of 5209 men and women, age 30 to 62 years, has produced the most extensive research on cardiovascular disease. Currently celebrating its 50th year of active research, the Framingham study has continued to identify major risk factors for the development of atherosclerosis (8).

INCIDENCE AND PREVALENCE

According to the American Heart Association, heart disease is the number one cause of death, disability, and loss of income in the United States. Coronary heart disease caused 481,287 deaths in 1995—1 of every 4.8 deaths. Some other facts are (9, 10):

- Coronary heart disease is the single largest killer of American men and women.
- In 1998, an estimated 1,100,000 Americans will have a new or recurrent coronary attack and about one-third will die.
- At least 250,000 people per year die of CAD within 1 hour of the onset of symptoms and before they reach a hospital. These are sudden deaths caused by cardiac arrest, usually resulting from ventricular fibrillation.
- 13,900,000 people alive today have a history of heart attack, angina pectoris, or both. Of this number, 7,100,000 are men and 6,800,000 are women.
- The risks of death from CAD are much greater for the least educated than for the most educated.
- From 1985 to 1995, the death rate from CAD declined 28.7%, but the actual number of deaths declined only 10.3%.
- 84% of people who die of CAD are age 65 or older.
- About 80% of CAD mortality in people under age 65 occurs during the first attack.
- In 48% of men and 63% of women who died suddenly of CAD, there were no previous symptoms of the disease.

PATHOPHYSIOLOGY

Arteriosclerotic disease is a progressive destruction of arterial structure and function. This destruction occurs in a series of changes caused by the development of plaques or lesions along the intimal layer of the vessel. These lesions are classified, in order of pathologic changes, into three types: fatty streak, fibrous plaque, and complicated plaque or lesion (1). Fatty streaks are found throughout the inner lining of the arterial tree in individuals from infancy through late adulthood. They are composed mainly of cholesterol and appear soft and yellow. It is not clearly known whether these lesions progress to a raised fibrous lesion or if they are reversible. Raised fibrous plaques are the typical lesions of arteriosclerosis. These lesions are yellowish-gray lumps that thicken and begin to impinge on the lumen of the artery.

The complicated plaques are fibrous plaques that have progressed through one or more pathological change, including possible calcification, necrosis, internal hemorrhage, and thrombus formation. The changes in the intima may cause degeneration of the medial layer with the resultant loss of the artery's distention capability. This weakened condition may create an aneurysm, which may rupture and cause hemorrhage.

These three types of lesions may coexist at various sites in the arterial structure. Pathological studies indicate that most lesions of the coronary arteries occur at proximal points in the two major coronary arteries at the bifurcation of the arteries. As CAD progresses, structural changes in the artery result in a decreased coronary blood flow and a decrease in oxygen distribution to the myocardium. The functional inability of the vessel to carry oxygen creates an imbalance of myocardial oxygen demand and supply, called ischemia. When ischemia is prolonged, the tissues can undergo irreversible injury that results in an MI. Ischemia and infarction are accompanied by pain, elevated serum enzymes, and symptoms related to the affected organ or tissues, such as decreased renal function with renal ischemia or muscle cramps with peripheral ischemia (1). A transition from ischemia to infarction is not inevitable and depends on several factors, including the rate of onset and duration of ischemia, the ability of the tissue to compensate for the decreased blood flow, the oxygen requirements of the particular tissue, and the amount of oxygen in the blood (1).

When ischemia develops gradually, the tissue can tolerate it because collateral circulation, which allows alternate pathways for blood to flow, can develop. Tissues adapt to the decreased oxygen supply by increasing their oxygen extraction from available blood flow (1).

Coronary artery disease does not always result from the arteriosclerotic process. Medical conditions and disabilities that have associated and secondary cardiac involvement include alcoholism, cerebrovascular disease, drug abuse, diabetes, Friedreich's ataxia, obesity, progressive muscular dystrophy, rheumatoid arthritis, and systemic lupus erythematosus (6).

SIGNS AND SYMPTOMS

Coronary artery disease creates the potential for four clinical syndromes: angina, MI, heart failure, and sudden cardiac death (10).

Angina pectoris is a reversible ischemic process caused by the temporary inability of the coronary arteries to supply sufficient oxygenated blood to cardiac muscle. The individual with angina experiences sudden anterior chest pain, described as a pressure sensation. This sensation has been described as a "viselike" tightening around the chest, as if a large, tight rubber band is wrapped around the individual. Other symptoms can include a burning sensation in the throat or jaw, discomfort between the shoulder blades, and shortness of breath (1). The frequency of attacks varies, depending on the degree of coronary insufficiency, effectiveness of treatment, and the physical and emotional characteristics of the individual (1).

The second manifestation of CAD is MI. A portion of cardiac muscle is destroyed because of sustained myocardial ischemia that results from acute occlusion of coronary vessels. Infarction also may result from hemorrhage or profound shock (1). The pathology of MI is similar to that of angina, and the clinical symptoms and signs are comparable. Individuals who have MIs often have a history of angina, although the MI may be the first sign of cardiovascular problems. About 15% of individuals are asymptomatic and have what are referred to as "silent MIs" (11), that is, episodes of ischemia, as documented by ECG, that are not associated with the chest discomfort of angina. As a result, there is no "warning system," and the individual may experience severe ischemia without realizing the need to stop activity. Some patients with silent MIs may have symptoms of dyspnea rather than angina. Complications of MI include: arrhythmia, heart failure, thrombolytic complications, and irreversible damage to the heart structure.

Arrhythmia, an irregularity or loss of normal heart rhythm, occurs in 90% of individuals who are diagnosed with MIs. They are the leading cause of sudden death in persons with CAD, although the effect of arrhythmias on the morbidity rate varies from benign to life-threatening (12). Early intervention has decreased the overall morbidity rate of acutely diagnosed patients (13). The types of arrhythmia vary with the area of the heart infarcted and the point on the conduction pathway where the tissue is damaged. Ninety-eight percent of arrhythmia disturbances can be detected by an ECG (1).

Heart failure, the second complication of an MI and the third clinical syndrome associated with CAD, occurs when the myocardium is unable to maintain adequate circulation of the blood for respiration and metabolism. Failure can occur in the right or left ventricle, or both (1). Several classifications of heart failure, including backward, congestive, forward, high output, and low output (14), exist. Backward heart failure occurs when reduced venous return to the heart results in venous stasis and congestion. Congestive heart failure occurs as a result of right-sided heart failure or pulmonary congestion caused by left-sided heart failure. This leads to systemic congestion that results in edema, an enlarged liver, and elevated venous pressure. Forward heart failure is a result of left ventricular failure after loss of ventricular contractility, after MI. High output heart

failure results from conditions that increase the amount of circulation, as with a large arteriovenous fistula or anemia. Low output heart failure refers to the failure of the heart to maintain adequate cardiac output because of insufficient venous return, as with hemorrhage (14).

The third complication associated with MIs is thrombolytic, of two types: venous and mural thrombi. Both result from an interruption in the flow of blood. Venous, or deep vein thrombi (DVT), develop in the calf as a result of forced inactivity. Mural thrombi form in the ventricular wall and, like venous thrombi, have potential for embolism, or the development of a "traveling" clot (1). "Pulmonary embolism" is the term used to indicate emboli that travel to the lung as a result of a venous thrombus. Although at one time this was a major complication and cause of death after MI, as a result of early rehabilitation efforts pulmonary embolism now accounts for less than 1% of total deaths (1). Mural emboli may dwell in visceral arteries, resulting in infarction of the brain, kidney, spleen, or intestine. They may also lodge in the extremities, creating sudden pain, numbness, and coldness in the affected part (1).

The fourth complication of an MI is heart structural damage. Possible structural damage includes ventricular aneurysm formation and rupture of papillary muscle, the ventricular wall, or the intraventricular septum. These complications may cause death or result in mild to severe heart failure. Surgical intervention may be required to repair the damage (1).

The fourth clinical syndrome associated with CAD is sudden cardiac death, commonly defined as an unexpected death in individuals without previous symptoms of heart disease. Cardiac death occurs as a result of sudden coronary artery occlusion that leads to ventricular fibrillation. Ventricular contraction is lost and death occurs in 4 minutes if the occlusion is sustained (15). In 1997, one in three individuals who had an MI died as a result of sudden cardiac death (9). The only known prevention for sudden cardiac death is prompt initiation of cardiopulmonary resuscitation (1).

In summary, arteriosclerosis and the ischemia infarction process are the basis for clinical manifestations of CAD. The clinical manifestations of CAD and its major complications must be understood so that individuals with this disease can be treated safely and effectively.

COURSE AND PROGNOSIS

Coronary artery disease is thought to be a progressive disease that can develop as early as the second decade of life. To assess the progression and prognosis of CAD, it is important to identify certain factors relative to the severity of the disease at the time of initial assessment. These factors predict coronary events, such as progression of symptoms, recurrent MI, or cardiac death. In a 10-year study of 601 nonsurgical patients having coronary artery occlusion with more than 50% narrowing, a significant prognostic factor was the number of coronary arteries involved (13). Single vessel, double vessel, and triple vessel disease were predicted to have 10-year survival rates of 63%, 45%, and 23%, respectively. Patients who had 50% or greater narrowing, specifically in the left main coronary artery, were predicted to have a 22% survival rate. Survival rates also were found to be related to ventricular function. Patients who experienced massive MIs and left ventricular dysfunction had lower survival rates than those with small infarcts and normal ventricular function. Other factors included severity of angina pectoris and subsequent functional impairment, evidence of left ventricular hypertrophy, conduction deficits during depolarization, and continued presence of risk factors such as smoking, diabetes, and hypertension.

DIAGNOSIS

Coronary artery disease is diagnosed through a variety of clinical and laboratory studies. The symptoms of angina, which indicate an ischemic condition, are usually the initial reasons for a person to seek medical attention. Ischemic symptoms are reversible events, but they also may indicate more serious cardiovascular pathology.

Diagnosis of angina is determined by the angina threshold (defined as the level of activity that initiates the sequelae of cardiac distress),

ECG changes, substernal pain that lasts from 1 to 3 minutes, dyspnea, variable pulse rate, and elevated blood pressure. The angina threshold is assessed through graded exercise testing, a measured exercise challenge designed to determine functional capacity during physical stress. Through a medical history, a physician is able to determine other factors that may precipitate angina, such as exposure to cold or eating. Persons with angina also may experience depressed left ventricular function as a result of the ischemic episode, which is evident by changes in the ECG.

Myocardial infarction that is the result of prolonged, severe ischemia is assessed by physical examination, laboratory tests, and the ECG (16). The physician observes the person for hallmark signs of cardiac dysfunction including pain, nausea, sweating, and dyspnea. The heart rate may be abnormally slow (bradycardia) or fast (tachycardia).

Of the three diagnostic tools, serum enzyme studies are the most conclusive (1). Serum enzyme levels are used for detecting MIs and other heart diseases and in determining recovery status. Significant enzymes include creatine phosphokinase (CPK) and lactic dehydrogenase (LDH).

Creatine phosphokinase levels increase after an MI during a 4-hour interval and peak at 36 hours. These levels continue to drop sharply and are back to normal in 2 to 4 days. Both CPK and LDH will elevate in an acute MI. Creatine phosphokinase is more sensitive to myocardial ischemia than any other enzyme. Because of the rapid degeneration of CPK when stored, testing should be done on the same day.

Lactic dehydrogenase elevates in the first 12 to 18 hours, peaks in 2 to 3 days, and returns to normal within 7 to 10 days. Its elevation also is related to the extent of the injury. An increase of more than 3000 units indicates a poor prognosis (17).

The occupational therapist should note serum enzyme levels when working with an individual. Any reelevation in these levels exceeding the normal time frame could indicate a new infarction or the extension of a previous one (1).

The occupational therapist selects a combination of low-level self-care activities in the initial evaluation. During these activities, the cardiovascular response is monitored by assessment of heart rate, blood pressure, ECG readings, signs and symptoms of cardiac dysfunction, and heart sounds. The primary purpose of this monitoring is to guide the therapist in treatment progression. One method of grading activity is to determine the energy expenditure of activities, measured by the amount of oxygen consumed, expressed as MET (basal metabolic equivalent) levels. One MET equals the amount of energy consumed when an individual is at rest in a semireclined position with extremities supported (semi-Fowler position) (6). This energy is equal to 3.5 mL of oxygen per minute per kilogram of weight (3.5/kg/min). When one changes posture, sits up,

ambulates, or performs activities, the metabolic demand and oxygen consumption increase (6).

Whereas various MET lists provide guidance for the therapist in selecting safe levels of activity, caution is required. A person who can achieve four MET levels during one activity may not be able to resume all potential activities in the four MET level list. Variables to consider include the person's pace, position, use of isometrics, environmental factors, muscles used, and emotional stress.

Resumption of activities must occur gradually, particularly in the initial, inpatient phase of recovery (stage I). Table 9.2 provides an example of a program of progressive activity with corresponding MET levels.

TABLE 9.2   Suggested Interdisciplinary Stages for Patients with Cardiopulmonary History or Precautions

STAGE/ MET LEVEL	ACTIVITIES OF DAILY LIVING	EXERCISE	RECREATION
Stage I (1.0–1.4 MET)	*Sitting:* Self-feeding, wash hands and face, bed mobility Transfers Progressively increase sitting tolerance	*Supine:* (A) or (AA) exercise to all extremities (10–15 times per extremity) *Sitting:* (A) or (AA) exercise to *only* neck and LEs Include deep breathing exercise	Reading, radio, table games (noncompetitive), light handwork
Stage II (1.4–2.0 MET)	*Sitting:* Self-bathing, shaving, grooming, and dressing in hospital Unlimited sitting *Ambulation:* At slow pace, in room as tolerated	*Sitting:* (A) exercise to all extremities, progressively increasing the number of repetitions NO ISOMETRICS	*Sitting:* Crafts, e.g., painting, knitting, sewing, mosaics, embroidery NO ISOMETRICS
Stage III (2.0–3.0 MET)	*Sitting:* Showering in warm water, homemaking tasks with brief standing periods to transfer light items, ironing *Standing:* May progress to self-grooming *Ambulation:* May begin slow-paced ambulation outside room on levels, for short distances	*Sitting:* W/C mobility limited distances *Standing:* (A) exercise to all extremities and trunk progressively increasing the number of repetitions *May include:* 1. Balance exercises 2. Light mat activities without resistance *Ambulation:* Begin progressive ambulation program at 0% grade and comfortable pace	*Sitting:* Card playing, crafts, piano, machine sewing, typing

(continued)

TABLE 9.2   Suggested Interdisciplinary Stages for Patients with Cardiopulmonary History or Precautions   (Continued)

STAGE/ MET LEVEL	ACTIVITIES OF DAILY LIVING	EXERCISE	RECREATION
Stage IV (3.0–3.5 MET)	*Standing:* Total washing, dressing, shaving, grooming, showering in warm water; kitchen/homemaking activities while practicing energy conservation (e.g., light vacuuming, dusting and sweeping, washing light clothes) *Ambulation:* unlimited distance walking at 0% grade, in and outside	*Standing:* Continue all previous exercise, progressively increasing 1. Number of repetitions 2. Speed of repetitions *May include* additional exercises to increase workload up to 3.5 METs, balance and mat activities with mild resistance *Ambulation:* Unlimited on level surfaces in or outside progressively increasing speed or duration for periods up to 15–20 minutes or until target heart rate is reached *Stairs:* May begin slow stair climbing until patient's tolerance up to two flights *Treadmill:* 1 mph at 1% grade, progressing to 1.5 mph at 2% grade *Cycling:* Up to 5.0 mph without resistance	Candlepin bowling Canoeing-slow rhythm, pace Golf putting *Light* gardening: weeding and planting Driving
Stage V (3.5–4.0 MET)	*Standing:* Washing dishes, washing clothes, ironing, hanging light clothes, and making beds	*Standing:* Continue exercises as in stage IV, progressively increasing 1. Number of repetitions 2. Speed of repetitions *May add* additional exercises to increase workload up to 4.0 MET *Ambulation:* As in stage IV, increasing speed up to 2.5 mph on level surfaces *Stairs:* As in stage IV and progressively increasing, if increasing to patient's tolerance *Treadmill:* 1.5 mph at 2% grade, progressing to 1.5 mph at 4% grade up to 2.5 mph at 0% grade *Cycling:* Up to 8 mph without resistance May use up to 7–10 lb of weight for UE and LE exercise in sitting	Swimming (slowly) Light carpentry Golfing (using power cart) Light home repairs
Stage VI (4.0–5.0 MET)	*Standing:* Showering in hot water, hanging or wringing clothes, mopping, stripping and making beds, raking	*Standing:* As in stage V *Ambulation:* As in stage V— increasing speed to 3.5 mph on level surfaces *Stairs:* As in stage V *Treadmill:* 1.5 mph at 4 to 6% grade, progressing to 3.5 mph at 0% grade *Cycling:* Up to 10 mph without resistance May use up to 10–15 lb of weight in UE and LE exercises in sitting	Swimming (no advanced strokes) Slow dancing Ice or roller skating (slowly) Volleyball Badminton Table tennis (noncompetitive) Light calisthenics

MEDICAL/SURGICAL MANAGEMENT

The primary goal of medical management is to maintain myocardial integrity by controlling complications that might jeopardize the healing process. Prevention of myocardial ischemia and infarction, which will improve existing cardiac function, is critical in long-term treatment. A major element in the medical management of CAD is the use of pharmacological agents. Common therapies include the use of nitrates, blocking agents, antiarrhythmics, cardiac glycosides, calcium channel blockers, and hypertensives (1). The specific drugs used and their effects and complications are described in the Medications Appendix. Surgical intervention does not alter the process of arteriosclerosis (1). The primary purpose is to improve the quality of life, especially the person's tolerance for activity. Common surgical procedures include coronary artery bypass grafting (CABG), heart transplantation, and percutaneous transluminal coronary angioplasty (PTCA). These surgeries are recommended only in cases of severe, chronically disabling CAD, and their aim is revascularization of the myocardium.

Percutaneous transluminal coronary angioplasty involves the insertion of a "balloon"-tipped tube through a catheter into the coronary arteries to the point of the arteriosclerotic lesion. The balloon is then inflated to compress the lesion against the arterial wall (12) (Fig. 9.5).

A CABG procedure usually involves bypassing one or more obstructed arteries either by anastomosis—or surgical connection—of a vein graft from the aorta to the coronary artery at a point distal to the obstruction or by patch grafting to widen the obstructed artery (12). This surgery often results in significant reduction of pain, increased tolerance for activity, and ECG ischemic changes. However, much controversy exists regarding the effectiveness of CABG vs. conventional drug management in prolonging life, and it is currently a major issue in clinical research. Recently, surgeons have enhanced the success of angioplasty by implanting a device called an "intracoronary stent" into the arterial blockage. This device is a thin cylinder of crushed metal, inserted into the diseased artery, that has tiny, stainless steel scaffolds designed to reduce the chance that the artery will reclose after angioplasty—a major complication of CABG surgery. The use of stents has decreased the rate of restenosis by 10% and this rate is expected to improve (18). The use of multiple stents demonstrated no additional risk over single insertion, indicating that this procedure may be beneficial in multiple artery bypass grafts (19).

Heart transplantation is performed in end-stage CAD when no recovery is expected. In 1996, 2345 heart transplants were performed in the United States (9). The major complications of this procedure are infection and rejection. Protective isolation is prescribed to minimize infection; an immunosuppressive regimen is used to prevent

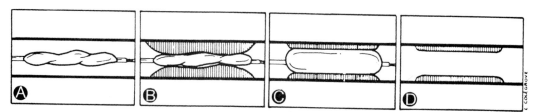

FIGURE 9.5. Percutaneous transluminal angioplasty. **A–B.** Deflated balloon-tipped catheter positioned within the atherosclerotic lesion. **C.** With controlled pressure, the balloon is rapidly inflated and deflated to compress the soft plaque into the vessel walls. **D.** After the balloon-tipped catheter is removed, the artery has improved patency. (Reprinted with permission from Brannon FJ, Geyer MJ, Foley MW. Cardiac Rehabilitation. Philadelphia: FA Davis, 1988.)

rejection. The first-year survival rate is 65%. Candidates for this surgery are usually younger than 50 to 60 years of age. They must be free of other chronic diseases, infection, and donor-specific antibodies. Emotional stability and a strong support system are required as well (16). A strong support system ideally includes the willingness and ability of family and significant others to provide the emotional and physical support the patient requires before and after the surgery.

IMPACT ON OCCUPATIONAL PERFORMANCE

The effects of CAD on occupational performance components are specific to each individual case. Age, the severity of the disease, complications of an infarct, and secondary diagnoses all are factors for consideration. It is likely that the person with an admitting diagnosis of MI also has a history of a cerebral vascular accident, diabetes, or rheumatoid arthritis.

For clarity, the discussion of occupational performance components and areas focuses on MI. The case studies, however, illustrate the effect of a secondary diagnosis, which is a common occurrence.

Sensorimotor: Neuromuscular and Motor Performance

From the onset of an MI, a person's neuromuscular and motor function can be affected. Muscle tone, strength, endurance, and activity tolerance are commonly evaluated and monitored during initial and later stages of cardiac rehabilitation. Fortunately, early mobilization after an MI lessens the negative effects of prolonged bed rest, which in previous years led to a debilitated neuromuscular status. In the last 20 years, cardiac rehabilitation programs have demonstrated that progressive activity programs under supervised conditions can prevent loss of neuromuscular function (3).

Some individuals, however, develop a "cardiac cripple" mentality as a result of an MI. This term refers to the inaccurate notion that because the heart has been damaged, resumption of normal activity is not possible or safe. The person takes on a sick role and lacks the motivation to improve health and function.

Regardless of the efforts of cardiac rehabilitation, anxiety from the event leads to fear of resuming previous activity. The impact of the resulting inactivity clearly can lead to deficits in neuromuscular function.

Cognitive

Coronary artery disease may affect cognitive function if cerebral arteries are occluded, causing interruption of cerebrovascular circulation. Cardiac dysfunction without cerebral artery involvement usually does not result in cognitive dysfunction.

Psychosocial Skills and Psychological Components

White stated 45 years ago that "after MI, the heart may recover more rapidly than the mental state which is so often a complication" (20). Anxiety and depression are the most common psychological responses on return home after an MI. A study of patients 6 months to 1 year after discharge found that 88% reported significant anxiety or depression, or both. Most reported frustration from forced inactivity (21). Even though the emotional distress after an MI decreases over time, early maladaptive behaviors are a strong predictor of overall adjustment problems during the course of the illness. Those persons who cannot manage anxiety and depression initially are more likely to have problems later (21).

Whereas the incidence of coronary disease is increasing in the female population, few studies exist regarding psychosocial adjustment in women (22). Where data are available, women demonstrate more difficulty adjusting to an MI than their male counterparts. Stern reported that 80% of women studied experienced anxiety or depression after an MI, fewer than half returned to work, and only 40% resumed sexual activity. These results could not be explained by age, severity of infarct, or presence of risk factors (23).

Clearly, further examination of women's response to heart disease is necessary, as well as additional studies on the psychosocial responses of the subgroups of the cardiac population. Differences in adjustment among social class and ethnic and racial groups have not been a topic of study in the research literature.

Increasing attention to the quality of survival has resulted in an appreciation of the profound effect of psychological factors on the patient's life. Heart disease often requires both the patient and family to make difficult changes in personality and lifestyle. The rehabilitation team must address these issues in the patient's overall educational program and discharge planning.

The impact of CAD on occupational performance areas is cross-categorical. The level of dysfunction, as in other conditions, is specific to the diagnosis, prognosis, occupational performance components involved, and the severity of involvement. For purposes of clarity, the impact of an MI on occupational performance areas is described.

Activities of Daily Living

The impact of an MI on activities of daily living is an immediate and critical concern of the occupational therapist. In cardiac rehabilitation protocols, activities such as grooming, oral hygiene, dressing, and eating are used as initial guides to determine the functional capacity of the post-MI patient. Depending on the extent of the MI, initiating and sustaining the physical endurance necessary to perform selected tasks may be difficult for the patient.

Functional mobility is not affected by an MI because of musculoskeletal impairment; rather impairment is the result of a lack of physical endurance. Much of the emphasis in cardiac rehabilitation is on progressive attainment of physical capacity. Carefully planned prescriptions of activities and exercises are developed to match physical capacity and endurance levels.

Resumption of sexual activity is a common concern after an MI. Anxiety and fear about the safety of sex must be addressed. As a guideline, physicians recommend a return to sexual activity if the person can walk up and down two flights of stairs without symptoms. In addition to concerns about resuming sexual activity, the individual may feel less attractive as a result of the MI. Perceived health status has been reported to have an impact on resumption of sexual activity. Gutmann reported that patients who saw themselves as ill or "damaged" were less likely to resume sexual relations than those who perceived more positive changes in their health. This same correlation was found for socialization (24).

Work Activities

Much of the literature on adjustment to an MI includes return to work in the context of vocation. Return to work in terms of home management, care of others, and educational activities has not been explored.

The degree to which an MI affects return to work depends mostly on physiological and psychological factors. In examining psychological barriers, Garrity (24a) explored factors that influence return to work. Patients who initially rated their health as poor at both the acute phase and 6 months after infarction were least likely to return to work. Gulledge also reported that early maladjustment makes vocational adaptation difficult (25). Patients who attribute their disease to work-related stress are less likely to return to work than those who do not make such an association (26).

Physiological variables also have major implications when examining the ability to return to work. Analysis of work by MET levels alone cannot determine complete physical capacity. Treadmill tests measure only lower extremity endurance and do not provide a valid assessment of work capacity. The most complete method of determining work capacity uses job analysis to determine which tasks demand the highest energy from the heart. Ogden has developed a task analysis that looks at six variables: rate, resistance, muscle groups used, involvement of trunk muscles, arm position, and isometric work.

Other aspects that must be examined include temperature, time, and emotional stress related to the task (27).

Leisure Activities

Leisure pursuits will be affected to the same degree that the person continues to experience the cycle of anxiety and depression. The health perception concept noted earlier also affects socialization and leisure activities. Those who continue to believe that they are ill will essentially "play the role" of a sick person. In this case, much of the leisure activity the person performs is passive.

CASE STUDIES

CASE 1

J. L. is a 54-year-old car salesman admitted to the emergency room 4 days ago after a 5-hour history of chest pain and discomfort in the shoulder, neck, and jaw. He complained of nausea and was diaphoretic and short of breath. He reported that he had felt fatigued for the last 2 weeks and experienced "heartburn" that was relieved with an antacid. J. L. was sitting at home and had finished his evening meal when the pain and shortness of breath occurred. He noted that the shortness of breath persisted even when he tried to lie down and rest.

Upon admission to the emergency department, he was observed for signs and symptoms of cardiac distress. Auscultation indicated an ectopic or irregular heart rate with a blood pressure rate of 140/110. Laboratory tests indicated elevation of CPK and LDH enzymes. Electrocardiographic studies revealed cardiac arrhythmias and confirmed evidence of an anterolateral MI with subsequent complications of left-sided heart failure and arrhythmias.

J. L. is married and has two teenage children. He was recently laid off from a long-held position at an automotive plant and had started a new job in auto sales 2 weeks prior to his hospitalization. The loss of his original job was stressful, and he was finding that he was not well suited for sales.

His wife had begun a parttime job as a bookkeeper, and managing her new job plus caring for teenage children kept her busy. She had never worked outside the home before because J. L. had refused to accept her desire to do so, and this was creating additional problems in the marriage.

The implications of left-sided heart failure include dyspnea, weakness, fatigue, and poor exercise tolerance (10). All these factors create the potential for a reduction in neuromuscular integrity, particularly the complications arising from congestive heart failure. J. L.'s current functional capacity is at the 1.5 MET level (Table 9.2). He has normal range of motion and muscle strength.

The immediate inactivity forced on J. L. by hospitalization has caused a loss of role functions. He feels anxious and is angry about the possibility of being unable to return to work and provide for his family's needs. He feels his current neuromuscular status will limit him in all his activities. He is reluctant to tell the cardiac rehabilitation team about his concerns about resumption of sexual activity. However, he angrily told his wife that "I guess you'll need to find someone else since I won't be able to please you." He stated that "I might as well go to a nursing home and lessen the burden on everyone." Whereas many of his friends and family have called him and sent him cards, he refuses to talk to them, asking to be left alone.

Most activities of daily living are affected by J. L.'s condition. A MET level of 1.5 indicates that he needs frequent rest periods to sustain activity. He can perform grooming, oral hygiene, and eating without discomfort, as these activities do not require sustained effort. Tasks such as dressing and toileting (bowel movements in particular) require more sustained, isometric work and may be more stressful. Issues around sexual activity are of concern because he believes he is unable to perform sexually.

Because of J. L.'s difficulty with his new job and the apparent stress he perceives from it, his return-to-work potential is affected. He is anxious about his ability to return to his new job and is distressed about his wife having to work to bring in needed income. A thorough analysis of the physical components of work demand cannot be completed until J. L. reaches the 5 MET level. At that time, a job analysis can be completed.

J. L. does not have a history of leisure interests and is not willing to explore new ones at this time. He refused to complete a leisure inventory assessment requested by the occupational therapist. He indicated that he was "too worried about his job and family to think about play."

CASE 2

M. M. is a widowed 92-year-old woman with congestive heart failure (status post 5 weeks) complicated by pulmonary congestion and a history of rheumatoid arthritis. She also is experiencing a recent and progressive visual loss because of acute glaucoma. Before her initial hospitalization and subsequent return home, M. M. was an active woman who enjoyed going for short walks, reading, visiting with friends, and her weekly bridge club. She had been independent in most of her activities of daily living, requiring assistance only for some household management requiring heavier maintenance, cleaning, and repairs.

M. M. cannot read, watch television, or engage in activities that require visual acuity because of her advancing visual loss. Her hearing and other senses are intact. As a result of congestive heart failure and arthritis, Mrs. M. is severely deconditioned and very weak. She complains of arthritic pain in her shoulders, elbows, hips, and knees. Overall passive and active range of motion is limited, predominantly in the proximal joints. Shoulder motion is limited to 100 degrees of flexion, 65 degrees of internal and external rotation, and 70 degrees of abduction. Hip range of motion is limited to 60 degrees of flexion. Knee flexion is limited to 30 degrees of active motion. Great care had to be taken in passive joint measurement because of her pain. Pronounced crepitation indicates diminished joint soft tissue integrity. Because of fatigue, she could not tolerate any additional activity after attempts to measure active range of motion.

M. M.'s cognitive status is intermittently intact and diffuse. She is easily aroused and will orient to others, yet a consistent pattern of verbal and tactile cues are required to maintain her attention. She recognizes family and staff without difficulty and can engage in meaningful conversation. Most of what seem to be attention deficits may be caused by physical fatigue making her want to close her eyes and sleep.

Although she demonstrates mild confusion when following instructions, she is generally aware of her errors, often seeking clarification of accuracy in performing a task or exercise. M. M. is able to recall short- and long-term events.

M. M. is a friendly, engaging woman who clearly enjoys the social contact from various visiting health team members. She asks about their families or jobs and shares information about her own family. Visits from other family members (e.g., grandchildren) are infrequent, because they all live out of state. When they have visited her, she reports it as very pleasant for her. M. M. lives with her daughter, who finds it difficult to meet all of her mother's physical needs. At times, her daughter expresses frustration and anger at the level of care her mother requires. M. M. senses this and is subsequently fearful and reluctant to request things from her daughter.

She expresses concern that she may never resume her previous activity level and notes that her days seem to get longer and longer as her level of inactivity continues. M. M. consistently expresses a concern that she is a major burden on her daughter and clearly hopes she can learn to be more self-sufficient to regain independence.

M. M. is dependent for all activities of daily living. A primary deficit is the lack of functional mobility. M. M. cannot independently change positions in bed and must be repositioned to prevent skin breakdown. She is currently confined to bed, except for being up in a chair for about 30 minutes each day. She cannot transfer from the bed without total assistance from two people. A neighbor helps her daughter put M. M. in the chair and back to bed. Because she is incontinent, she must wear diapers. She cannot bathe and depends on a daily bed bath, which is done 3 days a week by the home health aide and the other days by her daughter. M. M. can feed herself but often drops her utensils because of lack of endurance for grasping objects.

M. M. cannot complete any activities related to home management other than money management. She must depend on a cleaning person, who works 3 afternoons a week. Her daughter does her meal preparation and cleanup, shopping, and clothing care.

Owing to her lack of visual function, immobility, and generalized weakness, it is difficult for M. M. to pursue leisure interests. She cannot visit anyone outside the home at this time, and visits from others are limited. Thus, her opportunities for social interaction are almost nonexistent. She has enjoyed various handicraft activities in the past but feels she cannot perform these now because of her current condition (Table 9.3).

TABLE 9.3 Occupational Performance Profile

I. PERFORMANCE AREAS	II. PERFORMANCE COMPONENTS	III. PERFORMANCE CONTEXTS

A. Activities of Daily Living
  1. Grooming
  2. Oral Hygiene
  3. Bathing/Showering
  4. Toilet Hygiene
  5. Personal Device Care
  6. Dressing
  7. Feeding and Eating
  8. Medication Routine
  9. Health Maintenance
  10. Socialization
  11. Functional Communication
  12. Functional Mobility
  13. Community Mobility
  14. Emergency Response
  15. Sexual Expression
B. Work and Productive Activities
  1. Home Management
    a. Clothing Care
    b. Cleaning
    c. Meal Preparation/ Cleanup
    d. Shopping
    e. Money Management
    f. Household Maintenance
    g. Safety Procedures
  2. Care of Others
  3. Educational Activities
  4. Vocational Activities
    a. Vocational Exploration
    b. Job Acquisition
    c. Work or Job Performance
    d. Retirement Planning
    e. Volunteer Participation
C. Play or Leisure Activities
  1. Play or Leisure Exploration
	2. Play or Leisure Performance
	A. Sensorimotor Component
	  1. Sensory
	    a. Sensory Awareness
	    b. Sensory Processing
	      (1) Tactile
	      (2) Proprioceptive
	      (3) Vestibular
	      (4) Visual
	      (5) Auditory
	      (6) Gustatory
	      (7) Olfactory
	    c. Perceptual Processing
	      (1) Stereognosis
	      (2) Kinesthesia
	      (3) Pain Response
	      (4) Body Scheme
	      (5) Right–Left Discrimination
	      (6) Form Constancy
	      (7) Position in Space
	      (8) Visual–Closure
	      (9) Figure Ground
	     (10) Depth Perception
	     (11) Spatial Relations
	     (12) Topographical Orientation
	  2. Neuromusculoskeletal
	    a. Reflex
	    b. Range of Motion
	    c. Muscle Tone
	    d. Strength
	    e. Endurance
	    f. Postural Control
	    g. Postural Alignment
	    h. Soft Tissue Integrity
	  3. Motor
	    a. Gross Coordination
	    b. Crossing the Midline
	    c. Laterality
	    d. Bilateral Integration
	    e. Motor Control
	    f. Praxis
	    g. Fine Coordination/Dexterity
	    h. Visual–Motor Control
		c. Self-Control
		A. Temporal Aspects
		  1. Chronological
		  2. Developmental
		  3. Lifecycle
		  4. Disability Status
		B. Environment
		  1. Physical
		  2. Social
		  3. Cultural

(continued)

TABLE 9.3   Occupational Performance Profile (Continued)

I. PERFORMANCE AREAS	II. PERFORMANCE COMPONENTS	III. PERFORMANCE CONTEXTS
	i. Oral–Motor Control	

B. Cognitive Integration and Cognitive Components*
1. Level of Arousal
2. Orientation
3. Recognition
4. Attention Span
5. Initiation of Activity
6. Termination of Activity
7. Memory
8. Sequencing
9. Categorization
10. Concept Formation
11. Spatial Operations
12. Problem Solving
13. Learning
14. Generalization

C. Psychosocial Skills and Psychological Components
  1. Psychological
    a. Values
    b. Interests
    c. Self-Concept
  2. Social
    a. Role Performance
    b. Social Conduct
    c. Interpersonal Skills
    d. Self-Expression
  3. Self-Management
    a. Coping Skills
    b. Time Management

*Rule out if cerebral arteries involved.

POINTS FOR REVIEW

1. Describe how myocardial contraction occurs.
2. List the risk factors associated with CAD.
3. Describe the pathogenesis of arteriosclerosis.
4. What conditions other than arteriosclerosis can lead to CAD?
5. What happens to the heart muscle as a result of an MI?
6. How common is arrhythmia in patients diagnosed with MI?
7. Define heart failure and discuss the various classifications.
8. How early can CAD develop in one's life and why?
9. What are the primary methods used to diagnose an MI?

10. What tool does an occupational therapist use to assess energy expenditure?

11. What are common surgical procedures to treat CAD?

12. Discuss the impact of an MI on occupational performance.

REFERENCES

1. Brannon FJ, Geyer MJ, Foley MW. Cardiac Rehabilitation. Philadelphia: FA Davis, 1988.
2. Anthony CP, Thibodeau GA. Textbook of Anatomy and Physiology. St. Louis: CV Mosby, 1983:14–22.
3. Andreoli KG, Fowkes VK, Zipes DR, et al, eds. Comprehensive Cardiac Care: a Text for Nurses, Physicians, and Other Health Care Practitioners. St. Louis: CV Mosby, 1983.
4. Grollman S. The Human Body. 4th ed. New York: Macmillan, 1978:85–262.
5. Dubin D. Rapid interpretation of EKG's. Tampa, FL: C.O.V.E.R., Inc., 1974.
6. Foderaro D. Cardiac dysfunction. In: Pedretti L, ed. Occupational Therapy: Practice Skills for Physical Dysfunction. St. Louis: CV Mosby, 1985.
7. American Heart Association. Cardiopulmonary resuscitation: advanced life support. JAMA suppl, Aug. 1980.
8. Dawber TR. An approach to longitudinal studies in a community: the Framingham Study. Ann N Y Acad Sci 1963;107:539.
9. American Heart Association. 1997 Heart and Stroke Update. Dallas, TX: American Heart Association, 1998.
10. American Heart Association. Fact Sheet on Heart Attack: Stroke and Risk Factors. American Heart Association: Dallas, TX, 1998.
11. Vincent MO, Spence MI. Common Sense Approach to Coronary Care. St. Louis: CV Mosby, 1985: 160–243.
12. Underhill SL. Diagnosis and treatment of the patient with coronary artery disease and myocardial ischemia. In: Underhill SL, Woods SL, Snarjan ES, et al, eds. Cardiac Nursing. Philadelphia: JB Lippincott, 1982.
13. O'Sullivan SB. Coronary artery disease. In: O'Sullivan SB, Schmitz TJ. Physical Rehabilitation: Assessment and Treatment. Philadelphia: FA Davis, 1988.
14. Woods SL, Underhill SL. Coronary heart disease: myocardial ischemia and infarction. In: Patrick ML, et al, eds. Medical Surgical Nursing: Pathophysiological Nursing. Philadelphia: JB Lippincott, 1986.
15. Rothstein JM, Roy SH, Wolf SL. The Rehabilitation Specialists Handbook. Philadelphia: FA Davis, 1991.
16. Long C, ed. Prevention and Rehabilitation in Ischemic Heart Disease. Baltimore: Williams & Wilkins, 1980.
17. Wulf KS. Management of the cardiovascular surgery patient. In: Brunner LS, Suddarth SD, eds. Textbook of Medical Surgical Nursing. 5th ed. Philadelphia: JB Lippincott, 1984.
18. Bittl JA, Thomas P. Beyond the Balloon. Harvard Health Letter, Jan 21 (3) 4–6, 1996.
19. Squires S. Study discounts risks from multiple stents, Washington Post, April 21, 1998.
20. White PD. Heart Disease. New York: Macmillan, 1951.
21. Gundle MJ, Reeves BR, Tate S, et al. Psychosocial outcome after coronary artery surgery. Am J Psychiatry 1980;137:(1)591–594.
22. Stallones R. The rise and fall of ischemic heart disease. Psychosom Med 1987;49:109–117.
23. Stern MJ, Pascale L, Ackerman A. Life adjustment, postmyocardial infarction: determining predictive variables. Arch Intern Med 1977;137:1680–1685.
24. Gutmann MC, Knapp DN, Pollock ML, et al. Coronary artery bypass patients and work status. Circulation 1982;66:33–41.
24a. Garrity TF, Kotchen JM, McKean HE, Gurley D, McFadden M. The association between type A behavior and change in coronary risk factors among young adults. American Journal of Public Health 1990;80:1354–1357.
25. Gulledge AD. Psychological aftermaths of myocardial infarction. In: Gentry WD, Williams RB, eds. Psychological Aspects of Myocardial Infarction and Coronary Care. 2nd ed. St. Louis: CV Mosby, 1979.
26. Kushnir B, Fox KM, Tomlinson IW, et al. The effect of a pre-discharge consultation on the resumption of work, sexual activity and driving following acute myocardial infarction. Scand J Rehabil Med 1975;7:158–162.
27. Ogden LD. Guidelines for analysis and testing of activities of daily living with cardiac patients. Downey, CA: Cardiac Rehabilitation Resources, 1981.

CHAPTER 10

TRAUMATIC BRAIN INJURY

Gerry E. Conti

CRITICAL TERMS

Amnesia
Coma
Decerebrate
Decorticate

Diffuse axonal injury
Endotracheal
Myoclonus
Subdural hematoma

Perseveration
Rigidity
Spasticity

It had been a hot summer day, the work was hard, and the boss kept hanging around the garage. At last it was over. John picked up Kathy, his girlfriend of 4 years, and headed for the beach. Five hours and as many beers later, they sped home on familiar secondary roads. John negotiated the first part of an S-curve fine, but his reflexes were too slow to manage the second. Overcompensating, he lost control of the car, slamming it up against a tree.
Kathy was killed. John D., age 20, survived, with a traumatic brain injury.

ETIOLOGY

Traumatic brain injury (TBI), or head injury, involves a traumatic insult to the brain, capable of producing a complex matrix of physical, intellectual, emotional, social, and vocational changes. Many functions are compromised, including the ability to move in a coordinated manner, speak, remember, reason, and alter behavior (1). The combination of these changes makes the total disability far greater than any single deficit (2).

Acceleration, deceleration, and rotation are primary forces that act on the brain at the time of impact. Brain damage is caused in three ways.

Primary damage occurs at the time of injury and is caused by impact or unexpected loading. It may be either focal or diffuse. Focal damage is associated with direct impact of short duration. Such forces occur in the high speed impact of a motor vehicle accident and result in both coup and contrecoup injuries. Coup injuries occur at the initial site of impact; contrecoup damage is distant from the original site of injury. In this type of injury, direct damage is done as the cortex rotates on the brainstem while accelerating from the force of impact. The cortex strikes the skull, then reverses to accelerate in the opposite direction and hits the skull at a new location. This

165

continues until the force of impact has been absorbed (3, 4–6).

In addition to actual brain damage, the force may fracture the skull, injure the scalp, block the ventricles and blood vessels, and cause contusions or hematomas. The frontal and temporal lobes are particularly sensitive to contusion, hematoma, and other effects of direct damage.

Diffuse damage, called diffuse axonal injury (DAI), occurs with stretching and shearing of brain cell axons from each other at the time of impact. Although cell death usually does not occur, the transmission of normal neural impulses is disrupted. The cerebral hemispheres, mesencephalon, and brainstem are sensitive to DAI (3–6).

Secondary damage occurs shortly after impact, often within several hours or a day (7). Factors causing secondary damage include increased intracranial pressure, brain swelling, hemorrhage or infarction, and oxygen deprivation.

Physiological changes are the third cause of brain injury. These changes include hyperthermia, ischemic brain damage, electrolyte disturbances, hyperventilation, and abnormal responses of the autonomic nervous system (1, 4).

INCIDENCE AND PREVALENCE

Estimates suggest that between 1 and 2 million individuals with TBI are admitted annually to hospitals in the United States (3–10). It is the most common cause of death and disability for persons under age 38. Age, gender, environment, and ethnicity affect this incidence rate. At greatest risk are young men between the ages of 15 and 24, a group that is twice as likely as women to sustain a head injury. Other age groups that show an increased incidence of traumatic brain injury include adults older than age 75 and children younger than the age of 5. Inner city environments have high incidence rates, with African-American residents being twice as likely to be affected as whites (11).

Motor vehicle accidents are the most common cause of traumatic brain injury, accounting for more than half of all admissions. Gunshot wounds and falls are the next most common causes of TBI, with falls being the major cause for the elderly and the very young. Pedestrian accidents account for the fewest admissions for TBI (3, 12–14). A review of available studies suggests that alcohol is a prominent contributing factor in at least half of all cases (12).

Severity of injury is related to cause. Motor vehicle accidents are more likely to result in death or more severe disability; falls are more often associated with mild injury. Intoxication at the time of injury is significantly negatively correlated with outcome. Persons who were intoxicated when injured tend to be hospitalized longer and are discharged with a lower cognitive status than those not intoxicated at the time of injury (12). When all head injuries are considered, 70% result in mild injury, 20% in moderate to severe injury, and 10% are fatal (14). Other factors that correlate highly with outcome include age, length of coma, length of posttraumatic amnesia, and the area and extent of brain damage.

The costs, both individually and for society, are staggering: 50,000 to 70,000 TBI victims are discharged annually from acute care hospitals with little chance of resuming their previous social or economic lives. Another 50,000 to 70,000 begin the months-long process of rehabilitation, as a group incurring approximately $4 billion in hospitalization and treatment expenses. Add to this $75 billion to $100 billion per year in lost productive work skills for many persons with TBI (13).

SIGNS AND SYMPTOMS

The most obvious sign of recent traumatic brain injury is coma, or prolonged loss of consciousness. During this time, the patient may respond only minimally to cues from the external environment and does not obey commands, speak, or demonstrate eye opening (5).

As consciousness and cognition return, the patient displays a variety of symptoms and signs, which have been identified in the Rancho Los Amigos (RLA) cognitive scale (Table 10.1). This

TABLE 10.1 Rancho Los Amigos Cognitive Scale

I. No response: unresponsive to any stimulus
II. Generalized response: limited, inconsistent, nonpurposeful responses, often to pain only
III. Localized response: purposeful responses; may follow simple commands; may focus on presented object
IV. Confused, agitated: heightened state of activity; confusion, disorientation; aggressive behavior; unable to do self-care; unaware of present events; agitation appears related to internal confusion
V. Confused, inappropriate: nonagitated; appears alert; responds to commands; distractable; does not concentrate on task; agitated responses to external stimuli; verbally inappropriate; does not learn new information
VI. Confused, appropriate: good directed behavior, needs cuing; can relearn old skills as activities of daily living (ADLs); serious memory problems; some awareness of self and others
VII. Automatic, appropriate: appears appropriate, oriented; frequently robotlike in daily routine; minimal or absent confusion; shallow recall; increased awareness of self, interaction in environment; lacks insight into condition; decreased judgment and problem solving; lacks realistic planning for future
VIII. Purposeful, appropriate: alert, oriented; recalls and integrates past events; learns new activities and can continue without supervision; independent in home and living skills; capable of driving; defects in stress tolerance, judgment, abstract reasoning persist; may function at reduced levels in society

Prepared by Professional Staff Association, Rancho Los Amigos Hospital, Inc., Downey, California.
(Reprinted with permission from Duncan PW. Physical therapy assessment. In: Rosenthal M, Griffith ER, Bond MR, et al, eds. Rehabilitation of the Adult and Child with Traumatic Brain Injury. 2nd ed. Philadelphia: FA Davis, 1990:265.)

scale presents a typical progression pattern for the recovery of cognitive skills.

Level I is a period of dense unresponsiveness. In level II, the patient begins to respond ineffectively to pain. For example, a leg may extend in response to a pinch of the triceps tendon in the arm. Eye movement may be present, but the eyes do not appear to focus. Sounds and words may occur but often seem meaningless. With further recovery to RLA level III, the patient may be successful in moving an arm from pain and may now respond to a simple request to squeeze the therapist's hand. Verbal communication is still limited. The patient may respond unintelligibly or with automatic cursing. Self-initiation of verbal or motor response is limited. Action occurs only in response to strong cues from either the external environment (e.g., the therapist providing upper extremity range of motion) or the internal environment (e.g., an irritating urinary catheter).

At RLA level IV, the patient becomes confused and agitated. This phase may now involve intentional gross movement of the arms, legs, head, and trunk. Confusion and agitation predominate.

The patient appears to have heightened sensations and responds to routine stimuli in an explosive, exaggerated, and agitated manner. Disorientation to person, place, time, and circumstance is apparent. Retrograde amnesia, or memory loss for events immediately prior to injury, is observed as well. Brief conversations can be held, as basic speech patterns are now present; however, speech may be frequently interrupted by perseverative or profane phrases. At best, the patient can attend to any stimulus for only a short time. Physical discomfort and physical or mental fatigue occur quickly and may trigger an aggressive physical response (1).

With further improvement and movement through levels V through VIII, the patient changes from a confused state to an aware, intentional state and from random selection of behaviors, appropriate or inappropriate, to consistently more appropriate behavior (1).

With an increased cognitive and communicative capacity, additional deficits become apparent, including deficits of vision, perception, sensation and movement, and cognition. Abnormal or inappropriate behavioral responses also may appear. Visual deficits may include diplopia, blurred vision, visual field loss, and decreased oculomotor skills. Scanning abilities are frequently impaired (15). Apraxia, or the inability to perform purposeful movement despite normal coordination, muscle function, and sensation, may be present. The patient may be unaware of a personal body scheme (i.e., the internal physical model of one's body). Unilateral inattention or neglect is common and is suggestive of a parietal lobe lesion, with the patient unaware of sensation coming from one side of the body. Visual discrimination and spatial relations deficits also are common and can be seen in disorders of form perception and constancy, topographical orientation, figure ground perception, position in space, and spatial relations (15).

Abnormal postural reflexes, abnormal muscle tone, and decreased sensation are signs of ongoing motor dysfunction. Hypertonicity and movement disorders often are present. Hypertonicity appears either as rigidity or spasticity. The two types of rigidity most frequently seen in the early stages of recovery are decorticate and decerebrate posturing. In decorticate posturing, the lower extremities are intermittently or constantly held in a rigidly extended posture, whereas the upper extremities are tightly flexed. With decerebrate posturing, all extremities are rigidly extended. Spasticity appears as an increased involuntary muscle resistance to passive range of motion and voluntary movement. Head and total body control are impaired. Movement is uncoordinated and reflex-bound and may include ataxia, tremors, and myoclonus (15, 16).

As early cognitive signs of confusion and disorientation begin to decrease, underlying cognitive deficits appear. The ability to pay attention, sustain attention, and maintain divided attention is impaired (1). Retrograde amnesia typically continues to improve, but short-term and long-term memory problems become apparent. These ongoing memory deficits contribute significantly to ongoing disorientation and confusion (1, 17, 18). Higher-level cognitive skills, such as those needed

to select and execute plans, manage time, and regulate personal behavior, are impaired. These deficits are apparent as the patient shows difficulty identifying a goal, initiating a plan of action, and selecting appropriate steps and their sequence. Altering a plan in the face of new and conflicting feedback is difficult. Response time is slowed. Symptoms of limited time management include difficulty estimating or scheduling time and in changing schedules when necessary.

Behavioral problems caused by deficits in higher-level cognitive skills are of major concern. Impulsivity, perseveration, irritability, impaired judgement, and decreased inhibition are common behavioral consequences of frontal lobe lesions. Additionally, lability, apathy, or an altered sex drive may be noted. A lack of insight make these problems particularly difficult to manage (19–21).

COURSE AND PROGNOSIS

Response to and recovery from TBI tends to be highly individual, despite known neuropathological effects. Even so, identifying early factors that are predictive of recovery has been a major focus of research. The purpose has been to direct extensive medical and rehabilitation funds toward patients who could benefit most. Numerous methodological and theoretical problems, however, make the identification of such predictive factors difficult (6).

The Glasgow coma scale (GCS) is the most frequently used measure of consciousness. It evaluates three simple responses: eye opening, best motor response to stimulation, and best verbal response (7, 22, 23). Research has shown this scale to be a good predictor of both mortality and outcome. Individual scores in the three areas are added together to predict outcome (Table 10.2). A total GCS rating of 8 or below for a duration of 6 hours postinjury correlates with a 50% mortality rate or survival with moderate to severe injury. A GCS rating of 9–12 is associated with moderate injury, and 13–15 with mild impairment. Of the three GCS factors, the strongest predictor is the person's motor response. Patients who withdraw from painful

Table 10.2   Assessment of Conscious Level (Glasgow Coma Scale)[a]

	EXAMINER'S TEST	PATIENT'S RESPONSE	ASSIGNED SCORE
EYE OPENING (E)	Spontaneous speech	Opens eyes on own	E4
		Opens eyes when asked to in a loud voice	3
	Pain	Opens eyes upon pressure	2
	Pain	Does not open eyes	1
BEST MOTOR RESPONSE (M)	Commands	Follows simple commands	M6
	Pain	Pulls examiner's hand away upon pressure	5
	Pain	Pulls a part of body away upon pressure	4
	Pain	Flexes body inappropriately to pain (decorticate posturing)	3
	Pain	Body becomes rigid in an extended position upon pressure (decerebrate posturing)	2
	Pain	Has no motor response to pressure	1
VERBAL RESPONSE (talking) (V)	Speech	Carries on a conversation correctly and tells examiner where he/she is, who he/she is, and the month and year	V5
	Speech	Seems confused or disoriented	4
	Speech	Speaks so examiner can understand, but patient makes no sense	3
	Speech	Makes sounds that examiner cannot understand	2
	Speech	Makes no noise	1

[a]Coma score (E + M + V) = 3 to 15.
(Reprinted with permission from Miller JD, Pentland B, Berroll S. Early evaluation and management. In: Rosenthal M, Griffith ER, Bond MR, et al, eds. Rehabilitation of the Adult and Child with Traumatic Brain Injury. 2nd ed. Philadelphia: FA Davis, 1990:36.)

stimuli are much more likely to have only mild to moderate residual impairment (22, 23).

Other factors are used to estimate outcome. Posttraumatic amnesia of less than 1 hour suggests a mild injury, whereas amnesia lasting more than 1 day indicates a severe injury. A younger age at injury improves both chance of survival and overall outcome. The absence of pupillary light responses and abnormal eye movements indicate brainstem dysfunction, with an increased risk of death. Prolonged increased intracranial pressure is associated with death and severe disability (22, 23).

The Glasgow Outcome Scale (GOS) also is widely used as a predictive assessment. When used 6 months after injury, this scale is 90% accurate in outcome prediction. Predicted outcomes, however, are quite broad. The GOS outcomes include death, vegetative state, severe disability, moderate disability, and good recovery. Good recovery is defined to mean that the person is able to resume a normal social life and could return to work (7). Additional neuropsychological tests can enhance the accuracy of outcome prediction. When employment is the desired outcome, psychosocial skills show the strongest correlation with successful return to work (24).

Lastly, most recovery tends to occur during the first 6 months after onset (7). After the initial 6-month period, recovery may continue, but the rate of improvement often slows.

MEDICAL/SURGICAL MANAGEMENT

Medical management in the acute phase centers around preservation of life and the prevention of secondary damage. Maintaining an effective airway and circulatory function are critical life-preservation steps immediately after injury. An endotracheal tube may be placed. After arrival at the hospital and with medical stabilization, diagnostic tests are begun and the location and severity of all injuries identified. The patient typically receives a computerized axial tomography (CT) scan. If this reveals an intracranial hematoma, immediate surgical decompression is needed. Constant monitoring of consciousness occurs, as the duration and depth of coma are significant indicators of both mortality and morbidity (22).

Physicians from neurology, neurosurgery, internal medicine, or orthopaedics may direct overall medical management in the acute phase. More than 50% of patients with severe head injury have associated injuries. Hydrocephalus, or the abnormal accumulation of cerebrospinal fluid in the brain, is a serious complication for up to 75% of patients; 82% of those with TBI have one or more extracranial fractures as well, and 10% of these may be cervical spinal cord injuries. Medical management is then needed for both a brain injury and a high-level spinal cord injury (25, 26). Because of rigid abnormal posturing and other motor disturbance, up to 84% of patients develop contractures of the neck, trunk, arms, and legs. The longer the coma, the greater the potential for abnormal body posturing and development of contractures. About one-third of patients aspirate food into their lungs, causing pneumonia. These patients usually have a delayed or absent swallowing reflex (25, 26).

Intensive care medical management is constant. An indwelling urinary catheter is placed and closely monitored. A nasogastric tube is placed and used for high caloric feeding. Close attention to skin integrity is essential, and the patient's total body position is changed frequently. Twice-daily range of motion of all extremities helps prevent contractures. Suctioning of the endotrachial tube and vigorous respiratory therapy treatments help prevent additional pulmonary problems. Monitoring of the level of consciousness occurs frequently (22).

Rehabilitation in the intensive care unit may begin as soon as neurologic stability is achieved. Early rehabilitation centers around a program of graded and specific sensory stimulation, with the assumption that selective sensory input may speed or improve neurological recovery.

Medical stability, cognitive level, and the ability to benefit from intensive rehabilitation are used to identify the appropriate time for transfer to the rehabilitation phase (22). The patient's rehabilitation usually is directed by a physiatrist, a physician specializing in medical rehabilitation. The goals of the intensive rehabilitation program are to restore the patient to his or her optimal level of function in all areas and to minimize additional physical or psychosocial disability (22). Along with the patient's physician, the core rehabilitation team includes specialists in occupational therapy, physical therapy, speech and language pathology, nursing, neuropsychology, and social work. The long-term rehabilitation goals in occupational therapy are to reestablish sensorimotor integration and control, basic self-care skills and activities of daily living, and basic cognitive and communication skills. Where remediation is not possible or when maximal neurological recovery can be assumed to have occurred, compensation strategies are taught. As these goals are accomplished, the patient may be discharged from the hospital and allowed to meet higher-level goals on an outpatient basis. Outpatient occupational therapy long-term goals include all activities of daily living, community reintegration, and vocational rehabilitation (1).

Medications used with the traumatically brain-injured individual must be carefully selected and closely monitored because of their potentially deleterious side effects. Tegretol and phenobarbital are used to prevent or reduce seizure activity, but they further depress already slowed central nervous system responses. Increased muscle tone, or spasticity, may be treated with phenytoin, dantrolene sodium, or baclofen. Sleep disorders may be regulated by diazepam, which also may help moderate behavior (8, 9, 26). Diazepam has a strong depressant effect on the central nervous system and must be used with great caution in patients with TBI.

IMPACT ON OCCUPATIONAL PERFORMANCE

The deeply comatose patient—Rancho Los Amigos levels I through III—shows depressed function in all occupational performance components and is dependent in all occupational performance. With further recovery, improvement in all performance components occurs, and basic function within the self-care, home management, vocational activity, leisure activity, and community reintegration occupational performance areas may become possible. Table 10.3 lists all performance components, as all performance components are dramatically affected by a TBI.

TABLE 10.3   Occupational Performance Profile

I. PERFORMANCE AREAS	II. PERFORMANCE COMPONENTS	III. PERFORMANCE CONTEXTS
A. Activities of Daily Living*	A. Sensorimotor Component	A. Temporal Aspects
1. Grooming	1. Sensory	1. Chronological
2. Oral Hygiene	a. Sensory Awareness	2. Developmental
3. Bathing/Showering	b. Sensory Processing	3. Lifecycle
4. Toilet Hygiene	(1) Tactile	4. Disability Status
5. Personal Device Care	(2) Proprioceptive	B. Environment
6. Dressing	(3) Vestibular	1. Physical
7. Feeding and Eating	(4) Visual	2. Social
8. Medication Routine	(5) Auditory	3. Cultural
9. Health Maintenance	(6) Gustatory	
10. Socialization	(7) Olfactory	
11. Functional Communication	c. Perceptual Processing	
12. Functional Mobility	(1) Stereognosis	
13. Community Mobility	(2) Kinesthesia	
14. Emergency Response	(3) Pain Response	
15. Sexual Expression	(4) Body Scheme	
B. Work and Productive Activities	(5) Right–Left Discrimination	
1. Home Management	(6) Form Constancy	
a. Clothing Care	(7) Position in Space	
b. Cleaning	(8) Visual–Closure	
c. Meal Preparation/ Cleanup	(9) Figure Ground	
d. Shopping	(10) Depth Perception	
e. Money Management	(11) Spatial Relations	
f. Household Maintenance	(12) Topographical Orientation	
g. Safety Procedures		

(continued)

TABLE 10.3   Occupational Performance Profile (Continued)

I. PERFORMANCE AREAS	II. PERFORMANCE COMPONENTS	III. PERFORMANCE CONTEXTS

I. PERFORMANCE AREAS

    2. Care of Others
    3. Educational Activities
    4. Vocational Activities
       a. Vocational Exploration
       b. Job Acquisition
       c. Work or Job
          Performance
       d. Retirement Planning
       e. Volunteer Participation
C. Play or Leisure Activities
    1. Play or Leisure Exploration
    2. Play or Leisure
      Performance

II. PERFORMANCE COMPONENTS

    2. Neuromusculoskeletal
      a. Reflex
      b. Range of Motion
      c. Muscle Tone
      d. Strength
      e. Endurance
      f. Postural Control
      g. Postural Alignment
      h. Soft Tissue Integrity
    3. Motor
      a. Gross Coordination
      b. Crossing the Midline
      c. Laterality
      d. Bilateral Integration
      e. Motor Control
      f. Praxis
      g. Fine Coordination/Dexterity
      h. Visual–Motor Control
      i. Oral–Motor Control
  B. Cognitive Integration and Cognitive Components
    1. Level of Arousal
    2. Orientation
    3. Recognition
    4. Attention Span
    5. Initiation of Activity
    6. Termination of Activity
    7. Memory
    8. Sequencing
    9. Categorization
    10. Concept Formation
    11. Spatial Operations
    12. Problem Solving
    13. Learning
    14. Generalization
  C. Psychosocial Skills and Psychological Components
    1. Psychological
      a. Values
      b. Interests
      c. Self-Concept
    2. Social
      a. Role Performance
      b. Social Conduct
      c. Interpersonal Skills
      d. Self-Expression
    3. Self-Management
      a. Coping Skills
      b. Time Management
      c. Self-Control

*All occupational performance components and areas are affected: degree depends on level of coma, severity of injury, and progress during rehabilitation

CASE STUDIES

CASE 1

J. D., age 20, survived an automobile accident, with a moderate TBI. After 2 weeks in intensive care and 4 weeks in an acute medical unit, he is to begin intensive rehabilitation. His occupational therapist cannot get reliable information from him, so she relies on a medical record review for his medical history and a discussion with his mother to identify his previous occupational performance levels.

The medical record review reveals that J. D. sustained a right tibia-fibula fracture with the TBI. After 3 days of general unresponsiveness, he began to obey simple commands (RLA level III). From there he moved quickly to the agitated, confused state of level IV. At this point speech became intelligible and perseverative swearing was noted. Soft restraint of his arms became necessary, as he persisted in pulling out both his urinary catheter and his nasogastric tube.

The agitation has lessened somewhat, but he continues to be intermittently disoriented. He responds to therapeutic requests more quickly and positively in the morning. He persists in incorrectly calling the occupational therapist, "Kathy." Moderate to severe spasticity is present, and J. D. demonstrates poor sitting postural control. Right upper extremity movement is limited by spasticity, whereas the left upper extremity is slowed but functional. His eyes do not appear to focus, and he performs any activity better with an eye patch on.

His mother is very vague about his activities. She states that he has had three garage mechanic's jobs in the last 2 years. She says he seemed to get tired of routine and didn't get along well with his bosses. He moved into her two-bedroom apartment about 6 months ago so he could start saving money for a new car. He does not participate in any home-care tasks but does help with the rent. Leisure activities included fixing up his old car and "hot-rodding" around. J. D.'s mother does not care for many of his friends, but becomes tearful when asked about his relationship with Kathy. She says they were planning to be married in the fall.

At this time, J. D. is dependent in all areas of occupational performance. His greatest strength lies in the occupational performance categories of self-care and functional mobility. He requires moderate assistance and verbal cuing for shower-ing while seated in a shower chair and for putting on and removing his shirt. He can eat and needs verbal cuing only for task completion. Bed-to-wheelchair transfers now require only moderate physical assistance because of his fracture. J. D. has come a long way, but there is a longer way still to go.

CASE 2

C. R.'s family had the misfortune of being in the wrong place at the wrong time. Returning late one night, tanned and happy from 2 weeks at the lake, her husband could not avoid the oncoming car that went through a red light and sideswiped them. All family members were hurt, but C. R. most of all.

At the hospital, she was initially responsive to request, then became unresponsive during the third hour after injury. After surgical intervention for increased intracranial pressure, she regained awareness and achieved an RLA level IV within 2 weeks, at which time intensive rehabilitation began.

Surprisingly, she had no broken bones and her sensorimotor status improved rapidly. By the time of discharge from the hospital, she was walking in a slow but stable manner. Her primary physical problems involved decreased right upper extremity coordination and decreased endurance. Cognitively, she improved quickly to level VI. At the time of discharge, she had trouble with organization, sequencing, and task initiation. C. R. was delighted to leave the hospital and return home. She did not anticipate any problems in resuming her roles as wife, mother, and homemaker. She did not think that she could return to being a secretary at present.

At the time of admission to an outpatient rehabilitation program, she had deficits in a number of occupational performance areas. She can now type only 20 words per minute, and complains of eyestrain after 10 minutes of copy work. This does not bother her, as she says she does not plan to return to work in the near future, if at all.

She is neat and clean in appearance at all times. However, her clothes are all tight, as she gained 15 lb during her rehabilitation stay despite a strict diet. She has always been proud of her clean home but now does not clean it thoroughly. When pressed, she also admits that she has trouble organizing her day to accomplish all the tasks she had previously. Many tasks have been assumed by other family members. She is able to prepare simple meals, but the family has learned that she is often unable to read her recipe card correctly and that her memory problems make stove use a safety hazard.

C. R. was outgoing, assertive, and pleasant before her injury. At present, she seems content just to stay at home. She expresses no interest in going out with the family or in resuming any of her previous activities. When not involved, she sits in front of the television. Conversation is limited. She responds pleasantly and politely, but slowly, to questions. She seldom initiates conversation other than basic social remarks. When she speaks, it is usually of herself, and she no longer actively asks after others. Occasionally the noise created by two healthy children and their friends bothers her, and she becomes very angry. Her children now spend more time at their friends' homes than previously. C. R. recognizes that she is different and blames her change on her memory and vision problems. Although she cannot identify just how she is different, she does recognize those differences when they are pointed out. She would like to get better.

Comments

J. D. and C. R. are each just one person at one point in the continuum of recovery. Each patient with TBI has a very personal psychosocial background, an individual mechanism of injury, specific factors affecting recovery, and individualized time lines for recovery. At any point, recovery may slow or stop. The occupational therapist working with brain-injured patients must first identify and evaluate the many occupational performance roles and performance components affected by injury. Goals must be established either to remediate or maintain skills or to compensate for lost skills. Treatment priorities are then set, emphasizing performance skills initially, then gradually adding areas of occupational performance when improved skill levels make success feasible. All treatment must be established within the boundaries of the patient's physical and cognitive endurance, and frustration tolerance.

For the occupational therapist, patients with TBI represent a formidable but highly rewarding challenge. Principles of neurological recovery must be understood and applied, and effective treatment techniques must be identified and incorporated into meaningful activity. Despite the challenge, the rewards are great, for example, when a brain-injured person returns to a prized occupational role.

POINTS FOR REVIEW

1. Which age groups are most at risk for TBI?
2. Among those who suffer TBI, what is known to be a contributing factor?
3. What percentage of those with TBI are likely to require rehabilitation?
4. List factors that correlate with progress in rehabilitation outcomes.
5. Describe the damage to the brain due to the primary forces from impact.
6. What are the physiological changes, which occur after injury, that cause brain injury?
7. Outline the signs and symptoms that characterize the pattern of recovery from level I to level VII.
8. What is the GCS? What does it evaluate? Explain the scoring system.
9. Can outcome prediction be made based on the GCS scores? Explain.
10. What are the primary goals in medical management?
11. How soon would an occupational therapist begin intervention for someone with TBI, and what, in general, would be the goals of therapy?
12. Describe the impact of TBI on occupational performance in each of the levels of recovery as defined by the RLA scale.

REFERENCES

1. Sohlberg MM, Mateer CA. Introduction to Cognitive Rehabilitation. Theory and Practice. New York: Guilford Press, 1989.
2. Jennett B, Bond M. Assessment of outcome after severe brain damage. Lancet 1975;1:480–484.
3. Rimel RW, Jane JA, Bond MR. Characteristics of the head-injured patient. In: Rosenthal M, Griffith ER, Bond MR, eds. Rehabilitation of the Adult and Child with Traumatic Brain Injury. 2nd ed. Philadelphia: FA Davis, 1990:8–16.

4. Jennett B. Scale and scope of the problem. In: Rosenthal M, Griffith ER, Bond MR, et al, eds. Rehabilitation of the Adult and Child with Traumatic Brain Injury. 2nd ed. Philadelphia: FA Davis, 1990:59–74.

5. Bond MR. Standardized methods of assessing and predicting outcome. In: Rosenthal M, Griffith ER, Bond MR, et al, eds. Rehabilitation of the Adult and Child with Traumatic Brain Injury. 2nd ed. Philadelphia: FA Davis, 1990:59–74.

6. Katz DI. Neuropathology and neurobehavioral recovery from closed head injury. J Head Trauma Rehabil 1992;1(2):1–15.

7. Jennett B, Teasdale G. Management of Head Injuries. 6th ed. Philadelphia: FA Davis, 1984.

8. Manzi DB, Weaver PA. Head Injury. The Acute Care Phase. Thorofare, NJ: Slack, 1987.

9. Slater B. A Positive Approach to Head Injury. Guidelines for Professionals and Families. Thorofare, NJ: Slack, 1987.

10. National Head Injury Foundation. Every Fifteen Seconds. Washington, DC: 1993.

11. Whitman S, Coonley-Hoganson R, Desai BT. Comparative head trauma experiences in two socioeconomically different area communities: Chicago—a population study. Am J Epidemiol 1984;119:570–580.

12. Gordon WA, Mann N, Willer B. Demographic and social characteristics of the traumatic brain injury model system database. J Head Trauma Rehabil 1993;8(2):26–33.

13. Levati A, Farina M, Vecchi G, et al. Prognosis of severe head injuries. J Neurosurg 1982;57:779–783.

14. Horn LJ, Garland DE. Medical and orthopedic complications associated with traumatic brain injury. In: Rosenthal M, Griffith ER, Bond MR, et al, eds. Rehabilitation of the Adult and Child with Traumatic Brain Injury. 2nd ed. Philadelphia: FA Davis, 1990:107–126.

15. Zoltan B. Remediation of visual-perceptual and perceptual-motor deficits. In: Rosenthal M, Griffith ER, Bond MR, et al, eds. Rehabilitation of the Adult and Child with Traumatic Brain Injury. 2nd ed. Philadelphia: FA Davis, 1990:351–365.

16. Griffith ER, Mayer NH. Hypertonicity and movement disorders. In: Rosenthal M, Griffith ER, Bond MR, et al, eds. Rehabilitation of the Adult and Child with Traumatic Brain Injury. 2nd ed. Philadelphia: FA Davis, 1990:127–147.

17. Brooks DN. Cognitive deficits. In: Rosenthal M, Griffith ER, Bond MR, et al, eds. Rehabilitation of the Adult and Child with Traumatic Brain Injury. 2nd ed. Philadelphia: FA Davis, 1990:163–178.

18. Goethe KE, Levin HS. Behavioral manifestations during the early and long-term stages of recovery after closed head injury. Psychiatr Ann 1984:14(7):540–546.

19. Livingston MG. Effects on the family system. In: Rosenthal M, Griffith ER, Bond MR, et al, eds. Rehabilitation of the Adult and Child with Traumatic Brain Injury. 2nd ed. Philadelphia: FA Davis, 1990:225–235.

20. Rosenthal M, Bond MR. Behavioral and psychiatric sequelae. In: Rosenthal M, Griffith ER, Bond MR, et al, eds. Rehabilitation of the Adult and Child with Traumatic Brain Injury. 2nd ed. Philadelphia: FA Davis, 1990:179–192.

21. Miller JD, Pentland B, Berroll S. Early evaluation and management. In: Rosenthal M, Griffith ER, Bond MR, et al, eds. Rehabilitation of the Adult and Child with Traumatic Brain Injury. 2nd ed. Philadelphia: FA Davis, 1990:21–51.

22. Mack A, Horn LJ. Functional prognosis in traumatic brain injury. In: Horn LJ, Cope DN, eds. Physical Medicine and Rehabilitation: State of the Art Reviews. Philadelphia: Hanley & Belfus, 1989;3(1):13–26.

23. Sandel ME. Rehabilitation management in the acute care setting. In: Rosenthal M, Griffith ER, Bond MR, et al, eds. Rehabilitation of the Adult and Child with Traumatic Brain Injury. 2nd ed. Philadelphia: FA Davis, 1990:27–41.

24. Conti, G. Factors affecting return to work for the persons with traumatic brain injury. Unpublished manuscript: Eastern Michigan University, 1992.

25. Hanscom DA. Acute management of the multiply injured head trauma patient. J Head Trauma Rehabil 1987:2(2):1–12.

26. Eames P, Haffey WJ, Cope DN. Treatment of behavioral disorders. In: Rosenthal M, Griffith ER, Bond MR, et al, eds. Rehabilitation of the Adult and Child with Traumatic Brain Injury. 2nd ed. Philadelphia: FA Davis, 1990:410–432.

CHAPTER 11

SPINAL CORD INJURY

Laura Vincent Miller

CRITICAL TERMS

Autonomic dysreflexia
  (hyperreflexia)
Catheterization
Credé's method

Decubitus ulcers
Heterotopic ossification
Nonreflex neurogenic bladder
  or bowel

Peristalsis
Reflex arc
Scoliosis
Spinal shock

. . .of the many forms of disability which can beset mankind, a severe injury or disease of the spinal cord undoubtedly constitutes one of the most devastating calamities in human life.
—Sir Ludwig Guttmann,
*pioneer in twentieth century
management of spinal cord injury (1)*

The future lies in our own hands, and if a challenge should enter our life, it is important to remember we have tremendous strength, courage, and ability to overcome any obstacle.
—Douglas Heir, Esq., Attorney-at-Law
(personal communication)

The full impact of the preceding quotes may not strike the reader unless the whole story is known. The latter author, Doug Heir, sustained a spinal cord injury (SCI) at age 18. He dove into a pool to save a boy who appeared to be drowning. The boy was only playing, but Doug's injury rendered him quadriplegic. Now, more than a decade later,

Doug has become known for being many things, among them an author, U.S. delegate to the Soviet Union, cover athlete for Wheaties cereal, associate legal editor of the *National Trial Lawyer,* and a gold medalist in the 1989 Olympics in Seoul, Korea—an impressive list of accomplishments for someone who sustained "one of the most devastating calamities in human life!"

The goals of the health care team should include empowering clients to take charge of their futures. To accomplish this, the health professional must understand the complexities of the diagnosis. This chapter explores the ramifications of spinal cord injuries, beginning with a brief overview of the central nervous system (CNS) and surrounding structures.

OVERVIEW OF CNS AND RELATED STRUCTURES

The brain and spinal cord make up the CNS. The spinal cord receives sensory (afferent) information from the peripheral nervous system and transmits this information to higher structures (i.e., the thalamus, cerebellum, cerebral cortex) in the CNS. Descending motor (efferent) information, originating from the cortex, also is transmitted by the spinal cord back to the peripheral nervous system.

The consistency of the spinal cord has been compared to a ripe banana, and it is fortunate that the spinal cord and cerebral cortex are protected by bony structures. Whereas the skull protects the brain, the vertebral column protects the spinal cord. The vertebral column is composed of 33 vertebrae, with 7 cervical vertebrae in the neck region (C1–C7), 12 thoracic vertebrae in the chest region (T1–T12), 5 lumbar vertebrae in the midback region (L1–L5), 5 sacral vertebrae (S1–S5), which are actually fused in the lower back and pelvic region, and 4 fused coccygeal vertebrae that make up the coccyx, or tailbone (Fig. 11.1).

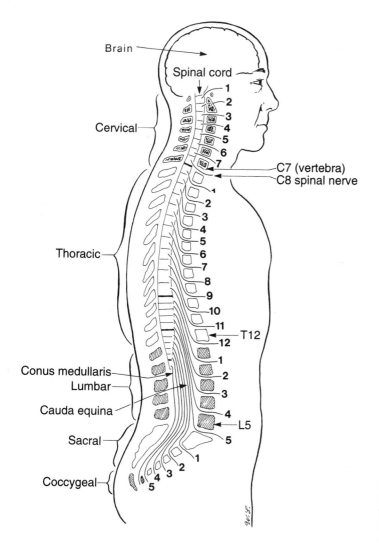

FIGURE 11.1 The spinal cord, spinal nerves, and vertebral column. (Reprinted with permission from the Rehabilitation Institute of Michigan.)

There are 31 pairs of spinal nerves, which exit from the spinal cord and branch to form the peripheral nervous system. The nerves exit through the openings formed between each two vertebrae. The spinal nerves are named according to the vertebrae above or below which they exit. Note that spinal nerves C1 through C7 exit above the corresponding vertebrae, whereas the remaining spinal nerves (C8–S5) exit below the corresponding vertebrae. Thus, although there are seven cervical vertebrae, there are eight cervical spinal nerves. The actual spinal cord ends just below the L1 vertebra. However, some spinal nerves continue, and exit beyond the point where the spinal cord ends. Because of their visual resemblance, this bundle of nerves is referred to as the cauda equina, which is Latin for "horse's tail" (2). The meningeal covering of the spinal cord, which contains the cerebrospinal fluid (CSF) that bathes the structures of the CNS, also extends past the end of the spinal cord to the L4 vertebral level. The CSF-filled meningeal space between L2 and L4, referred to as the lumbar cistern, is the site where spinal taps are performed, because the spinal cord is not present, yet CSF is accessible.

Sensory and Motor Tracts

The terms "tract," "pathway," "lemniscus," and "fasciculus" all refer to bundles of nerve fibers that have a similar function and travel through the spinal cord in a particular area. It is important to know the names, locations, and functions of these tracts to understand the possible outcomes of an SCI at a given level. The location of major tracts within a cross-section of the spinal cord can be seen in Figure 11.2.

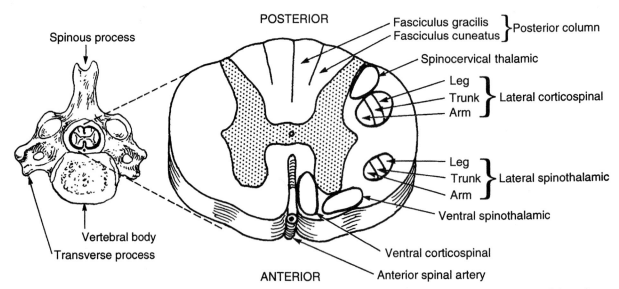

FIGURE 11.2 Cross-section of cervical spinal cord, shown in relation to surrounding vertebral structures. Selected ascending and descending pathways are illustrated. (Adapted from materials provided courtesy of Rehabilitation Institute of Michigan. Used with permission.)

Two basic types of nerve tissue make up the spinal cord. Gray matter is located centrally and resembles a butterfly in cross-sections of the cord. Gray matter is composed of cell bodies and synapses. White matter encompasses most of the periphery of the cord and contains the ascending and descending pathways. A more detailed description of the functions of the various sensory and motor pathways that travel through the white matter of the spinal cord is provided in Table 11.1. It may be helpful to remember that many pathways are named according to their origin and the location of their final synapse (e.g., spinocerebellar, corticospinal).

Specific motor and sensory information is carried by each pair of spinal nerves. In general, the cervical nerves (C1–C8) carry afferent and efferent impulses for the head, neck, diaphragm, arms, and hands. The thoracic spinal nerves (T1–T12) serve the chest and upper abdominal musculature. The lumbar spinal nerves (L1–L5) carry information to and from the legs and a portion of the foot, whereas the sacral spinal nerves (S1–S5) carry impulses for the remaining foot musculature, bowel, bladder, and the muscles involved in sexual functioning. A more detailed outline of muscles innervated by each level of the spinal cord and a dermatomal segmentation (sensory map) of the body are presented in Table 11.2 and Figure 11.3.

Reflex Arc

Most nerve impulses move up the spinal cord to the brain and back through the cord to the peripheral nerves. However, some impulses merely enter the cord through the dorsal nerve root, synapse, and exit by the ventral nerve root. This causes certain muscle functions or responses without direction from the brain. A simple example of this "looping" can be seen in the knee-jerk reflex. If the knee is tapped with a reflex hammer, the knee will extend without any influence from the brain. The stimulation by the hammer causes afferent impulses to enter the cord, synapse, and exit, causing a contraction of the muscle fibers

---

TABLE 11.1   Noninclusive Listing of Ascending and Descending Pathways

Ascending afferent (sensory) pathways	Function
Spinocerebellar	Nonconscious proprioception
Lateral spinothalamic	Pain, temperature
Ventral spinothalamic	Touch, pressure
Fasciculus gracilis/fasciculus cuneatus[a]	Two-point tactile discrimination, vibration, conscious proprioception, stereognosis
Spinocervicothalamic	Touch, proprioception, stereognosis, vibration

Descending efferent (motor) pathways	Function
Lateral corticospinal	Movement to extremities
Ventral corticospinal	Movement of neck and trunk
Vestibulospinal	Equilibrium
Reticulospinal	Autonomic functions: motor respiratory functions

[a]Called the "posterior column."

TABLE 11.2 Spinal Cord Innervations/Function

SPINAL CORD LEVEL	PRIMARY MUSCLE GROUPS	PRIMARY MOVEMENTS
C1–C3	Infrahyoid muscles Head/neck extension Rectus capitus (anterior and lateral) Sternocleidomastoid Longus colli Longus capitus Scaleni	Depression of the hyoid Neck extension, flexion, rotation, and lateral flexion

	ADDITIONAL PRIMARY MUSCLE GROUPS	ADDITIONAL PRIMARY MOVEMENTS
C4	Trapezius Upper cervical paraspinals Diaphragm	Shoulder elevation, scapular adduction and depression Independent breathing
C5	Rhomboids Deltoids Rotator cuff muscles (partially—some nerve supply is at C6 level) Biceps Brachialis (partially) Brachioradialis (partially)	Scapular downward rotation Weak shoulder external rotation, flexion, and extension Shoulder abduction and rotation Weak approximation of humeral head in glenoid fossa Elbow flexion
C6	Rotator cuff muscles (complete innervation) Serratus anterior (partially) Pectoralis (clavicular segments) Total innervation of elbow flexors Supinators Extensor carpi radialis Flexor carpi radialis	Full shoulder rotation, adduction, flexion, extension Scapular abduction Horizontal shoulder adduction Strong elbow flexion and supination Wrist extension (weak) Tenodesis action of hand Very weak wrist flexion
C7	Latissimus dorsi Pectoralis major (sternal portion) Triceps Pronator teres Flexor carpi radialis Flexor digitorum superficialis Extensor digitorum (partially) Extensor pollicis longus and brevis	Elbow extension Forearm pronation Wrist flexion Finger flexion (trace) Finger extension (weak) Thumb extension (weak)
C8	Flexor carpi ulnaris Extensor carpi ulnaris Flexor digitorum profundus and superficialis Flexor pollicis longus and brevis Abductor pollicis longus Adductor pollicis Opponens pollicis Lumbricals (partially)	Complete wrist extension, adduction, and abduction Finger flexion (stronger) Thumb flexion, abduction, adduction, opposition Weak flexion at MCP with IP extension

(continued)

TABLE 11.2 Spinal Cord Innervations/Function (Continued)

	ADDITIONAL PRIMARY MUSCLE GROUPS	ADDITIONAL PRIMARY MOVEMENTS
T1	Doral interossei Palmar interossei Abductor pollicis brevis Lumbricals (complete innervation) Erector spinae muscles (partially) Intercostal muscles (partially)	Finger abduction Finger adduction Thumb abduction (strong) MCP flexion with IP extension (strong) Thoracic spine extension Increased respiratory function with presence of intercostals
T4–8	Erector spinae muscles (partially) Intercostal muscles (partially) Abdominal muscles (beginning at T7)	Stronger thoracic spine extension Stronger respiratory function Thoracic flexion Weak trunk flexion
T9–12	Lower erector spinae muscles Lower intercostal muscles Abdominal muscles Quadratus lumborum (partially)	Strong thoracic spine extension Trunk flexion, extension, rotation, and stability Pelvic control and stability
L1–3	Quadratus lumborum (full innervation) Iliopsoas Erector spinae (lumbar segment)	Pelvic elevation Hip flexion Lumbar extension
L4–5	Lumbar erector spinae Hip adductors Hip rotators Quadriceps Hamstrings (partially) Tibialis anterior	Lumbar extension and stability Hip adduction Hip rotation Knee extension Knee flexion (weak) Ankle dorsiflexion (weak)
S1–2	Hip extensors Hip abductors Hamstrings (complete innervation) Plantar flexors Invertors of ankle Evertors of ankle	Hip extension Hip abduction and stability Knee flexion Ankle plantar flexion Ankle inversion and stability Ankle eversion and stability
S2–5	Bladder Lower bowel Genital innervations	Genitourinary functions Bowel functions

Abbreviations: MCP, metacarpophalangeal; IP, interphalangeal.

(Fig. 11.4). This activity is called a reflex arc. In persons with an intact spinal cord, afferent nerve impulses also travel to the brain almost instantaneously. This allows an awareness, or "feeling," of the initial stimulation (knee tap) and subsequent response (knee jerk). This concept is important to an understanding of SCIs. It explains why some individuals with SCI continue to have reflexes but do not have voluntary control of their muscles. It also explains why others have no reflexes at all below the level of their injury. This is discussed in much greater detail in the section on classification of injuries.

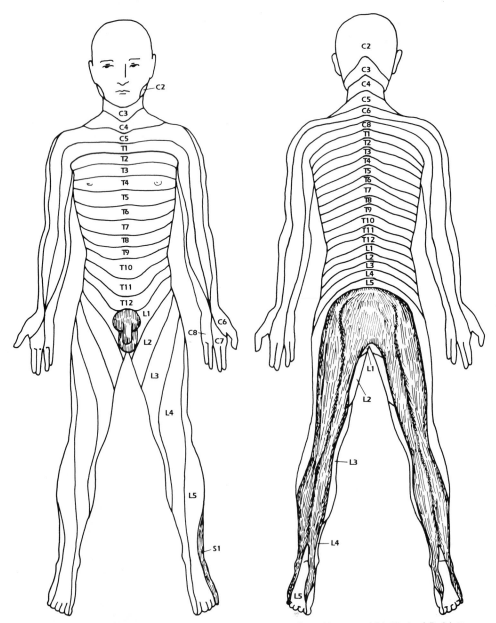

FIGURE 11.3 Dermatome map. (Reprinted with permission from Hammond M, Umlauf R, Matteson B, et al. Yes, You Can! A Guide to Self Care for Persons with Spinal Cord Injury. Washington, DC: Paralyzed Veterans of America, 1989.)

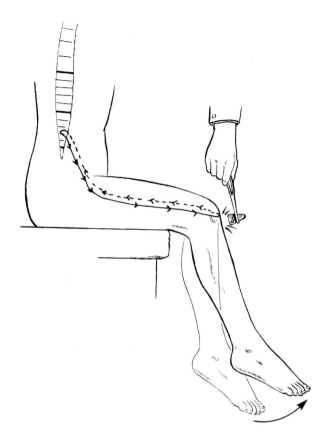

FIGURE 11.4   Knee-jerk reflex.

ETIOLOGY

Many statistics sources attempt to count the number of persons who have sustained SCIs. Unfortunately, the United States has only recently made strides in collecting comprehensive data on a national level. In 1985, the Centers for Disease Control and Prevention began promoting surveillance mechanisms at state and national levels for the collection and reporting of these data. Nonetheless, current data sources do provide a picture of the etiology and incidence of SCI in this country.

The leading cause of SCI in the United States is motor vehicle accidents, followed by falls and gunshot wounds (Fig. 11.5). Sports-related injuries account for most of the remaining SCIs, with diving being by far the most common (and preventable) cause (Table 11.3).

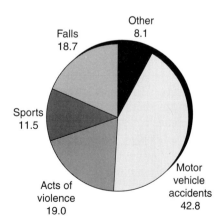

FIGURE 11.5   Etiologic distribution of spinal cord injury. (Reprinted with permission from the National Spinal Cord Injury Statistical Center. 1997 Annual Statistical Report. Birmingham, AL: University of Alabama at Birmingham, 1997.)

TABLE 11.3	Sports-Related Spinal Cord Injuries
SPORT	**PERCENTAGE**
Diving	66.0
Football	6.1
Snow skiing	3.8
Surfing	3.1
Trampoline	2.6
Other winter sports	2.3
Wrestling	2.3
Gymnastics	2.2
Horseback riding	2.0
Other	9.6

Reprinted with permission from Stover SL, Fine PR, eds. Spinal Cord Injury: The Facts and Figures. Birmingham, AL: The National Spinal Cord Injury Statistical Center, University of Alabama at Birmingham, 1986.

Analyzing the etiology of spinal cord injuries makes for well-targeted prevention programs. Public awareness of the effects of using substances while operating a vehicle is certainly heightened. Tougher penalties for driving under the influence of altering substances have been enacted, and many states have adopted seat belt and child restraint legislation. Grant monies have even been awarded to hospital-based programs that evaluate the home environments of senior citizens. Their recommendations may reduce the risk of falls—a major cause of SCI in the elderly. An innovative program sponsored by the Southeastern Michigan Spinal Cord Injury System tells high-risk youths about the consequences of interpersonal violence and presents strategies to avoid those tragic outcomes. This program is brought to elementary and high schools, where weapons are, unfortunately, too prevalent.

INCIDENCE AND PREVALENCE

Incidence rates for SCI in the United States are estimated at 40 cases/million population/year,

excluding those who die at the scene of an accident (3). Given a U.S. population of 254 million persons, this translates to about 10,000 new cases of SCI every year. But who is the "average" person with SCI? The statistics indicate it is an 18-year-old white male involved in an auto accident, but this can vary widely, both geographically and seasonally. Seasonal sports cause fluctuations in etiology statistics, and some urban hospitals are reporting that more than 40% of their SCI cases are caused by gunshot wounds.

Although much of the literature focuses on trauma, there are many nontraumatic causes of spinal cord damage. Developmental conditions, such as spina bifida, scoliosis, and spinal cord agenesis, may yield the same clinical signs as traumatic SCI. Many acquired conditions, such as bacterial or viral infections, benign or malignant growths, embolisms, thromboses, hemorrhages—even radiation or vaccinations—can lead to damage of spinal cord tissue.

CLASSIFICATION OF INJURY

The two major classifications of spinal cord injuries are complete and incomplete. A complete SCI occurs with a complete transection of the cord. In this case, all ascending and descending pathways are interrupted, and there is a total loss of motor and sensory function below the level of injury. The injury also may be referred to as an upper motor neuron (UMN) injury, if the reflex arcs are intact below the level of injury but are no longer mediated by the brain. Upper motor neuron lesions are characterized by a) a loss of voluntary function below the level of the injury, b) spastic paralysis, c) no muscle atrophy, and d) hyperactive reflexes (Fig. 11.6).

Complete injuries below the level of the conus medullaris (Fig. 11.1) are referred to as lower motor neuron (LMN) injuries, because the injury has affected the spinal nerves after they exit from the cord. In fact, injuries involv-

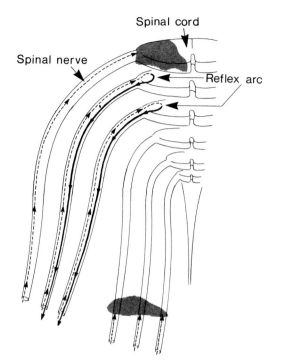

FIGURE 11.6 A diagrammatic representation of the reflex arc. The shaded lesion above denotes a UMN lesion, with the exception of the spinal nerve entering at the level of the lesion. The shaded lesion below represents an LMN lesion. (Reprinted with permission from the Rehabilitation Institute of Michigan.)

ing spinal nerves after they exit the cord at any level are referred to as LMN injuries. In these injuries, the reflex arc cannot occur, because impulses cannot enter the cord to synapse. As a result, LMN injuries are characterized by a) a loss of voluntary function below the level of the injury, b) flaccid paralysis, c) muscle atrophy, and d) absence of reflexes.

Upper motor neuron and LMN injuries may be complete or incomplete. There also may be a mixture of UMN and LMN signs after an incomplete lesion in the lower thoracic/upper lumbar region. The following section discusses incomplete injuries in greater detail.

Incomplete Injuries

If damage to the spinal cord does not cause a total transection, there will still be some degree of voluntary movement or sensation below the level of injury. This is known as an incomplete injury, which may be further categorized according to the area of the spinal cord that was damaged and the clinical signs that are present.

Anterior Cord Syndrome

This syndrome results from damage to the anterior spinal artery or indirect damage to anterior spinal cord tissue (Fig. 11.7). Clinical signs include:

Loss of motor function below the level of injury.
Loss of thermal, pain, and tactile sensation below the level of injury.
Light touch and proprioceptive awareness are generally unaffected.

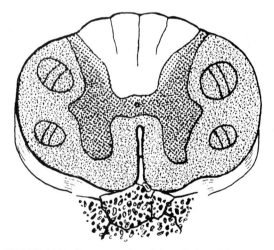

FIGURE 11.7 A cross-section of the spinal cord illustrating the damage that causes anterior cord syndrome. The anterior artery is involved, resulting in damage to most areas, with the exception of the posterior columns. (Reprinted with permission from the Rehabilitation Institute of Michigan.)

Brown–Séquard's Syndrome

This syndrome occurs when only one side of the spinal cord is damaged (Fig. 11.8). A hemisection of this nature frequently is the result of a stab or gunshot wound. The clinical signs of Brown–Séquard's syndrome generally include:

Ipsilateral loss of motor function below the level of injury.

Ipsilateral reduction of deep touch and proprioceptive awareness. (There is a reduction rather than loss as many of these nerve fibers cross.)

Contralateral loss of pain, temperature, and touch.

Clinically, a major challenge presented by Brown–Séquard's syndrome is that the extremities with the greatest strength have the poorest sensation.

Central Cervical Cord Syndrome

In this lesion, the neural fibers serving the upper extremities are more impaired than those of the lower extremities (Fig. 11.9). This occurs because the fibers that innervate the upper extremities

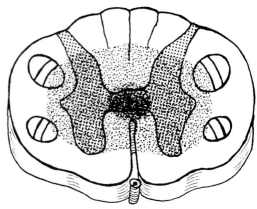

FIGURE 11.9 Cross-section of the cord, illustrating the damage resulting in central cervical cord syndrome. (Reprinted with permission from the Rehabilitation Institute of Michigan.)

travel more centrally in the cord and, as the name of the syndrome implies, the central structures are the ones that are damaged (Fig. 11.2). Injury to the central portion of the spinal cord is often seen, along with structural changes in the vertebrae. Most commonly, hyperextension of the neck, combined with a narrowing of the spinal canal, results in this type of injury. Because arthritic changes can lead to spinal canal narrowing, this syndrome is more prevalent in aging populations. The signs of central cord syndrome often include:

Motor and sensory functions in the lower extremities less involved than in the upper extremities.

A potential for flaccid paralysis of the upper extremities, as the anterior horn cells in the cervical spinal cord may be damaged. Because these are synapse sites for the motor pathways, an LMN injury may result.

Cauda Equina Injuries

Cauda equina injuries do not involve damage to the spinal cord itself, but rather to the spinal nerves that extend below the end of the spinal cord (Fig. 11.1). Injuries to the nerve roots and spinal nerves that comprise the cauda equina are

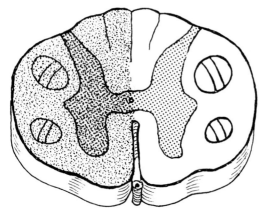

FIGURE 11.8 Cross-section of the cord, illustrating the damage that results in Brown–Séquard's syndrome. (Reprinted with permission from the Rehabilitation Institute of Michigan.)

generally incomplete. Because this type of injury actually involves structures of the peripheral nervous system (exiting spinal nerves), there is some chance for nerve regeneration and recovery of function if the roots are not too severely damaged or divided. These injuries are usually the result of direct trauma from fracture dislocations of the lower thoracic or upper lumbar vertebrae. Clinical signs of cauda equina injuries include:

Loss of motor function and sensation below the level of injury.

Absence of a reflex arc, as the transmission of impulses through the spinal nerves to their synapse point is interrupted. Motor paralysis is of the LMN type, with flaccidity and muscle atrophy seen below the level of injury.

In both complete and incomplete injuries, the terms "quadriplegia," "tetraplegia," and "paraplegia" may be used to further describe the impact of the injury. Quadriplegia refers to lost or limited function of all extremities as a result of damage to cervical cord segments. The American Spinal Injury Association (ASIA) prefers the term "tetraplegia" over quadriplegia. Tetraplegia refers to impairment or loss of motor or sensory function in the cervical segments of the spinal cord that is the result of damage of neural elements within the spinal canal. Tetraplegia causes impairment of function in the arms as well as in the trunk, legs, and pelvic organs. It does not include brachial plexus lesions or injury to peripheral nerves outside the neural canal (4). Paraplegia, which refers to lost or limited function in the lower extremities and trunk depending on the level of injury, occurs after lesions to thoracic, lumbar, or sacral cord segments. Spinal cord injuries are frequently classified further, based on the "ASIA Impairment Scale" (5), which contains the following categories:

A = Complete: no motor or sensory function is preserved in the sacral segments S4–S5.
B = Incomplete: sensory but not motor function is preserved below the neurological level and extends through the sacral segments S4–S5.

C = Incomplete: motor function is preserved below the neurological level, and the majority of key muscles below the neurological level have a muscle grade less than 3.
D = Incomplete: motor function is preserved below the neurological level, and the majority of key muscles below the neurological level have a muscle grade of greater than or equal to 3.
E = Normal: motor and sensory function is normal.

A manual muscle test is performed to assess the strength of muscles and aid in the determination of the extent and nature of injury. Usually, strength is graded on a six-point scale (6–9):

0 = Total paralysis
1 = Palpable or visible contraction
2 = Active movement, full range of motion (ROM) with gravity eliminated
3 = Active movement, full ROM against gravity
4 = Active movement, full ROM against moderate resistance
5 = (Normal) active movement, full ROM against full resistance
NT = Not testable

POSTTRAUMATIC PROGRESSION

The period of altered reflex activity immediately after a traumatic SCI is known as spinal shock. As a result of injury, spinal cord segments below the level of the lesion are deprived of excitatory input from higher CNS centers. What is observed clinically during this phase is a flaccid paralysis of muscles below the level of injury and an absence of reflexes (10). The bladder is also flaccid, requiring catherization, and there is no voluntay control of the bowel. Depending on the level of the injury, the person with an SCI may require a ventilator because of lost or temporarily interrupted innervation to the diaphragm, intercostals, and abdominal muscles.

Spinal shock generally lasts from 1 week to 3 months after injury. Once spinal shock subsides, the areas of the spinal cord above the level of the lesion operate as they did premorbidly. Below the level of the lesion, reflexes will resume if the reflex arc is intact. This is an important concept to understand. Unlike a plant, which may die entirely if its stem is cut in half, the spinal cord is still alive and functional above and below the level of injury. The problem is one of communication; the brain cannot receive sensory information beyond the lesion site and cannot volitionally control motor function below that point.

After spinal shock subsides, there is often an increase in spasticity, especially in the flexor muscle groups. The reflex arc "fires" and the brain is unable to interfere. After this phase, there may be a period of 6 to 12 months after injury when an increase in the spasticity of the extensor groups is common. Usually, after 1 year postinjury, the wide fluctuations in tone will cease.

COMPLICATIONS

An array of complications can greatly affect the prognosis of a person who has sustained an SCI. Some of the more common medical complications are addressed in this section.

Autonomic Dysreflexia (Hyperreflexia)

As implied by its name, autonomic dysreflexia, or hyperreflexia, involves an exaggerated response of the autonomic nervous system (ANS). You may recall that a function of the ANS is the integration of body functions in the "fight-or-flight" response—heart rate, blood vessel constriction/dilation, regulation of glands, and smooth muscle. The condition usually occurs in persons with spinal cord injuries above the T6 level. Signs to look for include a sudden, pounding headache, diaphoresis, flushing, "goosebumps," and tachycardia followed by bradycardia. All of this is caused by an irritation of nerves below the level of injury. Common sources of irritation include an overfull bladder or bowel, urinary tract infections (UTIs), or decubitus ulcers. Even

irritations such as ingrown toenails can trigger the response. All these would be bothersome to a person with an intact spinal cord—he or she would feel uncomfortable and act to remedy the situation. But the person with a spinal cord injury lacks this "feeling," and autonomic dysreflexia is the body's way of warning that something is wrong below the level of the injury.

The most important aspect of managing autonomic dysreflexia is to find the cause and alleviate it. This may require emptying the bladder, checking for blockages or "kinks" in the urinary drainage tubing, checking for bowel impaction, or evaluating for other factors. It helps to decrease blood pressure if the person assumes an upright position. Most persons with tetraplegia will experience an episode of autonomic dysreflexia at least once, but if the signs of autonomic dysreflexia appear frequently, medication may be indicated. Although autonomic dysreflexia may appear suddenly, it must be managed promptly. Because the blood pressure may elevate dramatically, there is risk of stroke or death if the situation is ignored or mismanaged.

Postural Hypotension

In contrast to autonomic dysreflexia, blood pressure decreases in postural hypotension. This condition, often seen in persons who have sustained cervical or thoracic SCIs, also may be referred to as orthostatic hypotension (11). Blood tends to pool distally in the lower extremities as a result of reduced muscle tone in the trunk and legs. The symptoms of postural hypotension frequently occur when a person attempts to sit up after prolonged periods of bed rest. Symptoms include lightheadedness, dizziness, pallor, sudden weakness, and unresponsiveness. Preventive measures include the use of antiembolism hosiery and abdominal binders, which externally assist circulation. Also, assuming an upright position slowly can help avoid these symptoms. If symptoms do occur, a semireclined or reclined position should be maintained until the symptoms subside.

Respiratory Complications

Persons with spinal cord injuries at or below the level of T12 generally have a normal respiratory status. Injuries above that level, however, compromise the respiratory system to some degree. The abdominal musculature is innervated by segments T7 through T12; the intercostal muscles are served by segments T1 through T12; and the diaphragm is innervated by C4. Persons with complete injuries above C4 usually need a respirator. Some may be candidates for a phrenic nerve stimulator if the nerve shows the ability to conduct an impulse. Generally, persons with complete injuries at C4 and below are not using respirators, but respiratory complications may persist. Breathing may be shallow, and the ability to cough productively may be weak. Various deep-breathing and assisted-coughing techniques may be taught, along with other procedures to keep the lungs clear.

Deep Vein Thromboses

Deep vein thromboses (DVT) can be a serious complication in many types of medical conditions. They are a potential complication in SCI for three main reasons: reduced circulation caused by decreased tone, frequency of direct trauma to legs causing vascular damage (e.g., repeated trauma during transfer or bed mobility activities), and prolonged bed rest. Edema is often seen in SCI for the same reasons. Clinical signs of DVT may include swelling in the lower extremities, localized redness, and a low-grade fever. However, a DVT may be relatively asymptomatic on bedside evaluation. Vigilant medical screenings for DVT should be performed in all cases of SCI. An undetected and unmanaged DVT may result in an embolism and death.

Thermal Regulation

You have already seen that damage to the spinal cord can disrupt the ANS, possibly resulting in autonomic dysreflexia. Thermal regulation is another function of the ANS that can be disturbed after SCI. Maintaining the appropriate body temperature often is a problem for persons whose injuries are above T6. During the first year after injury, the body tends to assume the temperature of the external environment. This condition is called poikilothermia (12). In time, some adjustment usually occurs. Cold weather often causes discomfort, as blood vessels below the level of injury do not constrict sufficiently to conserve the body's heat. Conversely, excessive sweating may occur above the level of injury in warmer weather but not below, which hampers the body's efforts to prevent hyperthermia. Because of this, extreme temperatures should be avoided, and attention should be given to the extent and type of clothing worn in all conditions.

Spasticity

In persons who have UMN lesions, increased tone appears in muscles below the level of injury after spinal shock subsides. Virtually all patients with cervical cord injuries experience spasms; 75% of those with thoracic lesions, less than 58% of those with lumbar injuries, and less than 25% of those with cauda equina injuries report spasms (13). An increase in spasticity can be triggered by a variety of factors including infections, positioning, pressure sores, UTIs, and heightened emotional states. Spasms are not necessarily disadvantageous. The ability to trigger their spasms can help some individuals maintain muscle bulk, circulation, bowel and bladder management, transfers, and other self-care activities. Excessive spasticity, however, may result in contractures, pain, and a reduced ability to participate in activities. At this point, medical or surgical options may be recommended.

Heterotopic Ossification (Ectopic Bone)

Heterotopic ossification (HO) refers to the abnormal formation of bone deposits on muscles, joints, and tendons. It occurs most often in the hip and knee and less frequently in the shoulder and elbow. It has been estimated that 20% of all persons with SCI have some degree of ectopic bone growth (14).

Clinical signs of HO may include heat, pain, swelling, and a decrease in active or passive range of motion. These signs should always alert the clinician, as they may indicate other serious complications, such as DVT. Many facilities that specialize in the care of patients with SCI routinely provide prophylactic medications that have shown promise in halting this abnormal calcification. In extreme cases in which range of motion is permanently and severely limited by HO, surgery may be indicated.

Urinary System Complications

Urinary tract infections are a common and dangerous complication of SCI. Prior to modern medical management, many persons with SCI who survived the initial trauma died within a few years after injury, with one of the most common causes being kidney failure due to chronic UTI. For several reasons, patients with SCI are more prone to UTI or bladder infections. The bladder is composed of smooth muscle, innervated by sacral segments of the spinal cord. As such, it is affected by a loss of sensory and motor function, as are other parts of the body, depending on the level and extent of injury. The nature of bladder function will depend on whether the injury caused LMN or UMN deficits (Fig. 11.10). Injury at point A yields a UMN bladder, also referred to as a reflex or spastic bladder. In this case, the bladder can contract and void reflexively. Although this action is involuntary, some persons with SCI can trigger the reflex through various stimuli, much as the knee-jerk reflex is triggered by tapping with a reflex hammer. That is because impulses can still enter the cord below the level of injury, synapse, and exit.

Persons with a UMN bladder may use various types of catheters and additional techniques to ensure that the bladder does not become distended or retain urine. They generally cannot rely on sensation to alert them that the bladder has exceeded its normal capacity; rather, they must rely on an established voiding schedule.

An LMN bladder may also be referred to as a nonreflex or flaccid bladder. This type of bladder function is usually seen during the spinal shock phase and may remain if the injury has affected the cauda equina area. An injury at point B or C (Fig. 11.10) can result in an LMN bladder. With

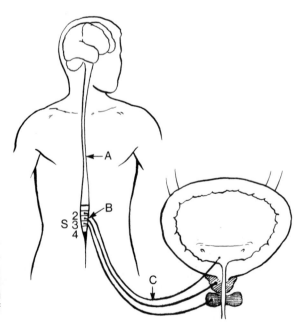

FIGURE 11.10 Bladder and corresponding spinal segment innervations. Injuries at point **A** would result in a UMN, or spastic bladder. Injuries at points **B** or **C** would result in LMN, or flaccid, bladder function. (Reprinted with permission from the Rehabilitation Institute of Michigan.)

this type of injury, a reflexive emptying of the bladder cannot occur, as the reflex arc is destroyed. Because the bladder is flaccid and does not spontaneously empty, urine will accumulate continuously. Patients with an LMN bladder must catheterize according to a schedule or must apply external pressure to the abdomen with their fists, which forces urine from the bladder. This application of external pressure is called Credé's method.

With either type of bladder (UMN or LMN), voiding must occur routinely and completely. Chronic overstretching of the bladder will reduce its ability to void adequately. Residual urine is a breeding ground for infections that can spread to all structures in the urinary system, including the ureters and kidneys. Chronic infections can lead to renal calculi (kidney stones), kidney failure and, potentially, death. Warning signs of a UTI include urine that appears cloudy or has excessive particles, dark or foul-smelling urine, an elevated fever, chills, or an increase in spasticity. The best treatment of UTI is prevention—adhering to an effective voiding schedule, using clean or sterile techniques, maintaining a proper diet and adequate fluid intake, and prompt attention to warning signs.

Complications Associated with the Bowel

Normally, elimination occurs when stool is present in the rectum. Nerves in the rectal musculature are stimulated, triggering a reflexive peristalsis and a relaxation of the rectal sphincters. A bowel movement may be prevented at this step of the process if the brain "overrides" this reflex, sending down an impulse to tighten the sphincter muscles until an appropriate time. We have all experienced the sensation of urgency caused by a full rectum, but perhaps we have not fully appreciated our brain's ability to allow us to forestall the inevitable until a socially acceptable time.

Unfortunately, an SCI can interfere with bowel function in much the same way as it impedes the bladder. The bowel can become spastic or flaccid. A reflex bowel can be caused by a lesion at point A (Fig. 11.11). In this case, stool can be eliminated reflexively if nerves located in the rectum are stimulated. This stimulation may be done manually through digital stimulation or in conjunction with the use of suppositories. Establishing and following

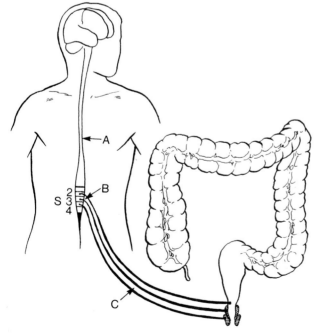

FIGURE 11.11 The bowel and corresponding spinal segment innervations. Injuries at point **A** would result in a UMN, or spastic bowel. Injuries at points **B** or **C** would result in LMN, or flaccid, bowel function. (Reprinted with permission from the Rehabilitation Institute of Michigan.)

a regular schedule for bowel management can prevent incontinence.

The bowel is usually flaccid during the phase of spinal shock and may remain in that state if the injury involves the areas illustrated at points B and C (Fig. 11.10). As with the flaccid bladder, the flaccid bowel cannot be stimulated to empty reflexively. Stool may often remain in the rectum after attempts at evacuation, and it may be necessary to remove it manually to prevent impaction.

Constipation or impaction may result if elimination does not occur regularly. Aside from the standard discomfort associated with this, autonomic dysreflexia may be triggered in persons with lesions above the T6 level.

Diarrhea is another complication that can be particularly frustrating for the person with an SCI who is trying to establish a set schedule for bowel management. This condition is always frustrating, but the majority of the general population has the benefit of intact sensation to provide a warning. The best prevention for diarrhea in the person with SCI is to make sure to use (not overuse) laxatives if they are prescribed, eat a proper diet, and follow a scheduled bowel program that reduces the chance of impaction, which can result in diarrhea.

Dermal Complications

The skin is the largest organ of the body, and it performs essential functions in maintaining your health. Skin assists in thermal regulation, insulating us in cold weather and sweating to prevent hyperthermia during hot conditions. Aside from literally keeping the body together, skin acts as a barrier to the external environment. At the cellular level, skin provides the site for O_2/CO_2 exchange through the capillary system. Keeping skin intact is essential and requires conscious effort by a person with SCI, as sensations that would normally provide warning of potential skin damage, such as pain and extremes in temperature, are not perceived below the level of injury.

Damage to the skin as a result of pressure sores, or decubitus ulcers, is a major reason for hospital readmissions in SCI populations. The mechanism is continued pressure due to lack of movement. Circulation is impaired because of the pressure, and capillary exchange is impeded. This can result rapidly in tissue necrosis. The severity of pressure sores can be classified in four stages.

Stage I. Clinical signs are reddened or darkened skin. Damage is limited to more superficial (epidermal and dermal) layers. At this stage, tissue breakdown can be halted merely by removing pressure until the skin returns to its normal color.

Stage II. The skin now appears reddened and open. A blister or scab is present. The scab is not a sign of healing; rather, the tissue beneath it is necrotic. This involves the epidermal and dermal layers, as well as deeper adipose tissue. Wound dressings may be involved at this stage, and it is imperative that pressure be kept off the site.

Stage III. The skin breakdown is deeper, and the wound is now draining. Muscle may be visible through the open wound. An ulcer is developing in the necrotic tissue. In addition to wound dressings, surgical intervention may be indicated if more conservative treatment is unsuccessful.

Stage IV. All structures, from the superficial levels to the bone, are destroyed. Infection and bone decay occur. Surgical intervention is likely, and the person with a pressure sore at this stage often must spend weeks after a skin graft with pressure totally removed from the involved site (15).

Pressure sores are preventable with diligent attention and preventative strategies. A person with SCI can use, or instruct another person to assist with, a variety of pressure relief methods. Also, visual skin inspections should be performed at least twice daily, taking particular note of areas most prone to breakdown. These would include areas where bony prominences (e.g., the sacrum, ischium, calcaneus, and scapula) can add to pressure. Proper nutrition also should be heeded, as healthy skin is less apt to break down and is more responsive to healing in early stages of pressure sore development.

Other dermal complications, such as burns or frostbite, are prevented by attentiveness and common sense. Even commonly encountered things, such as space heaters or exposed pipes under a sink, can cause severe burns to patients with SCI without their immediate knowledge. It is important to be aware of the environment and to rely on other, intact senses to avoid injury.

COURSE AND PROGNOSIS

A prognosis implies that one can forecast or predict the outcome and chances for recovery from a particular disease or traumatic injury. That is somewhat challenging for SCIs. Although some aspects of SCI are highly predictable (e.g., specific muscle functions impaired with a complete lesion at C5), other aspects are much more vague.

Part of the ambiguity lies in the definitions of the term "recovery." One definition is to "get back," or regain, which tends to be the patient's focus. Another definition for "recover" stresses compensation, which is often the thrust of the health care professional working with SCI. Whereas we will discuss the physiological prognosis of SCI, the clinician should always be aware, and acknowledge the validity, of the patient's perspective on recovery. To "get back" and to "compensate for" are dramatically different terms. When discussing prognosis with a person who has survived an SCI, the clinician should always be truthful but must also be acutely aware of the impact of what the patient is hearing. Perhaps the most crucial indicators of a patient's functional outcome are personal characteristics such as motivation, use of support systems, and coping mechanisms. The clinician must be skilled at fostering these strengths while at the same time providing accurate information to the patient.

Physiologically, although extensive research is ongoing, there is no way to induce functional axonal regeneration within a damaged human spinal cord. Recent research headlines have reported that the use of steroid—specifically, methylprednisolone—may improve neurological outcomes of patients with SCI if administered within the first 8 hours after injury (16). Experimental drugs, such as GM-1 ganglioside and 4AP, are touted as aiding in the preservation of damaged nerves and insulating them from the toxic level of chemicals the body releases during trauma (17). However, whether these neurological gains actually result in significant functional improvements for persons with SCI is not yet proven. Additional research is being aimed at a variety of strategies, including pharmacological and enzyme therapy, cloning of nerve cells, fetal tissue transplants, and the highly sophisticated altering of the cellular environment to encourage actual regeneration. As stated earlier, the spinal cord is alive above and below the level of injury; one goal of current research is to encourage functional reconnection of the disrupted pathways.

A different picture is presented with cauda equina injuries or injuries involving the nerve root. These types of injuries carry the potential for regeneration if the nerve roots are not severely damaged or divided. The degree of regeneration that can be expected is very difficult to predict, which must be done on an individual basis after extensive medical testing.

Aside from research on actual spinal cord regeneration, significant work also is being done with highly technical devices to compensate for paralysis. Functional electrical stimulation (FES) is one example. Persons with UMN injuries have experienced increases in their functional abilities (improved upper extremity function, standing ability, ambulation) with the external application of electrodes that stimulate muscle contraction. Although some may feel that the FES apparatus is cumbersome, unsightly, time consuming, and difficult to apply, refinements are ongoing. Many persons with SCI feel that, although not ideal, the technology provides an appealing alternative to outcomes from traditional methods of rehabilitation. Recently, the Food and Drug Administration approved the Freehand System, a neuroprosthetic device that may be surgically implanted in a person with tetraplegia (18). This system combines internal electrodes, stimulators, sensors, and transmission coils within an external control box. It allows a person with tetraplegia to achieve a degree of prehension function, enhancing such activities of daily living (ADL) as eating, writing, and phone and computer use.

Overall, although actual regeneration of the cord does not appear to be on the immediate scientific horizon, the advances in all phases of SCI management are promising. Everyone has the right to hope for what is not yet reality, without being said to have "unrealistic expectations." Assisting someone to be hopeful, while simultaneously working to maximize today's function, is to truly master the art of the therapeutic relationship.

IMPACT ON OCCUPATIONAL PERFORMANCE

Occupational performance relates to a person's ability to engage in activities that are essential and meaningful. Occupational performance includes work activities, play or leisure activities, and ADL.

Obviously, an SCI can have a catastrophic effect on a person's ability to function in these areas, because it can affect performance components that support the ability to participate in these activities. Occupational performance components relevant to SCI include sensory integration and neuromuscular, motor, and psychosocial components. (See Table 11.4 for a summary of the occupational performance components affected by SCI.) The importance of understanding the theory of occupational performance cannot be overstated. We cannot begin to holistically treat a person with SCI

TABLE 11.4   Occupational Performance Profile

I. PERFORMANCE AREAS	II. PERFORMANCE COMPONENTS	III. PERFORMANCE CONTEXTS

A. Activities of Daily Living
  1. Grooming
  2. Oral Hygiene
  3. Bathing/Showering
  4. Toilet Hygiene
  5. Personal Device Care
  6. Dressing
  7. Feeding and Eating
  8. Medication Routine
  9. Health Maintenance
  10. Socialization
  11. Functional Communication
  12. Functional Mobility
  13. Community Mobility
  14. Emergency Response
  15. Sexual Expression
B. Work and Productive Activities
  1. Home Management
    a. Clothing Care
    b. Cleaning
    c. Meal Preparation/Cleanup
    d. Shopping
    e. Money Management
    f. Household Maintenance
    g. Safety Procedures
  2. Care of Others
  3. Educational Activities
	A. Sensorimotor Component
	  1. Sensory
	    a. Sensory Awareness
	    b. Sensory Processing
	      (1) Tactile
	      (2) Proprioceptive
	      (3) Vestibular
	      (4) Visual
	      (5) Auditory
	      (6) Gustatory
	      (7) Olfactory
	    c. Perceptual Processing
	      (1) Stereognosis
	      (2) Kinesthesia
	      (3) Pain Response
	      (4) Body Scheme
	      (5) Right–Left Discrimination
	      (6) Form Constancy
	      (7) Position in Space
	      (8) Visual–Closure
	      (9) Figure Ground
	     (10) Depth Perception
	     (11) Spatial Relations
	     (12) Topographical Orientation
	  2. Neuromusculoskeletal
	    a. Reflex
	    b. Range of Motion
	    c. Muscle Tone
	    d. Strength
	    e. Endurance
	    f. Postural Control
	    g. Postural Alignment
	    h. Soft Tissue Integrity
		A. Temporal Aspects
		  1. Chronological
		  2. Developmental
		  3. Lifecycle
		  4. Disability Status
		B. Environment
		  1. Physical
		  2. Social
		  3. Cultural

(continued)

TABLE 11.4   Occupational Performance Profile (Continued)

I. PERFORMANCE AREAS	II. PERFORMANCE COMPONENTS	III. PERFORMANCE CONTEXTS

4. Vocational Activities
  a. Vocational Exploration
  b. Job Acquisition
  c. Work or Job
    Performance
  d. Retirement Planning
  e. Volunteer Participation
C. Play or Leisure Activities
  1. Play or Leisure Exploration
  2. Play or Leisure
    Performance
	3. Motor
	  a. Gross Coordination
	  b. Crossing the Midline
	  c. Laterality
	  d. Bilateral Integration
	  e. Motor Control
	  f. Praxis
	  g. Fine Coordination/Dexterity
	  h. Visual–Motor Control
	  i. Oral–Motor Control
	B. Cognitive Integration and Cognitive Components
	  1. Level of Arousal
	  2. Orientation
	  3. Recognition
	  4. Attention Span
	  5. Initiation of Activity
	  6. Termination of Activity
	  7. Memory
	  8. Sequencing
	  9. Categorization
	  10. Concept Formation
	  11. Spatial Operations
	  12. Problem Solving
	  13. Learning
	  14. Generalization
	C. Psychosocial Skills and Psychological Components
	  1. Psychological
	    a. Values
	    b. Interests
	    c. Self-Concept
	  2. Social
	    a. Role Performance
	    b. Social Conduct
	    c. Interpersonal Skills
	    d. Self-Expression
	  3. Self-Management
	    a. Coping Skills
	    b. Time Management
	    c. Self-Control	

*NOTE: All Occupational Performance Areas are affected depending on degree of disability until we can visualize the impact that this diagnosis has on the various aspects of that person's life. The following sections explore occupational performance areas and components to present a comprehensive view of the impact of SCI.

Activities of Daily Living

Grooming, Oral Hygiene, Eating, Bathing, Dressing

For a person with quadriplegia, grooming, oral hygiene, and eating may be extremely laborious. The use of extensive adaptive devices or reliance on a caregiver may be necessary because of deficits in sensory and neuromuscular performance components. Persons with paraplegia are generally independent in these tasks, but they must often "think ahead," making sure that items are available and sufficient time is allocated.

Bathing and dressing present major challenges for persons with quadriplegia. With higher-level injuries (C1–C4), total assistance is required. At lower levels of injury, with extensive adaptive equipment and assistance from others in some task components, the person with quadriplegia can be a more active participant. It is extremely important for the person's own goals to be acknowledged. A recent study revealed that a person with a complete C6 injury required from 20 to 60 minutes to dress independently (19), yet none of the 10 patients in the study reported dressing themselves routinely after discharge from the hospital. Assistance was sought from others, because of feelings that the task was too time consuming and exhausting. The question becomes, "Is this functional?" If a person is attempting reentry into the work force or return to school, is it "functional" to spend an entire hour, as well as all the physical energy, in just getting dressed? Or is it a sign of greater autonomy to delegate some tasks to a caregiver to allow participation in activities that are more meaningful?

Secondary conditions aside, individuals with paraplegia are usually independent in bathing and dressing. Many even have the strength to transfer to the bottom of a tub without assistive devices.

Toileting

Managing altered bowel and bladder function is a challenge for everyone with SCI. The two aspects to this challenge are the actual physiological management and the various techniques and equipment used in the toileting process.

Medications may be required for physiological management. Stool softeners are used, as well as suppositories to assist in evacuation. A goal of effective bowel management is to eliminate reliance on medications. For persons with injuries at C7 or below, independence in toileting can usually be achieved with an array of equipment that may include suppository inserters, digital stimulators (devices that trigger reflexes to relax the rectal sphincter in UMN injuries), catheterization devices, leg separators, mirrors, and adapted commode chairs that allow access to the perianal area for bowel-training procedures.

Aside from medications and equipment, additional strategies include maintaining a specific schedule for elimination, eating a healthy diet that promotes regularity, assuming positions that facilitate elimination, and the use of Credé's method. If toileting appears to be tiring, then it has been portrayed correctly! But many persons with SCI become adept at its management. It may be a very different picture, though, when a person attempts these procedures in a community environment (i.e., rest rooms at work or school).

The person with a higher-level cervical injury faces another scenario. Although the bowel- and bladder-management concepts are the same, neuromuscular deficits limit performance of the tasks, even with adaptive equipment. Generally, persons with injuries above the C6 level require a caregiver to perform functions such as suppository insertion, digital stimulation, catheterization, and general perianal care. The person with SCI must indicate who the caregiver will be, particularly for tasks that are socially sensitive. Even though family members may be willing to assist, it is perfectly justifiable for the person to request someone else as a caregiver. Some persons may have no reservations about who assists them, whereas others may feel strongly that it would negatively affect established roles. Whatever the case, whenever feasible, the preferences of the person should be the deciding factor in selecting caregivers for various tasks.

Personal Device Care

The extent of personal and adaptive devices required by an individual with an SCI can generally be predicted by level of injury (Table 11.5). Additional complications, such as reduced range of motion resulting from contractures, may require use of more extensive devices than are typically seen at a particular level. Usually, personal device care is performed by others for those with injuries at C4 and above. Those with injuries at the C5 level and below have progressively more ability to assist in personal device care and use, but this fluctuates greatly depending on the individual's endurance, motivation, resources, and priorities.

Health Maintenance

Fostering a healthy lifestyle is critical, but often challenging, after an SCI. Most persons with an SCI are advised to follow life-long exercise programs to preserve and enhance range of motion and strength, as well as to promote good cardiovascular fitness and weight management. Many individuals report weight gains in the months after injury, as their energy demands are greatly altered in great part by use of a wheelchair for mobility. Attention also must be given to proper nutrition for weight management, impact on skin integrity, and bowel and bladder management. As

mentioned earlier, routine attention to skin condition is crucial to avoiding dermal complications. A health maintenance routine may require the assistance of others, depending on the level of injury, for such activities as setting up weights and equipment, performing passive range of motion, and aiding in skin inspection.

Socialization, Functional Communication, and Emergency Response

In pure SCIs, no cognitive deficits can preclude a person from socializing in an appropriate contextual manner. What is challenging, though, are the variety of barriers that may inhibit socialization. Architectural, environmental, and transportation barriers, reduced endurance, and increased reliance on others may discourage or actually prevent someone from traveling to the places where they socialized before their injury. Psychological barriers also may prevent reintegration into a premorbid social support system, and these "barriers" are as real as physical ones.

In all but the highest of injuries, verbal communication is functional. Persons with injuries at C7 or below are generally independent with a variety of forms of communication (e.g., writing, keyboard use, phone use) without the use of adaptive equipment. Above this level, however, adaptive devices are needed.

Requesting assistance in emergencies is possible at virtually all levels of injury, depending on the environment and adaptive equipment available. For persons with higher-level injuries, adaptive phone devices, emergency call systems, and environmental control units make contact with emergency agencies feasible. At the level of C4 and above, however, the availability of a caregiver 24 hours a day remains the most appropriate safety option. Individuals with injury below this level may use a phone independently but may be limited in other emergency responses, such as exiting a dwelling or attending to the physical needs of another injured person.

TABLE 11.5 Expected Functional Outcomes of Various Levels of Complete Injury (Noninclusive)

LAST SPINAL CORD LEVEL INTACT (SPARED)	EXPECTED FUNCTIONAL OUTCOME
C1–C3	Requires 24-hour availability of caregiver Generally ventilator-dependent Requires maximal assistance of another for pressure relief, or requires an adapted switch and reclining chair May propel power chair independently with adapted switches (pneumatic, chin, head, mouthstick); requires maximal assistance for set-up Maximal assistance needed for transfers, positioning, bed mobility, dressing, feeding, hygiene, grooming, and bowel/bladder care Dependent with driving
C4	Requires 24-hour availability of caregiver Generally not using ventilator; continued difficulty with productive coughing and deep breathing Pressure relief, wheelchair propulsion, transfers, bed mobility, dressing, hygiene, bowel/bladder care, and driving comparable to C1–C3 level Adaptive feeding and grooming devices are available; they are very time-consuming and exhaustive for a person at this level and generally do not result in task independence
C5	May require 24-hour availability of caregiver Decreased respiratory endurance, but not using ventilator A strong person with a C5 injury may be independent in pressure relief by leaning side to side; a weaker person may require maximal assistance. Independent on level surfaces with a power chair and occasionally wrist/forearm supports; a manual wheelchair with rim adaptations may be used by a strong person for short distances Moderate to maximal assistance is required for all transfers, and generally a sliding board is used Moderate assistance is required for bed mobility A strong person with a C5 injury may assist with some dressing, hygiene, and grooming activities with the aid of adapted equipment. Feeding is generally possible with the use of adapted utensils and set-up. Driving is generally not feasible at this level, but an exceptionally strong person may be able to drive with specially adapted steering, braking, and acceleration hand controls
C6	Amount of assistance needed from another person varies from moderate to very limited with just a few specific activities Some decrease in respiratory capacity and productive cough Has potential for independence in pressure relief Independently uses a manual wheelchair on level surfaces, gradual inclines, and down a curb backward. May require an electric chair for long distances or rough terrain. Ability to transfer varies. Some strong persons with C6 injuries are able to transfer independently with the use of a sliding board to a car, chair, bed, commode, or tubseat. Has the potential for independent bed mobility and positioning with rails, power controls, and trapeze With some adapted devices, usually independent with hygiene, shaving, and grooming. Potential for independence in bathing and bowel/bladder care with equipment. Generally independent with U.E. dressing, and potential for independence in L.E. dressing with adaptive devices. Independent with feeding, although a wrist–hand orthosis (WHO) and set-up may be required Generally able to drive independently using hand controls and adaptive devices.

(continued)

LAST SPINAL CORD LEVEL INTACT (SPARED)	EXPECTED FUNCTIONAL OUTCOME
C7–C8	May be able to live independently without attendent care Some decreased respiratory endurance Independent in pressure relief Independently uses manual wheelchair Generally able to transfer without a sliding board; very strong persons may be able to transfer to the floor and tub bottom independently Generally independent with positioning, bed mobility, hygiene, feeding, shaving, hair care, dressing, bathing, cooking, and light housekeeping. (Independent with bowel/bladder care using adaptive equipment/techniques) Drives independently with hand controls/steering adaptations Can stand in parallel bars once assisted to upright position, with the use of knee–ankle–foot orthoses (KAFOs)
T1–T3	Can live independently Respiratory capacity and coughing abilities significantly improved All transfers generally independent Independent with all self-care; may require assistance with heavy household cleaning Finger dexterity, strength, and coordination are functional Drives independently with hand controls. Can get own wheelchair in and out of car Able to stand with minimal assistance, KAFOs, and use of walker or parallel bars. Ambulation is generally not practical due to reduced balance and high energy expenditure.
T4–T8	Can live independently Respiratory status stronger than T1–T3 level; only slightly decreased Pressure relief, wheelchair use, positioning, bed mobility, and self-care all independent. May continue to require assistance with heavy cleaning Driving: comparable to T1–T3 level Generally able to ambulate short distances with the use of a walker or Loftstrand crutches and KAFOs. Can stand independently with the use of a walker. May be able to manage curbs or stairs, but generally requires assistance. Ambulation requires high energy output.
T9–T12	Respiration is functional Pressure relief, wheelchair use, transfers, positioning, bed mobility, self-care, homemaking (except heavy tasks) all independent Able to drive with hand controls Can generally ambulate short community distances with KAFOs and Loftstrand crutches
L1–L3	Same as T9–T12 level with the addition of improved ambulation distances; a wheelchair may still be required for long distances
L4–L5	Same as above, with exceptions Driving independent without adaptive devices Generally able to ambulate with ankle–foot orthoses (AFOs) and canes Wheelchairs generally not needed
S1–S2	A person with a S2-spared injury has the potential to ambulate without devices or orthoses A wheelchair is required. Hip extensors/abductors, knee flexors, and ankle plantar flexors are weak at the S1 level of injury. As with all other preceeding levels, bowel and bladder function is impaired but managed independently at this level through adapted devices/techniques

Developed with material from the Rehabilitation Institute of Michigan, 1996.

Functional Mobility

Persons with complete injuries at the T3 level and above usually rely on wheelchairs for household and community mobility. Those with injuries at C6 or above may require additional assistance in wheelchair management, or they may use an electric wheelchair with adapted controls. Acquiring an electric wheelchair may be a function of financial resources, not just need. Persons with complete injuries at T4 and below often can ambulate short distances with ambulation devices (walkers, Loftstrand crutches) and orthotic devices. Persons with sacral injuries often can ambulate community distances without orthoses or devices.

Sometimes it is not so much the ability or inability of the person with SCI but the inaccessibility of the environment that limits functional mobility. Whereas the home environment can be modified through creative thought, planning, and finances, the community environment is much harder to change. Many states have laws related to accessibility, but enforcement and compliance are less than ideal. Many physically challenged persons are fighting discriminatory situations (e.g., inaccessible public transportation, restaurants, offices, classrooms) in court. As these individuals become more numerous and visible, more legislation will be introduced to ensure their rights. A lighter side of the inaccessibility issue was recalled recently by Ed Roberts, founder of the first Center for Independent Living. He reminisced that early protestors in the disability rights movement were released from police custody because paddy wagons and jail cells were inaccessible (20)! In the vast majority of situations, however, an inaccessible environment is frustrating, demeaning, and personally violating. The health care team can do its part by helping physically, emotionally, or cognitively challenged persons to be aware of their rights, as well as by providing them with information on advocacy groups.

An extension of the functional mobility category includes driving. A strong C5-injured person may be able to drive with specially adapted low-effort steering, braking, and acceleration hand controls. Usually, those with injuries below the C5 level cannot drive because of physical and respiratory limitations. Persons with C6 injuries and below may be able to drive independently using hand controls and adaptive steering devices. A van with an electric lift may be recommended for someone who has difficulty maneuvering a wheelchair in and out of a car or van. Again, finances more than need may dictate the type of transportation used.

Sexual Expression

As with bowel and bladder function, most persons with SCI experience alterations in their ability to perform sexually as compared with their premorbid status. The nerves that innervate the genital area (both motor and sensory components) originate at the sacral spinal cord levels, so in the great majority of cases, sexual function is affected.

For the most part, the person can participate in a variety of sexual activities despite SCI, although the level of sensation and motor response will vary, depending on the extent and level of injury. Medications, surgical implants, and sexual enhancement devices may be recommended by specialists, but this is highly individualized.

Advances in the field of fertility have improved the chances for a spinal cord-injured male to father a child. Although fertility rates for men with SCI are estimated at less than 10% (21), techniques such as electrostimulation to induce ejaculation in paraplegics have proven successful in many cases (22). Men may be well advised to delay a decision about surgical penile implants until at least 1 year after injury. This allows time to evaluate the full impact of the SCI on sexual function and to determine the extent, if any, of sensory or motor return in an incomplete injury. The reproductive capabilities of women are generally unaltered by an SCI, and women and their partners should be made aware that the potential for pregnancy exists.

Addressing sexual function should be an integral part of each person's treatment plan, but a distinction should be made between purely physiological sexual performance—arousal, orgasm, ejaculation—and sexuality, which is the totality of a person's attractiveness, personality, and self-perception as a sexual being. Sexuality does not have to rely on physiology. Whereas performance may be hampered as a result of an SCI, one's sexuality can be quite healthy and intact. The health-care provider must make accurate information available and identify sources of more detailed information or expertise. It is entirely at the discretion of the person with an SCI to explore, or not explore, options available to them.

Work Activities

Home Maintenance

Tasks such as household maintenance, meal preparation, shopping, cleaning, clothing care, and safety procedures are included within the general category of home maintenance. Usually, persons with a C6-level injury or above require assistance with all of these activities and need some attendant care. Persons with injuries at C7 or lower can live independently (without attendant care) in accessible environments. Heavier home-maintenance tasks may be performed by others, but most routine activities can be accomplished with adaptive techniques and equipment.

Care of Others

An SCI can certainly make caring for others difficult, particularly if the injured person had been the primary care-giver for a child, spouse, or parent. Although a major goal of those with SCI is mastering self-care, a concurrent goal may be the introduction of activities (e.g., diapering, bathing a child) that can allow them to assume some premorbid roles. Often, many of these previous responsibilities must be delegated to others. In these cases, it is ideal if the person with SCI retains the responsibility for the verbal direction of care.

Education

Persons with SCI can generally resume educational activities, even while still inpatients in rehabilitation facilities. Many specialty hospitals retain the services of teachers from local school districts, and educational instruction is often scheduled along with other therapies for elementary, secondary, and high school students, allowing smoother reintegration after discharge.

College students would most likely be able to resume their studies. Depending on their level of injury, however, persons may reevaluate their course of study to prepare for a more feasible career.

Adaptive writing devices, page turners, tape recorders, and computers have made returning to the classroom less intimidating. Laws have also improved the accessibility of public buildings, such as schools. It is challenging for the student to manage bowel and bladder schedules, adjustment of clothing, eating devices, and so forth, but with planning and the assistance of others, if needed, many individuals have successfully returned to the classroom.

Vocational

It is appropriate for a person with any level of SCI to begin to formulate vocational options, even as an inpatient, with the members of the health-care team. Individual situations are so variable—premorbid occupation, level of injury, educational level, other vocational interests, family support, cognitive abilities, motivation, financial resources—making it impossible to say whether a person with a certain level of SCI can or cannot be gainfully employed. However, legislation mandates that work sites be accessible, within reason. Also, many employers recognize the importance of a trained employee and will make additional accommodations to return a valued person to the workplace.

As we move from an industrial to an information society, the job market will change, with positions requiring less menial labor (and being better compensated) than previously. Job requirements for this "new society" will include analytical thought, problem solving, and creativity, all of which are certainly intact after a spinal cord injury!

Leisure Activities

For most people, leisure pursuits are an integral part of a meaningful life. Although an SCI can alter the way in which one participates in leisure activities, it does not have to change the intensity of participation.

Sports, both individual and team, are excellent leisure pursuits that are growing in popularity for persons with SCI. Virtually any sport can be undertaken, from basketball to tennis to archery. True, adaptive equipment and modified regulations help make some sports more feasible and competitive for persons with SCI, but most athletes use "adaptive" equipment. How long would a catcher last in baseball without a mitt and a mask? Adaptive equipment need not detract from the legitimacy of the contest. It is heartening to see that, even internationally, the wheelchair athlete is recognized for excellence, with designated events in the Olympic games. Persons with SCI who want to participate have numerous avenues open to them.

Aside from sports, opportunities for social activities from square dancing to traveling abound. Travel agencies and tour groups have recognized the market created by the wheelchair traveler and have responded. Most hospitals with specialized SCI rehabilitation units have well-established programs that help persons get involved with special interest groups. Often, during the acute phase of SCI, persons cannot envision themselves participating again in the things they enjoy. The health care professional must be available for these individuals to encourage renewed interest in favorite leisure activities.

Several resources related to leisure activities, as well as other issues, have been discussed in this chapter. The reader is encouraged to consult the References and Suggested Readings at the end of this chapter for more information. Additionally, Table 11.5 gives an overview of specific expected outcomes for each level of SCI.

CASE STUDIES

CASE 1

M. L. is a 19-year-old woman who sustained an SCI during a motor vehicle accident while on her honeymoon. Her husband was thrown from the vehicle but received only minor injuries. M. L. was transported by EMS to the local emergency department. She was diagnosed with a C5–6 vertebral subluxation and a C6 crush injury, resulting in a complete C6 spinal cord injury. She also sustained a left clavicular fracture. She received nasal O_2 for respiratory support. Once stabilized, she was transferred to the specialized trauma center near her home. A halo vest was applied, which stabilized her cervical spine. No operative procedures were indicated at that time. After 22 days, her endurance improved so that she could tolerate sitting upright in a chair for up to 1 hour. She was transferred to the nearby rehabilitation facility's SCI unit. During her 12 weeks there, the only complications she experienced were two episodes of autonomic hyperreflexia (apparently secondary to hard stool in the lower rectum) and a mild UTI. Spasticity developed in her wrists, elbows, and lower extremities.

Before her injury, M. L. was a college student in a liberal arts curriculum. She and her new husband had recently signed a 1-year lease on an upstairs apartment close to the university. She had been totally independent in all of her ADL and home-management activities. Her leisure pursuits included recreational team sports (particularly softball) and more sedentary activities like reading and gourmet cooking. She was also involved with her family, particularly two sisters and her parents, who live close by.

Many occupational performance components are significantly affected by M. L.'s injury. Her sensorimotor deficits are consistent with those anticipated for a C6 complete quadriplegia.

M. L. is challenged by the psychosocial/psychological issues facing her as a result of her SCI. She feels that her role has changed significantly, especially in her relationship with her husband. He has been willing to assist her in those activities in which she is physically limited; however, his assistance in some activities—particularly bowel management—has been difficult for her to accept. This has been a source of frustration for her, and she has discussed with him the possibility of hiring an attendant on a limited basis to assist with specific activities. He resists this idea, stating that it is his desire and duty to care for her. He took a temporary leave of absence from the family-owned landscaping company where he is employed when she was discharged 2 weeks ago. There is no definite timetable for his return. M. L. also is concerned about her ability to express herself sexually, as well as her potential to have children in the future. She attended classroom sessions on these topics in the rehabilitation facility, but she did not seek any individual counseling. M. L. states that she probably wasn't ready to hear anything specific then, but she now wishes she had someone of whom she could ask questions.

M. L. has not begun to consider her work activities or return to school. Even before her accident, she had been undecided about a career path. She has expressed interest, however, in exploring possible alternatives.

M. L. has stated that eventually she might like to get involved in team sports again. In the 2 weeks since her discharge, though, her main leisure pursuits have been reading and watching television.

POINTS FOR REVIEW

1. What are the major causes of SCI?

2. Why is it so important to analyze the etiology of SCI?

3. What are the two major classifications of SCI and what do they mean?

4. What is a UMN injury and what are its characteristics?

5. Describe the syndromes associated with incomplete injuries.

6. What is tetraplegia?

7. How does the ASIA classify SCI?

8. Trace the progression of an SCI from acute to postspinal shock.

9. At what level of injury will people have respiratory complications? Explain.

10. Describe changes in muscle tone that may occur with SCI.

11. Why is it important for persons with SCI to have routine bladder voiding?

12. What are the complications associated with bowel function?

13. What are the major reasons for hospital readmissions for persons with SCI?

14. In discussing prognosis with a person with an SCI, what will his or her focus often be, as opposed to that of the health care professional?

15. Is there potential for regeneration of a damaged spinal cord in humans? What current research is being conducted in this effort?

16. Describe the impact of an SCI on occupational performance for someone who has tetraplegia.

REFERENCES

1. Guttmann L. Spinal Cord Injuries. Oxford, England: Blackwell Scientific, 1976.

2. Hanak M, Scott A. Spinal Cord Injury: An Illustrated Guide for Health Care Professionals. New York: Springer Publishing, 1983.

3. Woodruff BA, Baraon RC. A description of nonfatal spinal cord injury using a hospital based registry. Am J Prev Med 1994;10:10–14.

4. American Spinal Injury Association/International Medical Society of Paraplegia. International Standards for Neurological and Functional Classification of Spinal Cord Injury. Chicago: American Spinal Injury Association, 1992:5.

5. American Spinal Injury Association/International Medical Society of Paraplegia. International Standards for Neurological and Functional Classification of Spinal Cord Injury. Chicago: American Spinal Injury Association, 1992:27.

6. Aids to Investigation of Peripheral Nerve Injuries. Medical Research Council War Memorandum. 2nd ed. Revised. London, HMSO, 1943.

7. Brunnstrom F, Dennen M. Round table on muscle testing. Annual Conference of American Physical Therapy Association, Federation of Crippled and Disabled, Inc., New York, 1931:1–12.

8. Hislop H, Montgomery J, Connelly D, eds. Muscle Testing: Techniques of Manual Examination. 6th ed. Philadelphia: Saunders, 1995.

9. Lovett RW. The Treatment of Infantile Paralysis. 2nd ed. Philadelphia: P. Blakiston's Son, 1917:136.

10. Yashon D. Spinal Injury. 2nd ed. East Norwalk, CT: Appleton-Century-Crofts, 1986:35–36.

11. Bloch RF, Basbaum M. Management of Spinal Cord Injuries. Baltimore: Williams & Wilkins, 1983: 153–154.
12. Hanak M, Scott A. Spinal Cord Injury: an Illustrated Guide for Health Care Professionals. New York: Springer Publishing, 1983:30.
13. Burke DC, Murray DD. Handbook of Spinal Cord Medicine. New York: Raven Press, 1975:67.
14. Hernandez AM, Fjorner JV, DeLaFuente T, et al. The paraarticular ossifications in our paraplegics and tetraplegics: a survey of 704 patients. Paraplegia 1978;16:272–275.
15. Cassell BL. Treating pressure sores stage by stage. RN 1986;49:36.
16. Bracken M, Holeord TR, Shepard MJ, et al. A randomized, controlled trial of methylprednisolone or naloxone in the treatment of acute spinal cord injury. N Engl J Med 1990;322(20):1405–1411.
17. Pipp TL. Mobilizing hope. Detroit News, September 15, 1997:1–2B.
18. NeuroControl Corporation, Cleveland, 1997.
19. Weingarden S, Martin C. Independent dressing after spinal cord injury: a functional time evaluation. Arch Phys Med Rehabil 1989;70:518–519.
20. Price D. Building lives with no barriers. Detroit News Washington Bureau, March 18, 1990:17–23A.
21. Berczeller PH, Bezkor MF. Medical Complications of Quadriplegia. Chicago: Year Book Medical Publishers, 1986:165.
22. Perkash I, Martin D, Warner H, et al. Electroejaculation in spinal cord injury patients: simplified new equipment and technique. J Urol 1990;143:305–307.

SUGGESTED READINGS

General Texts Relating to SCI

American Spinal Injury Association/International Medical Society of Paraplegia. International Standards for Neurological and Functional Classification of Spinal Cord Injury. Chicago: American Spinal Injury Association, 1992.

Berczeller PH, Bezkor MF. Medical Complications of Quadriplegia. Chicago: Yearbook Medical Publishers, 1986.

Buchanan LE, Nawoczenski DA. Spinal Cord Injury: Concepts and Management. Baltimore: Williams & Wilkins, 1987.

Ozer MN. The Management of Persons with Spinal Cord Injury. New York: Demos Publications, 1988.

Treischmann R. Spinal Cord Injuries: Psychological, Social and Vocational Rehabilitation. 2nd ed. New York: Demos Publications, 1988.

Whiteneck G, Lammertse D, Manley S, et al. The Management of High Quadriplegia. New York: Demos Publications, 1989.

Yashon D. Spinal Injury. 2nd ed. East Norwalk, CT: Appleton-Century-Crofts, 1986.

Patient/Family Resources

Corbet B. Options: Spinal Cord Injury and the Future. Denver: A. B. Hirschfield, 1980.

Hammond M, Umlauf RL, Matteson B, et al. Yes You Can! A Guide to Self Care for Persons with Spinal Cord Injury. Washington, DC: Paralyzed Veterans of America, 1989.

Phillips L, Ozer A, Axelson P, et al. Spinal Cord Injury: A Guide for Patient and Family. New York: Raven Press, 1987.

General Neuroanatomy

Barr ML. The Human Nervous System: An Anatomic Viewpoint. 3rd ed. New York: Harper & Row, 1979.

Liebman M. Neuroanatomy Made Easy and Understandable. 3rd ed. Rockville, MD: Aspen Publishers, 1986.

Functional Electrical Stimulation

Kralj A, Bajd T. Functional Electrical Stimulation: Standing and Walking after Spinal Cord Injury. Boca Raton: CRC Press, 1989.

CHAPTER 12

BURNS

Nancy Cox

CRITICAL TERMS

Allograft	Debridement	Mesh graft
Autograft	Eschar	Partial thickness burn
Cellulitis	Epithelialization	Sheet graft
Collagen	Hypertrophic scar	

She awoke coughing and choking. Her eyes were open, but she was unable to see anything except blackness and smoke. She crawled toward the door, down the hall, and found her way out to the front lawn of the house. Later when asked, she did not remember how she got out of the burning house. She does recall being on her hands and knees, coughing and hearing a neighbor say, "This lady over here is burned," and realizing that the neighbor was referring to her. This is the story told to an occupational therapy student after he asked his patient what she remembered about the house fire.

ETIOLOGY

Agents responsible for burns may be thermal, chemical, or electrical (1). In the United States, scalds are the most frequent source of burn injuries that require hospital admission (2). Thermal injuries sustained in household fires are the leading cause of burn fatality in the United States (3). Household fires account for approximately 4% of annual hospital admissions (3). Approximately 1100 deaths occur from electric current each year. Within this group of burns, approximately one-third occur in the home (3). Causes of burn injuries vary; however, the good news is that, overall, instances of burns are on the decline in the United States. Based on U.S. Vital Statistics reports, deaths attributed to fire, flames, and hot liquids have dropped an estimated 40% from 1971 to 1991 (4).

Decreases in the national incidence of thermal injuries are attributed to many variables. These include the development of a national network of burn centers, wide dissemination of fire and burn prevention devices and programs, and regulation of consumer product and occupational safety (4).

THE INTEGUMENTARY SYSTEM

Skin is the largest organ of the human body (5). The functions of the skin are many:

- Serves as a thermoregulatory system
- Transmits sensory feedback from the environment
- Serves as a barrier to external objects/organisms
- Provides cosmetic function
- Serves as part of the immune system (5)

Structurally the skin is composed of two distinctively different layers—the epidermis and the dermis (6). Subcutaneous fat lies beneath the epidermis and dermis (6) (Fig 12.1).

The Epidermis

The epidermis is the outermost layer of the skin and is composed of four layers. These layers are: the stratum corneum, stratum granulosum, stratum spinosum, and basal cell layer of keratinocytes (5). The epidermis replaces itself in 45 to 75 days by generating new cells at the basal cell layer and sloughing off dead cells at the most superficial layer, the stratum corneum (7). Melanocytes are cells located primarily in the epidermis and they provide skin pigmentation (7). Other structures within the skin that are lined with epidermis are hair follicles and sebaceous and eccrine sweat glands (7). Eccrine sweat glands are found throughout the body and have a primary role in regulation of body temperature (8). The interface between the epidermis and dermis is referred to as the basement membrane (9). Microscopic rete pegs interconnect the two primary subdivisions of the skin at the basement membrane (7).

The Dermis

The dermis is composed of two divisions—the papillary and reticular layers (5). The dermis is composed primarily of the protein collagen, which provides the skin with its tensile strength (10).

The papillary dermis is the most superficial of the two dermal divisions (5). The papillary dermis encloses the skin's microcirculatory blood and lymphatic plexuses (5). The reticular dermis is described as being primarily avascular and is comprised of dense connective and collagenous tissue (5). Beneath the reticular dermis lies subcutaneous fat, fascia, muscle, and bone. Signs and symptoms that occur with differing levels of tissue destruction determine the depth of the burn. The following section contains a description of the signs and symptoms that signal the depth of the burn.

DETERMINING DEPTH AND SEVERITY OF BURN

Four major factors influence the degree of cutaneous involvement with burn injuries: duration of exposure, temperature, heat source, and skin thickness (11). Burn wound classification has been divided into three subdivisions, based on depth: superficial, or first degree; partial thickness—either superficial or deep, second degree; and full thickness, or third degree. A diagrammatic representation of the level of burns is provided in Figure 12.1.

Superficial, or First Degree, Burns

Burns at this level are limited to the epidermis and are characterized by erythema, edema, and pain (11). Superficial burns will heal in 3 to 7 days without scarring, if infection is prevented. These wounds are painful because the nerve endings that propagate sensory afferents are not damaged.

Superficial Partial Thickness, or Second Degree, Burns

Limited to the epidermis and papillary dermis, superficial partial thickness burns are characterized by erythema, edema, pain, and blistering (12). These wounds are painful and will blanch to touch. Healing will occur in 14 to 21 days with negligible scarring, if infection is prevented (13).

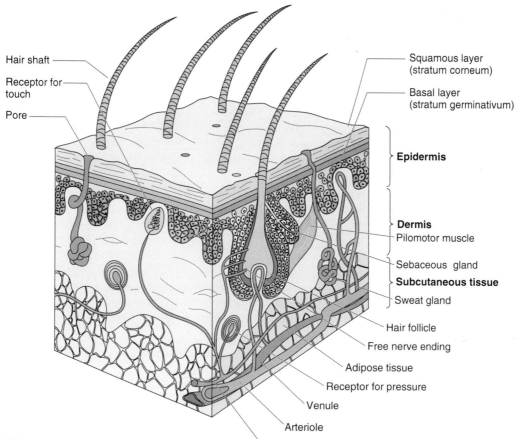

FIGURE 12.1 The skin. (Reprinted with permission from Clark G, Wilgis E, Aiello B, et al. Hand Rehabilitation, A Practical Guide. 2nd ed. New York: Churchill Livingston, 1997:30.)

Deep Partial Thickness, or Second Degree, Burns

This level of burn involves the epidermis and papillary and reticular layers of the dermis. These burns appear mottled and white. They do not blanch to touch in the areas where the reticular dermis is involved, because the microvasculature supply has been destroyed. The patient will complain of pain in areas where the dermis remains intact, but the burn will be anesthetic in the deeper areas of reticular involvement (11). Deep partial thickness burns will heal in 4 to 6 weeks if there is no infection and the total body surface area (TBSA) involved is not too great (14). Deep partial thickness burns that heal will develop hypertrophic scarring and burn scar contractures if left untreated (14).

Full Thickness, or Third Degree, Burns

These burns are characterized by destruction of the epidermis, dermis and subcutaneous fat, and they may involve fascia, muscle, and bone. The burn wound is not painful, because the sensory afferents have been destroyed. The wounds appear white and leathery, and no blisters are present in the full thickness area. Full thickness wounds involving a large TBSA will require skin grafting to close the area. Full thickness wounds that are allowed to heal from the periphery of uninvolved skin will take a considerable time to close and hypertrophic scarring will occur (13).

In 1981 the American Burn Association published guidelines to differentiate between burns

TABLE 12.1 Classification of Burn Severity

Minor burn
15% TBSA or less of a first and second degree burn in an adult
10% TBSA or less of a first and second degree burn in a child
2% TBSA or less of a third degree burn in child or adult not involving eyes, ears, face, or genitalia

Moderate burn
15 to 25% TBSA second degree burn in an adult
10 to 20% TBSA second degree burn in a child
2 to 10% TBSA third degree burn in child or adult not involving eyes, ears, face, or genitalia

Major burn
Greater than 25% TBSA second degree burn in an adult
Greater than 20% TBSA second degree burn in a child
Greater than 10% TBSA third degree burn in child or adult
All burns involving eyes, ears, face, hands, feet, or genitalia
All inhalation injuries
Electrical burns
Complicated burn injuries involving fractures, head injury, or other major trauma
All patients who are at high risk, with preexisting conditions such as cerebrovascular accidents,
    psychiatric disability, emphysema and other lung diseases, cancer, diabetes, etc.

defined as minor, moderate, and major (15). The intent in publishing guidelines was to help health care providers determine whether a person with a burn could be treated in an outpatient, rather than an inpatient, setting. Burn injury classifications—minor, moderate, and major— are shown in Table 12.1 (15).

Minor burn injuries, as defined by the American Burn Association, may be treated in an outpatient setting. Regular follow-up appointments are scheduled to assess the patient's progress. Persons with moderate burns should be admitted. The individual and his or her family need to learn necessary care to facilitate wound closure. Burns defined as major should be referred to, and treated in, a center that specializes in the treatment of severe burn injuries. At present, 138 such centers have been designated in the United States (3). Burn centers are staffed with multidisciplinary teams to address the medical, psychosocial, and rehabilitative needs of burn victims.

INCIDENCE AND PREVALENCE

According to the American Burn Association, 2,000,000 people in the United States receive med-

ical treatment for burn injuries each year (16). Of these, the following information is known (17):

- 500,000 will receive medical treatment in an emergency department
- 70,000 require hospitalization as a result of the thermal injury
- 7,800 die as a result of their burn injury
- 67% are male
- 30 to 40% of these patients are younger than age 15

DIAGNOSIS

Despite the advent of technological advances to define burn wound depth, such as laser Doppler flowmetry, nuclear magnetic resonance imaging, and thermography, the standard technique for determining burn depth is still clinical observation by an experienced physician (18). With burn wounds, it is imperative to recognize that they can change; a burn wound that appears to be a superficial partial thickness injury on day 1 may become a deep partial thickness wound on day 3. The physician is guided by the signs and symptoms of superficial, partial, and full thickness burns to formulate a medical plan of intervention.

MEDICAL/SURGICAL MANAGEMENT

In the initial evaluation of a burn injury, the physician must assess the depth, location, and extent of involvement of the body. The estimation of TBSA is a critical factor in determining the severity of thermal injury (15). Two methods of determining TBSA are widely used: the rule of nines and the Lund and Browder chart see Figures 12.2 and 12.3. The Lund and Browder chart was developed to assess more accurately the area of involvement in persons younger than age 10 (14).

Burn recovery consists of three stages: emergent, acute, and rehabilitative. The emergent stage is the period from the initial insult until 48 to 72 hours after injury. During this phase, fluid resuscitation is initiated when burns are more than

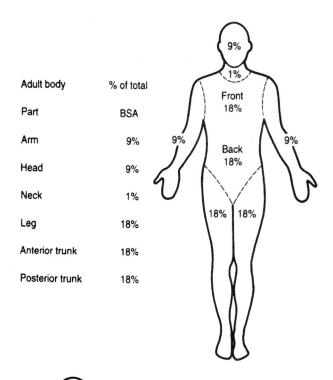

Adult body	% of total
Part	BSA
Arm	9%
Head	9%
Neck	1%
Leg	18%
Anterior trunk	18%
Posterior trunk	18%

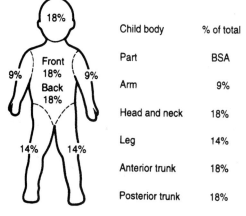

Child body	% of total
Part	BSA
Arm	9%
Head and neck	18%
Leg	14%
Anterior trunk	18%
Posterior trunk	18%

FIGURE 12.2 Estimation of burn size using the Rule of Nines. (Reprinted with permission from Hernden D. Total Burn Care. London: WB Saunders, p. 35.)

Age	0–1	1–4	5–9	10–14	15
A – $\frac{1}{2}$ of head	$9\frac{1}{2}$%	$8\frac{1}{2}$%	$6\frac{1}{2}$%	$5\frac{1}{2}$%	$4\frac{1}{2}$%
B – $\frac{1}{2}$ of one thigh	$2\frac{3}{4}$%	$3\frac{1}{4}$%	4%	$4\frac{1}{4}$%	$4\frac{1}{2}$%
C – $\frac{1}{2}$ of one leg	$2\frac{1}{2}$%	$2\frac{1}{2}$%	$2\frac{3}{4}$%	3%	$3\frac{1}{4}$%

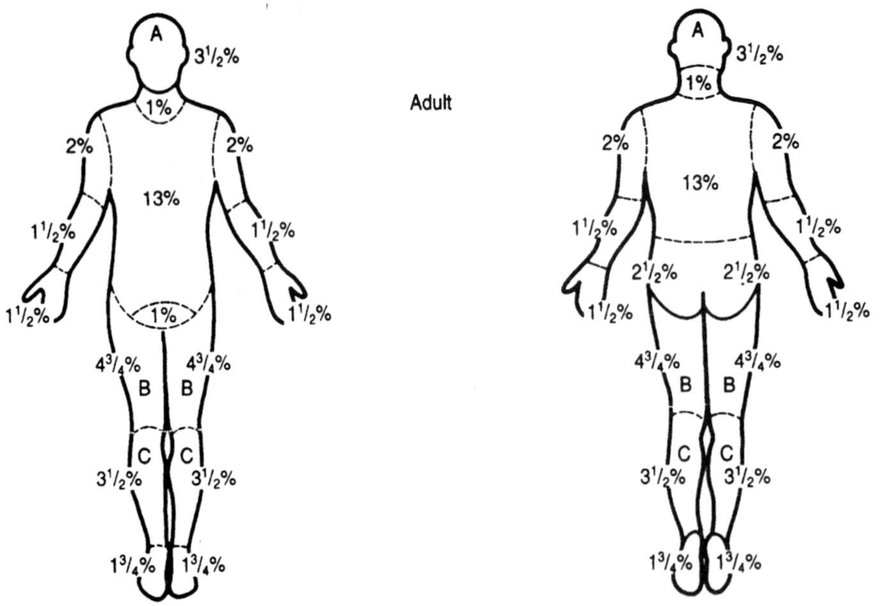

FIGURE 12.3   Estimation of burn size using the Lund and Browder method. (Reprinted with permission from Hernden D. Total Burn Care. London: WB Saunders, p. 36.)

20% TBSA. Fluid resuscitation is initiated to prevent the occurrence of hypovolemic shock. Hypovolemic shock occurs as a result of decreases in cardiac output, plasma volume, and extracellular fluids. Intravenous fluids are initiated to prevent the onset of hypovolemia. Before the 1940s, hypovolemic shock was identified as the leading cause of death from burns (18). In present-day medical practice, 50% of burn deaths occur within the first 10 days after initial injury for those with burns over extensive TBSA, and one of the most significant contributors to burn mortality continues to be inadequate fluid resuscitation (18).

Once the person is stabilized, the acute stage of intervention proceeds. This stage begins at 72 hours after the initial injury and continues until the burn wound is closed. Burn wounds are considered closed when they have been grafted or have healed spontaneously. Spontaneous epithelialization will occur in partial thickness wounds, if infection is prevented, through the provision of appropriate wound care (19). The cells that form over an open wound to provide a protective barrier are called "epithelium." Epithelialization is the process whereby the epithelium moves from the edges of the uninvolved tissue and remaining skin appendages, such as hair follicles and sweat glands, to cover the wound. It is a physiological process that allows superficial partial thickness wounds to close without surgical intervention.

Wound care to promote wound closure is the primary focus in the acute phase.

The objectives of wound care are to prevent bacterial wound invasion, remove dead tissue (eschar), prepare the wound for skin grafting, if indicated, and promote wound closure. Wound care is typically provided in hydrotherapy or during a shower. The patient's wounds are either immersed or sprayed with water to facilitate removal of the burn dressing and topical antimicrobial medication. These substances are applied directly to the cleansed burn wound to suppress the growth of or to kill bacteria (20). Silver sulfadiazine, sodium hypochlorite (NaClO), silver nitrate ($AgNO_3$), mafenide acetate (Sulfamylon), povidone-iodine, and gentamicin sulfate are topical antimicrobials currently used (20). Silver sulfadiazine is the topical antimicrobial agent that is used most often worldwide (21). After the topical agent is applied, a gauze covering or wrap is placed over the wound. Dressing changes occur in a clean and sterile environment once or twice daily.

All wounds have bacterial growth; however, the level of this growth is critical. Small pieces of the patient's burned tissue are microscopically examined to determine the level of bacterial growth in the wound. Bacterial counts higher than 100,000 organisms/gram of tissue will lead to wound sepsis (22). The clinical signs of burn wound sepsis are hypothermia or hyperthermia, congestive heart failure (CHF) in a patient with no prior history, mental confusion, and the onset of respiratory distress (22). Burn wound sepsis is treated with topical antimicrobial agents and antibiotic medications (20).

Surgical excision or debridement is used to remove infected tissue and to prepare the wound bed for skin grafting. Debridement is done by either tangential or fascial excision. When the bacterial count is less than 100,000 organisms/gram of tissue, the wound may be grafted. Burn wound excision is performed in the operating room under sterile conditions, typically with the patient under general anesthesia. Tangential excision of the burn wound is sequential removal of necrotic, or dead, layers of tissue until there is bleeding (23). This procedure is used for patients with partial thickness injuries. It is usually performed with an instrument called a dermatome, which allows the surgeon to remove very small layers of tissue at a time. The instrument is typically set at 0.005 to 0.01 inch, thus preserving viable underlying tissue (24). Fascial excision is used for deep, full thickness injuries (23). In this procedure, all nonviable tissue is removed, down to the fascial layer of muscle or deeper—through muscle—if necessary. Once necrotic tissue has been removed, the physician determines what type of grafting will be needed to close the wound.

Biological and synthetic materials are used for skin grafting or wound coverage. An autograft is biological tissue taken from the patient and transferred to his or her wound for long-term coverage. Individuals with large, deep, partial and full thickness burns will require autografting for wound closure. The autograft is harvested from the patient's unburned skin and may either be split or full thickness. Split thickness skin grafts (STSG) are generally 0.007 to 0.016 inches in thickness (25). The area where the skin is harvested is called the donor site. Split thickness skin grafts may either be sheet or meshed grafts, but sheet grafts are preferred because they contract (shrink) less than meshed grafts. Sheet grafts are used to cover the face, hands, neck, and joint surfaces. Meshed autografts are made with an instrument called a mesher. Skin grafts are meshed to try to enlarge a piece of skin to cover a greater area. Meshed grafts have small holes, referred to as interstices, punched into them. Interstices will heal from the surrounding autograft and underlying epidermal appendages. Full thickness skin grafts (FTSG) are harvested from the donor site down to, but not including, the subcutaneous fat (25). They are from 0.025 to 0.030 inches thick (25) and are used for areas of the body that require more durable skin, such as the soles of the feet or palmar surface of the hand. Once STSGs and FTSGs are applied, they are usually secured in place with sutures or staples.

Homografts or allografts are biological tissues used to cover burn wounds. A homograft is tissue taken from the same species and used as a temporary covering. They provide the patient with a barrier against fluid loss, decrease his or her pain because the nerve endings are covered, decrease the total number of dressing changes, provide a barrier against the influx of microorganisms, and promote wound closure (26). Homografts are harvested from cadavers and will eventually be rejected by the recipient, usually within 14 days of application (27). Homografts can be applied at bedside or in the operating room.

The autografted area will be immobilized for 4 to 5 days postoperatively (26). Immobilization protects the skin graft from shearing forces and allows for the growth of capillaries that promotes adherence (26). Splints and other positioning devices are used to prevent deformity positions. After burn wound coverage is completed, the patient moves into the rehabilitative stage of recovery.

The rehabilitative stage is described as the time from wound coverage until the burn scar has matured. Burn scar maturation extends from 2 to 24 months after the initial injury (28). Hypertrophic scarring and scar contractures are associated with burn scar maturation in deep partial and full thickness burns. The major unresolved problems in the rehabilitative phase are poor cosmetic results and functional impairment (29).

Complications

The incidence of hypertrophic scarring and burn scar contractures can be sharply decreased through proper positioning, splinting, range-of-motion activities, stretching, and the provision of pressure garments. Despite considerable scientific investigation, the pathophysiology of hypertrophic scarring is still unknown (30). The goal of pressure garment therapy is to prevent or diminish hypertrophic scars (31). Research has shown that pressure garments must be worn 23 hours daily to decrease the incidence of hypertrophic scars. Customized garments are made to be worn over the involved area. The patient should begin wearing them within 2 weeks after wound closure (32). The garments should provide at least 15 mm Hg of capillary pressure to prevent undesired changes in the scar tissue (32).

The formation of burn scar contractures is another complication for persons with partial and full thickness burns. As with hypertrophic scarring, burn scar contracture formation is not completely understood (33). Despite the uncertainties related to the formation of burn scar contractures, it appears they develop as a result of excessive wound tension (33). The anatomical regions associated with the highest incidence of contractures are, in order of occurrence: the head and neck, axilla, and hand (33). Splinting, positioning modalities, and pressure therapy help to decrease the incidence of both hypertrophic scarring and burn scar contractures (33).

IMPACT ON OCCUPATIONAL PERFORMANCE

The impact of a burn injury on a person's occupational performance depends on the size, location, and depth of the burn. Table 12.2 lists all the occupational performance components and areas. Those in bold print are the components and areas that may be affected. A person who has sustained a burn can have any combination of the listed deficits.

The major performance component compromised by a burn is sensorimotor. Tactile sensory processing, pain response, range of motion, and soft tissue integrity are the areas most affected. If an individual has sustained a deep partial thickness or full thickness burn, it can be assumed that the reticular dermis is damaged and the collagen and elastin fibers have been disrupted. These areas of burn injury will form hypertrophic scars. Hypertrophic scarring that crosses a joint or comes close to a joint will reduce the range of motion at that joint. Until scar tissue is mature, it will continue to contract unless an opposing force stops it. It is important during the acute and rehabilitative phases of treatment to evaluate

TABLE 12.2   Occupational Performance Profile

I. PERFORMANCE AREAS	II. PERFORMANCE COMPONENTS	III. PERFORMANCE CONTEXTS

A. Activities of Daily Living
  1. Grooming
  2. Oral Hygiene
  3. Bathing/Showering
  4. Toilet Hygiene
  5. Personal Device Care
  6. Dressing
  7. Feeding and Eating
  8. Medication Routine
  9. Health Maintenance
  10. Socialization
  11. Functional Communication
  12. Functional Mobility
  13. Community Mobility
  14. Emergency Response
  15. Sexual Expression
B. Work and Productive Activities
  1. Home Management
    a. Clothing Care
    b. Cleaning
    c. Meal Preparation/
      Cleanup
    d. Shopping
    e. Money Management
    f. Household
      Maintenance
    g. Safety Procedures
  2. Care of Others
  3. Educational Activities
  4. Vocational Activities
    a. Vocational Exploration
    b. Job Acquisition
    c. Work or Job
      Performance
    d. Retirement Planning
    e. Volunteer Participation
C. Play or Leisure Activities
  1. Play or Leisure Exploration
  2. Play or Leisure
    Performance
	A. Sensorimotor Component
	  1. Sensory
	    a. Sensory Awareness
	    b. Sensory Processing
	      (1) Tactile
	      (2) Proprioceptive
	      (3) Vestibular
	      (4) Visual
	      (5) Auditory
	      (6) Gustatory
	      (7) Olfactory
	    c. Perceptual Processing
	      (1) Stereognosis
	      (2) Kinesthesia
	      (3) Pain Response
	      (4) Body Scheme
	      (5) Right–Left Discrimination
	      (6) Form Constancy
	      (7) Position in Space
	      (8) Visual–Closure
	      (9) Figure Ground
	     (10) Depth Perception
	     (11) Spatial Relations
	     (12) Topographical Orientation
	  2. Neuromusculoskeletal
	    a. Reflex
	    b. Range of Motion
	    c. Muscle Tone
	    d. Strength
	    e. Endurance
	    f. Postural Control
	    g. Postural Alignment
	    h. Soft Tissue Integrity
	  3. Motor
	    a. Gross Coordination
	    b. Crossing the Midline
	    c. Laterality
	    d. Bilateral Integration
	    e. Motor Control
	    f. Praxis
	    g. Fine Coordination/Dexterity
	    h. Visual–Motor Control
	    i. Oral–Motor Control
		A. Temporal Aspects
		  1. Chronological
		  2. Developmental
		  3. Lifecycle
		  4. Disability Status
		B. Environment
		  1. Physical
		  2. Social
		  3. Cultural

(continued)

TABLE 12.2   Occupational Performance Profile   (Continued)

I. PERFORMANCE AREAS	II. PERFORMANCE COMPONENTS	III. PERFORMANCE CONTEXTS

	B. Cognitive Integration and Cognitive Components
	  1. Level of Arousal
	  2. Orientation
	  3. Recognition
	  4. Attention Span
	  5. Initiation of Activity
	  6. Termination of Activity
	  7. Memory
	  8. Sequencing
	  9. Categorization
	  10. Concept Formation
	  11. Spatial Operations
	  12. Problem Solving
	  13. Learning
	  14. Generalization
	C. Psychosocial Skills and Psychological Components
	  1. Psychological
	    a. Values
	    b. Interests
	    c. Self-Concept
	  2. Social
	    a. Role Performance
	    b. Social Conduct
	    c. Interpersonal Skills
	    d. Self-Expression
	  3. Self-Management
	    a. Coping Skills
	    b. Time Management
	    c. Self-Control	

Components and areas in boldface may or may not be affected, depending on depth of the burn in combination with percentage and location of TBSA affected.

range of motion and skin tightness daily. Tactile sensation will be diminished or absent depending on burn depth and will require evaluation and subsequent education.

A burn will also affect psychosocial skills and psychological components. The appearance of hypertrophic scars and the possible loss of body parts will affect the person's self-concept. Loss of function will compromise role performance. Pain and deformity will challenge an individual's premorbid coping skills and techniques. The combination of these affected components may lead to depression. The extent to which occupational performance areas are affected depends on the severity of the burn and the body areas involved. For example, a small, less than 10% TBSA, partial thickness burn injury affecting the dominant anterior forearm and extending onto the wrist and palm will initially impair all activities of daily living, most work and productive activities, and all play/leisure pursuits. These impairments are caused by edema in the dominant upper extremity, loss of range of motion at the elbow, wrist, and hand, and pain throughout the whole upper extremity; however, they will not result in long-term functional deficits. A larger, greater than 30% TBSA, deep partial thickness or full thickness burn will have long-term implications in all performance areas. The area of burn location will determine specific performance areas affected.

CASE STUDIES

CASE 1

R. W., 8 months old, sustained a 10% TBSA burn injury when he was 6 months old. His 2-year-old brother accidentally set R. W.'s shirt on fire when playing with a cigarette lighter. R. W.'s mother is 19 years old and stays at home to take care of the two boys. R. W.'s father is also 19 and works two jobs to support his family. They have no health insurance coverage and are awaiting Medicaid approval to cover the medical costs.

R. W. has a circumferential full thickness burn injury to his left hand and wrist. On his left forearm, he has a circumferential deep partial thickness burn that extends from his antecubital area to his midarm. He has a half-dollar–size deep partial thickness burn on the lateral anterior surface of his left foot.

R. W. underwent initial debridement and autografting on his fourth day after injury. His entire left upper extremity and the area on his left foot were autografted and immobilized in custom-fabricated splints. Active range of motion was initiated 4 days after surgery. He had full flexion and extension at his left elbow but limited range of motion at his wrist and the digits of his left hand. Edema, pain, and necrotic tissue at each digit tip limited range of motion. The autografts adhered to his left foot and left forearm and elbow but had sloughed off his digits and portions of his hand. Further debridement and autografting, in two separate operations, were necessary. Ultimately, digits 1 to 5 were amputated at the metacarpophalangeal joints.

R. W.'s mother found it difficult to visit with her younger son while he was hospitalized. She found it difficult to care for her 2-year-old son and to attend to R. W.'s needs. Consequently, his mother did not visit regularly and when she did, it was for short periods. After 8 weeks of hospitalization, R. W. was ready for discharge. When he was admitted in the emergency department, a Child Protective Services form was filed and a case subsequently opened. At discharge, R. W. was cleared to go home, but the case was still under investigation. Outpatient therapy was set up for three times a week.

At the time of discharge, R. W. had several sensorimotor deficits including the areas of sensory processing, neuromusculoskeletal, and motor. Tactile sensory processing of input was diminished because of the depth of burn, and he experienced hypersensitivity. He was required to wear his wrist flexion and elbow extension splints, except during structured playtime. This was necessary as he was developing significant scarring.

Neuromusculoskeletal components of range of motion, strength, postural alignment, and soft tissue integrity were all affected. R. W. had loss of range of motion of left wrist flexion and left forearm supination. Full elbow extension could only be achieved with passive range of motion and a long sustained stretch. He would not initiate active range of motion with his left upper extremity except at the shoulder.

Affected motor components included gross coordination, crossing the midline, bilateral integration, motor control, and fine coordination/dexterity. During therapy sessions, when R. W.'s splints were removed, he was only beginning to use his left upper extremity to prop or weight shift. He would not use his left arm in any bilateral tasks, such as rolling, scooting, or any precrawling positions.

Activities of daily living and play or leisure activities are the occupational performance areas that have been affected. Feeding, eating, and functional mobility are the areas that are important for R. W. He uses his right upper extremity for finger feeding but will not attempt to use his left arm to assist with holding his bottle. He often will attempt to use his feet to substitute for his left upper extremity. R. W. uses only his right arm during functional mobility tasks and often cries with frustration when he fails.

As previously noted, R. W. does not use bilateral upper extremity movement. When sitting, he will use his lower extremities to assist with toy manipulation and for toy stabilization, as his left foot has healed and is not hypersensitive. He is becoming proficient with this method of play. His preferred play position is sitting. However, he cannot assume this position on his own.

CASE 2

R. M., a 62-year-old electrician, sustained a 40% TBSA flash burn from an electrical box explosion at work. He has deep partial thickness burns to the dorsa of both hands and to his midchest to lower abdomen. Partial thickness burns are located on his bilateral palmar surfaces, circumferentially around his forearms, face, anterior and right lateral sides of his neck, and his upper chest. It is 6 days since his injury and 4 days since his operative procedure of debridement and a combination of allografting and autografting. R. M. has allografts on both forearms and his upper chest. Autografts are located on the dorsa of his hands and his midchest to abdomen. His donor sites are located on his anterior and lateral thighs. He has been immobilized in bilateral intrinsic plus-position hand splints since surgery. Today is the first day he can initiate range of motion with his hands. He has participated in therapy for facial exercises since the day of his admission.

R. M. has been married for 43 years. He has three adult sons, two of whom live out of state. His wife works outside the home as a realtor. She does not like the sight of blood and cries when she visits. R. M. has expressed concerns about what his skin is going to look like, when his pain is going to decrease, and who will take care of him when he goes home.

All of R. M.'s occupational performance areas are affected. He is dependent for all activities in all performance areas because of both the loss of function in his hands and the pain from his donor sites. This injury also has affected his sensorimotor and psychosocial skills and psychological components. Depth of burn, pain, and edema all affect his tactile and visual sensory processing, range of motion, and his soft tissue integrity. R. M. has already begun to express concern regarding his self-concept, role performance, and coping skills. He has been a highly independent person and does not like asking others for help. Needing assistance to feed himself is very difficult for R. M. He also has expressed concern at how his wife will be able to assist him, as she has difficulty looking at his wounds, especially his face. As an electrician, he prides himself on his strength and ability to manipulate small electrical systems. He realizes that he has to take his rehabilitation one step at a time and will begin with achieving independence with basic self-care tasks.

POINTS FOR REVIEW

1. What are the five functions of the integumentary system?

2. Describe the four layers of the epidermis and the two layers of the dermis.

3. Describe each of the three classifications of a burn wound, based on depth.

4. Identify the details of the three classifications of burns according to severity.

5. What occurs at each of the three stages of burn recovery?

6. What major complications may occur after a burn?

REFERENCES

1. Johnson CL, O'Shaughnessy EJ, Ostergren G. Burn Management. New York: Press, 1981.
2. Baker SP, O'Neill B, Karpf RS. The Injury Fact Book. Lexington: DC Heath, 1984.
3. Pruitt BA, Mason AD. Epidemiological, demographic and outcome characteristics of burn injury. In: Herndon DN, ed. Total Burn Care. Philadelphia: WB Saunders, 1996.
4. Brigham PA, McLoughlin E. Burn incidence and medical care use in the United States: estimates, trends, and data sources. J Burn Care Rehabil 1996;17(2):95–104.
5. Odland GF. Structure of the skin. In: Goldsmith LA, ed. Biochemistry and physiology of the skin. New York: Oxford University Press, 1983.
6. Jakubovic HR, Ackerman B. Structure and function of skin: development, morphology and physiology. In: Moschella SL, Hurley HJ, eds. Dermatology. Philadelphia: WB Saunders, 1985.
7. Falkel JE. Anatomy and physiology of the skin. In: Richard RL, Staley MJ, eds. Burn Care and Rehabilitation: Principles and Practice. Philadelphia: FA Davis, 1994.
8. Patterson JW, Blaylock WF. Dermatology. New York: Medical Examination, 1987.
9. Pinnell SR, Marud S. Collagen. In: Goldsmith LA, ed. Biochemistry and Physiology of the Skin. New York: Oxford University Press, 1983.

10. Linares HA. Pathophysiology of the burn scar. In: Herndon DN, ed. Total Burn Care. Philadelphia: WB Saunders, 1996.

11. Zalar GL, Harber LC. Cutaneous reactions to heat. In: Moschella SL, Hurley HJ, eds. Dermatology. Philadelphia: WB Saunders, 1985.

12. Artz DP, Moncrief JA. The Treatment of Burns. Philadelphia: WB Saunders, 1969.

13. Johnson C. Pathologic manifestations of burn injury. In: Richard RL, Staley MJ, eds. Burn Care in Rehabilitation: Principles and Practice. Philadelphia: FA Davis, 1994.

14. Warden GD. Outpatient management of thermal injuries. In: Boswick JA. The Art and Science of Burn Care. Rockville: Aspen, 1987.

15. Warden GD, Kravitz M, Schnelby A. The outpatient management of moderate and major thermal injury. J Burn Care Rehabil 1981;2:159–161.

16. Herndon DN, Rutan RL, Rutan TC. Management of the pediatric patient with burns. J Burn Care Rehabil 1993; 4(1):3–7.

17. American Burn Association. Hospital and prehospital resources for optimal care of patients with burn injury: guidelines for development and operation of a burn center. J Burn Care Rehabil 1990;11(2):98–100.

18. Warden GD. Burn shock resuscitation. World J Surg 1992;16:16–23.

19. Sorenson B. Closure of the burn wound. World J Surg 1978;2:167–174.

20. Heggers J, Linares HA, Edgar P, et al. Treatment of infections in burns. In: Herndon DN, ed. Total Burn Care. Philadelphia: WB Saunders, 1996.

21. Robson MC. Bacterial control in the burn wound. Clin Surg 1979; 6(4):515–522.

22. Robson MC. Infection in the surgical patient: an imbalance in the normal equilibrium. Clin Surg 1979;6(4):493–503.

23. Heimbach DM. Early excision and grafting. Surg Clin North Am 1987;67(1):93–106.

24. Muller MJ, Nocolai M, Wiggins R, et al. Modern treatment of a burn wound. In: Richard RL, Staley MJ, eds. Burn Care and Rehabilitation: Principles and Practice. Philadelphia: FA Davis, 1994.

25. Miller SF, Staley MJ, Richard RL. Surgical management of the burn patient. In: Richard RL, Staley MJ, eds. Burn Care and Rehabilitation: Principles and Practice. Philadelphia: FA Davis, 1994.

26. Alsbjorn BF. Biologic wound coverings in burn treatment. World J Surg 1992;16(1):43–46.

27. Greenhalgh DG, Staley MJ. Burn wound healing. In: Richard RL, Staley MJ, eds. Burn Care and Rehabilitation: Principles and Practice. Philadelphia: FA Davis, 1994.

28. Hurren JS. Rehabilitation of the burned patient: James Laing memorial essay for 1993. Burns 1997;21:126.

29. Monafo WN, Bessey PQ. Benefits and limitations of burn wound excision. World J Surg 1992;16(1):37–42.

30. Mann R, Yeong EK, Moore M, et al. Do fitted pressure garments provide adequate pressure? J Burn Care Rehabil 1997;18:247–249.

31. Staley MJ, Richard RL. Scar management. In: Richard RL, Staley MJ, eds. Burn Care and Rehabilitation: Principles and Practice. Philadelphia: FA Davis, 1994.

32. Kraemer MD, Jones T, Deitch EA. Burn contractures: incidence, predisposing factors, and results of surgical therapy. J Burn Care Rehabil 1988;9(3):261–264.

33. Larson DL, Abston S, Evans EB, et al. Techniques for decreasing scar formation and contractures in the burned patient. J Trauma 1971;2(10):809–822.

CHAPTER 13

PROGRESSIVE NEUROLOGICAL DISORDERS

Diane K. Dirette

CRITICAL TERMS

Agnosia	Dysarthria	Neurogenic bowel/bladder
Cogwheel rigidity	Electroencephalogram	Nystagmus
Demyelination	Myelin	Optic neuritis
Dysesthesia	Myelogram	Orthostatic intolerance

Shortly after the birth of her second child, J. started getting the sensation of pins and needles in her legs. Within a couple of weeks, she noticed some weakness in her arms and legs. She was having difficulty walking for long distances and began to worry that she might drop her 2-year-old son or even her newborn. When the children napped in the afternoon, she found herself slumped on the couch for a much-needed rest. Convinced that this was just part of her postpartum recovery, J. did not inform her doctor of this difficulty. However, when she found herself struggling one day to focus on the words of her son's bedtime story, she decided to seek medical advice.

Over time, J. found out she had a progressive neurological disorder (PND) called multiple sclerosis (MS). Progressive neurological disorders are a group of diseases that affect various areas of the central nervous system (CNS), are chronic in nature, and cause a deterioration of function over time. This chapter discusses three of the most common PNDs: MS, Parkinson's disease, and amyotrophic lateral sclerosis (ALS).

Multiple sclerosis is a PND in which the immune system attacks the myelin sheath of neurons in the CNS (1–4). The location of demyelination varies from person to person. The visual, motor, sensory, cognitive, psychological, and bowel and bladder systems can be affected.

Parkinson's disease is a PND caused by dysfunction of the substantia nigra, a system of nerve cells in the basal ganglia (5). Dysfunction in the substantia nigra leads to reduced amounts of dopamine in the corpus striatum, a group of nerve cells in the deep gray matter of the cerebral hemisphere (6, 7). This leads to deficits in the speed and quality of motor movements, postural stability, cognitive skills, and affective expression (6, 8).

Amyotrophic lateral sclerosis is a PND that causes progressive degeneration of the motor neurons in the corticospinal pathways, the motor nuclei of the brainstem, and the anterior horn cells of the spinal cord (9, 10). Degeneration of motor neurons leads to progressive atrophy of muscles, usually beginning with the loss of strength in the small muscles of the hands or feet (3, 9). When the motor neurons are affected, the reflexes can become hyperactive. Progressive loss of muscle movement, difficulty speaking and swallowing, loss of emotional control, and reduced body temperature regulation (3, 9) are common.

ETIOLOGY

There is no known cause of any of these three PNDs, but recent research indicates that etiology is a combination of interrelated factors (5, 11). These include genetic predisposition, viruses, and environmental influences.

A genetic predisposition is suspected because these diseases are more prevalent among families and certain racial groups. For example, twins studies have shown that if one twin has MS, the other is more likely to have it as well, if the pair is identical rather than fraternal (4). Immediate relatives of a person who has MS are 12 to 20 times more likely than an unrelated person of the same ethnicity living in the same climate to have the disease develop. Also, as many as 50% of people with Parkinson's disease have an affected relative.

Viruses and their resulting autoimmune response also may be involved as an external cause of these PNDs. Specific viruses have not been isolated, but particular interest has been focused on a viral subgroup called retroviruses. What causes them is unknown, and they can remain silent for years before the onset of disease.

Environmental factors, including exposure to such toxins as lead or pesticides, also have been associated with a higher incidence of PND (7, 11, 12). None of these factors, however, have been isolated as the single cause.

INCIDENCE AND PREVALENCE

The incidence and prevalence of these three PNDs vary depending on the diagnosis. Currently, an estimated 250,000 to 350,000 people in the United States have MS (2), and the distribution of these individuals varies geographically. The closer a person lives to the equator, the less likely he or she is to have MS (4). For example, in the southern United States, the rate of incidence is 20 to 39/100,000. In the northern United States and Canada, the rate is more than 40/100,000 (4).

Worldwide, the prevalence of Parkinson's disease is estimated at 1% of the population, with an estimated 500,000 cases in the United States (6). These cases appear to be evenly distributed throughout the world, based on available diagnoses. Diagnostic data, however, vary from one medical care system to another.

The distribution of people with ALS is estimated to be 2/100,000 people worldwide, with the exception of Guam and the Kii peninsula of Japan where the rates are higher (9, 13, 14). The high rates in this area have been attributed to consumption of the seeds of a neurotoxic plant, *Cycas circinalis,* which causes an ALS-parkinsonism dementia. Ongoing investigation indicates the possibility of increasing prevalence of ALS worldwide (13).

The incidence of these PNDs also varies according to gender. Multiple sclerosis affects females more often than males at a ratio of 1.7:1 (2). Parkinson's disease has been reported to affect males slightly more than females, but recent studies report an equal distribution among the genders (6). Amyotrophic lateral sclerosis affects males more often than females with a ratio of 1.6:1 (9).

Multiple sclerosis occurs more frequently among people of European ancestry than other white racial groups. It is twice as common among Caucasians than other races; it is rare among Japanese or Chinese people (4). Parkinson's disease occurs in all races worldwide (6). However, in the United States, there is a lower incidence among African-Americans than Caucasians (7). Amyotrophic lateral sclerosis occurs uniformly worldwide.

SIGNS AND SYMPTOMS

Multiple Sclerosis

Some of the more common symptoms of MS include visual deficits, sensory disturbances such as dysesthesia or paresthesia, urinary incontinence or retention, muscle weakness and spasticity, gross and fine motor incoordination, fatigue, ataxia, dysphagia, dysarthria, and cognitive or emotional disturbances. Each person with MS has symptoms that result from lesions in specific areas of the CNS. The types of symptoms, their intensity, and their effects on the person's functional status are highly individualized (15). Table 13.1 includes a summary of common signs and symptoms.

Visual disturbances often are among the earliest signs of MS. They usually appear as a partial loss of vision (scotoma), double or blurred vision, or ocular pain. Sudden loss of vision with pain in or behind the eye is caused by optic neuritis. These early symptoms may subside after 3 to 6 weeks without any residual deficit. For others, visual loss may be insidious and painless. Nonetheless, nearly 80% of all persons who have MS have some loss of visual acuity.

Oculomotor control also may be affected, caused by lesions of the supranuclear connection to the oculomotor nuclei in the brainstem. As a result, the person loses horizontal eye movement either unilaterally or bilaterally.

The individual with MS can experience a variety of other sensory disturbances such as numbness; impairment of vibratory, proprioceptive, pain, touch, and temperature sensation; and distortion of superficial sensation. Because of these sensory losses, the person also may lose various perceptual skills such as stereognosis, kinesthesia, and body scheme (16).

Fatigue is the most common complaint and is often identified as the most debilitating symptom (3, 15). Increased energy is required for nerves to conduct their impulses in a demyelinated nervous system, making it difficult for the individual to initiate movement and perform sustained

---

TABLE 13.1   Common Signs and Symptoms of Multiple Sclerosis

Tactile awareness
*Numbness
*Disturbances in pain sensation
*Hypersensitivity

Motor
*Spasticity
*Limitations in tolerance/low energy
*Weakness
*Ataxiclike symptoms
*Intention tremor

Visual
*Double vision
*Pain behind the eyes

*Blurred vision
*Partial blindness/scotoma
*Nystagmus

Cognitive
*Memory loss or disturbance
*Difficulty with complex ideas
*Decreased attention span

Psychological
*Depression or euphoria
*Impulsivity
*Lability

Taken in part from Umphred DA, ed. Neurological Rehabilitation. 1st ed. St. Louis: CV Mosby, 1985:401.

activities. The individual also may experience muscle weakness. As the disease progresses, the person requires more frequent rest periods between activities, and decreased levels of activity lead to further debilitation.

Approximately 50% of individuals with MS experience some change in their cognitive ability. For some it is difficulty with verbal or spatial–motor memory (15). Others have disorders of judgment, decreased attention and concentration, various types of agnosia, or diminished ability to think conceptually (17).

An emotional component to this disease results in some individuals having bouts of depression, euphoria, or lability (17), thought to be caused by lesions in the frontal lobes of the brain.

Parkinson's Disease

The major symptoms of Parkinson's disease are resting tremor, cogwheel rigidity, bradykinesia, and postural changes (6, 7) (Table 13.2). The most obvious and familiar of these symptoms is tremor, which is usually noted initially in the hand on one side and sometimes in the foot. In the hand, the movement is frequently described as "pill-rolling." The tremors are usually variable. They disappear when the person is asleep or calmly resting and they increase under stress or intense mental activity (6).

Secondary symptoms of Parkinson's disease include gait disturbances, dexterity and coordination difficulties, involuntary immobilization, speech and swallowing difficulties, poor balance, oculomotor impairments, reduced facial expression, sleep disturbances, reduced bowel and bladder function, painful cramping, sexual dysfunction, low blood pressure, seborrhea, and fatigue (5–7). This array of symptoms varies among people with Parkinson's disease. Some people may not experience a specific symptom, whereas for another person, that symptom might be a major complaint.

Amyotrophic Lateral Sclerosis

The most common initial symptom of ALS is weakness of the small muscles of the hand or an asymmetrical foot drop (9). Night cramps, particularly in the calf muscles, also may be present. The signs and symptoms of ALS are progressive, most commonly in a distal to proximal pattern. The symptoms can be divided into three areas, including lower motor neuron, corticospinal tract, and corticobulbar tract dysfunction (Table 13.3).

The lower motor neuron dysfunction symptoms include focal and multifocal weakness, atrophy, cramps, and muscle twitching. Spasticity and hyperresponsive reflexes are associated with corticospinal tract dysfunction. Dysphagia and dysarthria are associated with corticobulbar dysfunction (9, 14).

TABLE 13.2   Primary and Secondary Signs and Symptoms of Parkinson's Disease

Primary signs and symptoms
Tremor (resting, pill-rolling)
Rigidity (cogwheel)
Bradykinesia (slowness of movement)
Postural changes (stooped, unsteady)

Secondary signs and symptoms
Gait disturbances (shuffle, reduced reflexes, falling)
Impaired dexterity and coordination
Involuntary immobilization (freezing)
Speech difficulties (soft, monotone, rapid)
Swallowing difficulties (drooling)

Poor balance
Oculomotor impairments (deficits in fixation, scanning, tracking)
Reduced facial expression
Sleep disturbances
Reduced bowel and bladder function
Painful cramping of muscles
Sexual dysfunction
Low blood pressure
Sensory disturbances (numbness, tingling, burning sensations)
Seborrhea (oily skin, dandruff)
Fatigue

TABLE 13.3 Signs and Symptoms of Amyotrophic Lateral Sclerosis

Lower motor neuron
Focal and multifocal weakness
Atrophy (progressive; distal to proximal)
Muscle cramping
Muscle twitching (fasciculation)

Corticospinal tract
Spasticity
Hyperreactive reflexes

Corticobulbar tract
Dysphagia (difficulty swallowing)
Dysarthria (impaired quality of speech production)

COURSE AND PROGNOSIS

Multiple Sclerosis

All three of these PNDs are progressive. Multiple sclerosis is usually diagnosed between the ages of 20 and 40 years (4). It is rarely seen in children or diagnosed in adults older than age 50. No two people with MS follow the same course, and each person experiences variability in symptoms over time (2). The clinical course of this disease can be roughly organized into four types or patterns. The first is benign, in which the person experiences one or two episodes of neurological deficits with no residual impairments. This person's chance of remaining symptom free increases with each non-symptomatic year. The next pattern of progression is relapsing–remitting–nonprogressive. In this pattern the person returns to the previous level of function after each exacerbation. With the third type, relapsing–remitting–progressive, however, the person has some residual impairments with each remission. Finally, there is the progressive pattern, which involves a steady decline in function without remissions and exacerbations. Individuals with MS may shift from one pattern to another, with no reliable predictors of these shifts (3, 18, 19).

Overall, about 60% of individuals with MS remain fully functional up to 10 years after their first exacerbation, and about 30% remain functional 30 years after their first attack (20). In a longitudinal study conducted in 1971, more than two-thirds of subjects were ambulatory 25 years after onset (21). In spite of the seriousness of this disease, it does not significantly decrease the person's life expectancy. A few people, however, do become severely disabled and die prematurely because of recurring infections or complications resulting from inactivity (16, 20).

Parkinson's Disease

Parkinson's disease is usually first diagnosed when a person is older than 50 years (7). The average onset age is about 60 years. It rarely affects people younger than age 40 (6).

As with MS, the progression of Parkinson's disease differs with each person. In general, Parkinson's disease is a slow, progressive disorder (5). The clinical scale by Hoehn and Yahr divides Parkinson's disease into five stages, as follows:

Stage I: Signs of Parkinson's disease are strictly one-sided, affecting one side of the body only.
Stage II: Signs of Parkinson's disease are bilateral and balance is not impaired.
Stage III: Signs of Parkinson's disease are bilateral and balance is impaired.
Stage IV: Parkinson's disease is functionally disabling.
Stage V: Patient is confined to bed or a wheelchair.

Progression through these stages is variable for each person. Usually, a person will have Parkinson's disease for 15 to 20 years before entering the most severe stages. There are also fluctuations within each stage. The loss of function is not a linear progression. Each person experiences some periods of improvement scattered throughout the progressive loss of function. Because of advances in medical treatment, life expectancy is not significantly affected by a diagnosis of Parkinson's disease.

Amyotrophic Lateral Sclerosis

The age of onset of ALS occurs between 16 and 77 years, but it is usually diagnosed when a person is between the ages of 50 and 70 years (14). The course of ALS is usually progressive and relatively rapid. The duration of survival after diagnosis is usually 1 to 5 years, with a mean survival of three years (9, 14). The younger a person is and the more mild the symptoms at the time of diagnosis, the longer the course. There is some evidence of a "resistance in ALS," in which a person may demonstrate improvements and live longer than 10 years. This is seen in approximately 10 to 16% of people with ALS (14).

DIAGNOSIS

All three of these PNDs require skilled practitioners to put together the pieces of the puzzles that lead to diagnoses. No definitive laboratory tests exist for the diagnosis of any of these PNDs. Often the diagnosis is made through observation of the clinical picture and elimination of other possible causes for the presenting symptoms.

Multiple Sclerosis

To make a definitive diagnosis of MS, the physician examines the person's medical history, symptoms reported by the person, and signs detected by various tests (2). These tests include magnetic resonance imaging (MRI) to detect plaques or lesions in two distinct areas of the central CNS, neurological examination, evoked potentials (visual, brainstem auditory and somatosensory), and spinal tap to assess cerebral spinal fluid proteins. The results of these diagnostic procedures help contribute to a diagnosis of MS, but they do not determine the diagnosis independently. Many other conditions can elicit positive results. The physician and the individual must work together to rule out other causes before a diagnosis can be made.

A definitive diagnosis of MS is made when the person has episodes of exacerbation and remission and slow or step-by-step progression over 6 months. There also must be evidence of lesions in more than one site in the white matter (as determined by MRI) and no other neurological explanation for the clinical picture (16).

Parkinson's Disease

To determine a diagnosis of Parkinson's disease, the physician observes the current symptoms, eliminates other diseases as the cause of those symptoms, and evaluates the person's response to medications used to treat Parkinson's disease (7). At least one of the primary symptoms (resting tremor, rigidity, bradykinesia, or postural instability) is always present. Several tests, such as computerized axial tomography (CAT) scan, MRI, or electroencephalogram (EEG), are used to eliminate the possibility of other neurological disorders. The physician may also use a positron emission tomography (PET) to detect a loss of dopamine, which is indicative of Parkinson's disease.

Amyotrophic Lateral Sclerosis

To make a definite diagnosis of ALS, the physician pieces together clinical symptoms, electromyogram (EMG) results, and tests to exclude other causes of the clinical presentation (9, 14). The EMG findings will include motor denervation and fasciculation (twitching) with intact sensory responses. A CT scan or MRI of the CNS may be used to rule out other causes of the symptoms. Blood tests are usually normal. Cerebrospinal fluid is often normal but may show raised protein levels.

MEDICAL/SURGICAL MANAGEMENT

For each of the PNDs discussed in this chapter, surgical intervention is not part of the routine care given. Several medications are used to alleviate the myriad of symptoms caused by each of these diseases (Table 13.4).

TABLE 13.4 Occupational Performance Profile

I. PERFORMANCE AREAS	II. PERFORMANCE COMPONENTS	III. PERFORMANCE CONTEXTS
A. **Activities of Daily Living**	A. **Sensorimotor Component**	A. **Temporal Aspects**
1. Grooming	1. Sensory	1. Chronological
2. Oral Hygiene	a. Sensory Awareness	2. Developmental
3. Bathing/Showering	b. Sensory Processing	3. Lifecycle
4. Toilet Hygiene	(1) Tactile	4. Disability Status
5. Personal Device Care	(2) Proprioceptive	B. **Environment**
6. Dressing	(3) Vestibular	1. Physical
7. Feeding and Eating	(4) Visual	2. Social
8. Medication Routine	(5) Auditory	3. Cultural
9. Health Maintenance	(6) Gustatory	
10. Socialization	(7) Olfactory	
11. Functional Communication	c. Perceptual Processing	
12. Functional Mobility	(1) Stereognosis	
13. Community Mobility	(2) Kinesthesia	
14. Emergency Response	(3) Pain Response	
15. Sexual Expression	(4) Body Scheme	
B. **Work and Productive Activities**	(5) Right–Left Discrimination	
1. Home Management	(6) Form Constancy	
a. Clothing Care	(7) Position in Space	
b. Cleaning	(8) Visual–Closure	
c. Meal Preparation/	(9) Figure Ground	
Cleanup	(10) Depth Perception	
d. Shopping	(11) Spatial Relations	
e. Money Management	(12) Topographical	
f. Household	Orientation	
Maintenance	2. Neuromusculoskeletal	
g. Safety Procedures	a. Reflex	
2. Care of Others	b. Range of Motion	
3. Educational Activities	c. Muscle Tone	
4. Vocational Activities	d. Strength	
a. Vocational Exploration	e. Endurance	
b. Job Acquisition	f. Postural Control	
c. Work or Job	g. Postural Alignment	
Performance	h. Soft Tissue Integrity	
d. Retirement Planning	3. Motor	
e. Volunteer Participation	a. Gross Coordination	
C. **Play or Leisure Activities**	b. Crossing the Midline	
1. Play or Leisure Exploration	c. Laterality	
2. Play or Leisure	d. Bilateral Integration	
Performance	e. Motor Control	
	f. Praxis	
	g. Fine Coordination/Dexterity	
	h. Visual–Motor Control	
	i. Oral–Motor Control	

(continued)

TABLE 13.4 Occupational Performance Profile (Continued)		
I. PERFORMANCE AREAS	**II. PERFORMANCE COMPONENTS**	**III. PERFORMANCE CONTEXTS**
	B. Cognitive Integration and Cognitive Components	
	1. Level of Arousal	
	2. Orientation	
	3. Recognition	
	4. Attention Span	
	5. Initiation of Activity	
	6. Termination of Activity	
	7. Memory	
	8. Sequencing	
	9. Categorization	
	10. Concept Formation	
	11. Spatial Operations	
	12. Problem Solving	
	13. Learning	
	14. Generalization	
	C. Psychosocial Skills and Psychological Components	
	1. Psychological	
	a. Values	
	b. Interests	
	c. Self-Concept	
	2. Social	
	a. Role Performance	
	b. Social Conduct	
	c. Interpersonal Skills	
	d. Self-Expression	
	3. Self-Management	
	a. Coping Skills	
	b. Time Management	
	c. Self-Control	

The medications most often prescribed to treat the symptoms of MS include antispasmodics, muscle relaxants, and anticonvulsants. The medications usually prescribed to treat the symptoms of Parkinson's disease include dopamine replacement medications, acetylcholine inhibitors, and antiviral compounds. The medications prescribed to treat the symptoms of ALS include antispasmodic medications, nonsteroidal anti-inflammatory medications, and antibiotics.

IMPACT ON OCCUPATIONAL PERFORMANCE

Each of these PNDs is progressive and can affect all occupational performance components and performance areas. The extent of this effect depends on the stage and severity of the disease. Table 13.4 lists all the components and areas that may be affected. In each case, a person may have any combination of the deficits listed.

Activities of Daily Living

Self-care skills are affected by changes in the person's sensorimotor skills. Changes are usually noted in gross and fine motor coordination, postural control, muscle tone, endurance, and sensation (except in ALS).

Toileting can become problematic for persons with MS or Parkinson's disease because of the loss of bladder and bowel control. The individual may experience any combination of the complications noted earlier in this chapter.

Eating may be difficult, either because the person loses the strength and coordination to self-feed or because of chewing or swallowing difficulties (dysphagia). The latter is caused by weakness or incoordination of the pharyngeal musculature, which also can make it difficult for an individual to ingest oral medications.

Dysarthria or imperfect articulation is caused by a lack of control of the tongue and other oral muscles essential to speech. This problem can affect the person's ability to communicate thoughts, needs, and desires and can limit social interaction. The individual may lose upper extremity function, making it difficult to compensate for speaking problems with written communication.

Functional mobility is another critical concern. Neuromuscular and motor problems make ambulation difficult or impossible, either independently or with assistive devices, even in an electrically propelled wheelchair. Acquiring alternate methods of mobility requires the ability to adapt. The person must be able to change motor patterns, requiring concurrent new and varied perceptual and cognitive strategies. At the same time, the individual is challenged psychologically to make the necessary adjustments to new and different types of mobility. As the person's function decreases, issues of home and work accessibility must be considered, and the necessary adaptations must be made to maintain critical occupational performance.

Because of depression and diminished self-concept, the person may no longer feel attractive, which causes problems in sexual expression. Also, loss of specific motor and sensory function can affect physical performance.

Communication, mobility, sexual dysfunction, and eating problems may all affect the person's normal socialization with individuals or groups. This leads to secondary psychosocial problems because of lifestyle changes. These PNDs require an initial social–psychological adjustment as well as continual readjustment because of erratic progression of symptoms. A person who was active and outgoing may have a diminished self-concept because of the inability to engage in activities that were once of interest and value. The result is a variety of role changes in the family or society.

Role expectations, which exist in every social situation, are ways of behaving or reacting that fit with one's self-image and the expectations of others. These include attitudes, activities, and patterns of decision-making, expressing feelings, and meeting the needs of significant others (22). Some individuals with loss of bladder control may avoid going out in public. Mothers may be unable to care for their children. Some may come to see themselves as no longer useful or attractive to others. Marriages may break up under the strain of living with PNDs. Occasionally, individuals with PNDs threaten suicide. An individual with a PND must think seriously about current role expectations and how these might be threatened by the PND (22).

Work

All performance components have the potential to affect work activities. Work is a crucial area of occupational performance and, for many adults, is an important part of self-identity.

As motor skills decline, the ability to perform specific work tasks also declines. "Invisible symptoms" such as fatigue, weak or blurred vision, and difficulties with bladder control often confound the issue. Co-workers may not understand why someone who does not look ill cannot work. Again, this affects the person psychologically, with changes in societal roles and self-concept. This is particularly true for an individual whose job requires a high degree of physical stamina and skill. For example, assembly workers or truck drivers may lose their jobs fairly early in the course of these diseases. An individual who has been the breadwinner of the family and whose identity is closely tied to physical strength and endurance may have serious adjustment problems. Cognitive deficits also may make it difficult for the person to function and continue to find satisfaction in work.

A normal work activity for many persons with PND is the care of others, including a spouse or significant other, children, or older, dependent adults. The individual with a PND may have increasing difficulty fulfilling this role. In fact, he or she may have to rely on these care receivers to provide support and care, creating a major role reversal. These changes in responsibilities can be very stressful for all concerned; they challenge everyone's ability to maintain the integrity of relationships.

Play and Leisure

Many leisure activities can be affected by the changes that result from PNDs. Alternative leisure activities must be explored as more and more performance deficits occur. A balance between work and play should be maintained as long as possible. However, if the person can no longer engage in usual work and daily living activities, it is even more critical to have meaningful and fulfilling leisure pursuits. These activities will grow in importance as a means of self-actualization and satisfaction.

Progressive neurological disorders may cause dysfunction in all performance components and occupational performance areas. Because of the unpredictable nature of the course of each PND, potential dependency issues are ongoing problems. The following cases illustrate how this condition changed three people's lives.

CASE STUDIES

CASE 1

Multiple Sclerosis

M. A. is a 28-year-old woman who was diagnosed with MS 5 years before this hospital admission. She was admitted because she noticed a progressive

deterioration of function during the past 6 months. The main problems she identifies are an increase in fatigue, difficulty with bowel and bladder function, and numerous falls from her wheelchair.

She is married and has two children, an 11-year-old girl and a 5-year-old boy. She is not employed outside the home. Her husband works full-time and has been very supportive. At the time of admission, he seemed overwhelmed.

M. A. tries to do her morning self-care but is finding it more difficult and frustrating. Getting dressed is particularly fatiguing, and she admits that at times she goes to bed fully dressed to avoid having to get dressed in the morning. She has been using a manual wheelchair for the past 3 years.

Her daughter is currently helping with the laundry, cooking, and simple cleaning. M. A. states that she has problems doing household tasks because she must hold onto something stable before reaching for, or lifting, an object.

She currently enjoys no leisure activities. At one time, she liked to knit, but it has become too frustrating to be pleasurable.

She complains of bladder urgency but often cannot void. She also has a mild dysarthria, spasticity of the lower extremities, weakness of the upper extremities (able to move against gravity against minimal resistance), poor sitting balance, poor fine and gross motor coordination, blurred vision, and loss of stereognosis and light touch.

When the occupational therapist spoke with her, it became apparent that she did not comprehend the nature and course of MS. She is feeling frustrated and depressed about her recent decline of function.

She is currently taking Tylenol, Senokot, Metamucil, Colace, heparin, and multivitamins and is using Dulcolax suppositories.

CASE 2

Parkinson's Disease

C. R. is a 72-year-old man with stage III Parkinson's disease. He has recently experienced a severe loss of balance and functional mobility. He reports difficulty moving quickly and gracefully. He also complains of poor handwriting, problems sleeping, and numbness in both hands.

C. R. is a single, retired accountant who lives independently in a two-story home. His bedroom and bathroom are on the second floor. There are four steps to enter the home. He has no children. He has one sister who lives within walking distance of his home. She, however, is suffering from arthritis and has difficulty offering much assistance.

C. R. has been caring for himself thus far, but his sister reports she is concerned about his safety, especially with activities such as cooking and bathing. She reports that he has fallen on several occasions recently and spends most of his time sitting in his chair in his living room.

His sister brings him meals as often as possible but is unable to bring meals in the morning or during bad weather. Her children live out of state and are only able to offer assistance to him during occasional visits when they try to do some of the major household chores such as painting, repairs, and cleaning.

C. R. was once interested in music and art. He played the piano and painted with watercolors. He reports that he has not participated in these leisure activities for "a long time." He also played tennis on a regular basis at the local club. He is still a member of the club but has not been there in more than a year.

C. R. is reportedly self-conscious of his illness and, therefore, does not like to go out in public very much. His sister, who has always been very close to her brother, expresses concern about his "depression and lack of motivation." She states that she has tried on several occasions to get him to go to local musical concerts or museums, but she feels he is just too depressed.

He is currently taking Sinemet and Artane. His sister, however, reports that he does not consistently take his medications because they "make him feel sick."

CASE 3

Amyotrophic Lateral Sclerosis

T. M. is a 48-year-old man who has recently been diagnosed with ALS. Six months before being referred to O. T. services, he began to experience some weakness in his hands and he began dropping objects, such as tools. He reports loss of strength in his arms and legs. The weakness in his legs has become so severe that he now uses a borrowed wheelchair part of the time. He complains of difficulty sleeping due to cramps in his legs. He also reports that he has lost almost 20 lb in the last 6 or 8 months.

T. M. is married and has two sons, ages 6 and 4. He independently owns and operates a lawnmower shop at which he sells and repairs lawnmowers. He reports significant difficulty performing the repair parts of his job because of weakness in his hands and arms. Most of the repairs have become backed up in the shop and he is considering hiring assistance or sending the work to another shop.

His wife is employed full-time as a legal secretary. She has helped with the business as much as possible by completing some of the bookkeeping after hours. She is very busy caring for their boys and trying to maintain the household. She appears to be very supportive of T. M., but also seems very burdened by her responsibilities.

T. M. has many interests in sports and outdoor activities. He has been racing in "Iron Man" triathalons and marathons for the last several years. He was a high school track and cross country star. He enjoys biking and camping. Every summer, he and his family take a 2-week trip to a remote location where they hike and camp.

He is also supportive of his sons' sports events and enjoys teaching them various sports. Last year, he was a soccer coach for his oldest boy's team.

The course and prognosis of ALS has been explained to T. M. and his wife and they have reportedly been discussing future plans. They are, however, "hoping for a miracle." At this time, he is taking pain relievers to reduce the pain from the cramping in his legs.

POINTS FOR REVIEW

1. What are the three most common PNDs?
2. Define each disorder.
3. What are the etiologies of these conditions?
4. The distribution of people with ALS is estimated to be higher in Guam and the Kii peninsula of Japan. Why is this?
5. What is the prevalence of Parkinson's disease?
6. Is there a difference in distribution by gender for PNDs?
7. Describe the signs and symptoms of MS.
8. Describe the signs and symptoms of Parkinson's disease.
9. Describe the signs and symptoms of ALS.
10. At what age is MS usually diagnosed?
11. How variable is the course among those diagnosed with MS?
12. What are the four types or patterns of MS?
13. If diagnosed with MS, do most people lose function quickly?

14. Does MS reduce one's life expectancy?

15. At what age is Parkinson's disease usually diagnosed?

16. List and describe the fives stages of Parkinson's disease as defined by Hoehn and Yahr's scale.

17. At what age is ALS diagnosed?

18. Is the progression of ALS similar to that of MS? How is it the same or different?

19. What factors confirm the diagnosis of MS?

20. How is a diagnosis of Parkinson's disease confirmed?

21. ALS is diagnosed primarily by what procedure?

22. What drugs are used most often to treat Parkinson's disease?

23. Describe the impact of each these three disorders on occupational performance.

REFERENCES

1. Pryse-Phillips W. The epidemiology of multiple sclerosis. In: Cook SD, ed. Handbook of Multiple Sclerosis. New York: Marcel Dekker 1990:1–24.

2. Kalb RC. Multiple Sclerosis: the Questions You Have, the Answers You Need. New York: Demos Vermande, 1996.

3. Maloney FP, Burks JS, Ringel SP, eds. Interdisciplinary Rehabilitation of Multiple Sclerosis and Neuromuscular Disorders. Philadelphia: JB Lippincott, 1985.

4. Matthews B. Multiple Sclerosis: The Facts. 3rd ed. Oxford: Oxford University Press, 1993.

5. Hutton JT, Dippel RL. Caring for the Parkinson Patient: A Practical Guide. Buffalo, NY: Prometheus Books, 1989.

6. Duvoisin RC, Sage J. Parkinson's Disease: A Guide for Patient and Family. Philadelphia: Lippincott-Raven, 1996.

7. Lieberman AN, Williams FL, Imke S, et al. Parkinson's Disease: The Complete Guide for Patients and Caregivers. New York: Simon & Schuster, 1993.

8. Taylor AE, Saint-Cyr JA, Lang AE. Parkinson's disease: cognitive changes in relation to treatment response. Brain 1987;110:35–51.

9. Beresford S. Motor Neurone Disease (Amyotrophic Lateral Sclerosis). London: Chapman & Hall, 1995.

10. Rusk HA. Rehabilitation Medicine. 3rd ed. St Louis: Mosby, 1971.

11. Armon C, Kurland LT, Beard CM, et al. Psychologic and adaptational difficulties anteceding amyotrophic lateral sclerosis: Rochester, Minnesota, 1925–1987. Neuroepidemiology 1991;10(3):132–137.

12. O'Sullivan SB, Cullen KE, Schmitz TJ. Physical Rehabilitation: Evaluation and Treatment Procedures. Philadelphia: FA Davis, 1981.

13. Durrleman S, Alperovitch A. Increasing trend of ALS in France and elsewhere: are the changes real? Neurology 1989;39:768–773.

14. Mitsumoto H, Hanson MR, Chad DA. Amyotrophic lateral sclerosis: Recent advances in pathogenesis and therapeutic trials. Arch Neurol 1988;45:189–202.

15. Delisa JA, Hammond MD, Mikulic MA, et al. Multiple sclerosis: part 1. Common physical disabilities and rehabilitation. Am Fam Physician 1985;32(4):157–163.

16. Umphred DA. Neurological Rehabilitation. 2nd ed. St Louis: CV Mosby, 1990.

17. Chusid JG. Correlative Neuroanatomy and Functional Neurology. 16th ed. Los Altos, CA: Lange Medical Publications, 1976.

18. Delisa JA, Miller RM, Mikulic MA, et al. Multiple sclerosis: part 2. Common functional problems and rehabilitation. Am Fam Physician 1985;32(5):127–132.

19. Ferguson JM. Helping an MS patient live a better life. Rehabilitation Nursing 1987;50(12):22–27.

20. Andreoli TE, Carpenter CC, Plum F, et al. Cecil Essentials of Medicine. Philadelphia: WB Saunders, 1986.

21. Percy AK. Multiple sclerosis in Rochester, Minnesota: a 60 year appraisal. Arch Neurol 1971;25:105.

22. Holland NJ, Kaplan SR. Social adaptations. In: Scheinberg LC, Holland NJ, eds. Multiple Sclerosis: A Guide for Patients and Their Families. New York: Raven Press, 1987:219–239.

CHAPTER 14

RHEUMATOID ARTHRITIS

Cynthia D. Batts Shanku

CRITICAL TERMS

Analgesia
Anemia
Ankylosis
Antibodies
Antinuclear antibodies
Apophyseal
Arthritis
Autoimmune disease
Bursitis

Carpal tunnel syndrome
de Quervain's disease
Epstein-Barr virus
Erythemas
Erythrocyte sedimentation rate
 (ESR)
Inflammation
Juvenile rheumatoid arthritis

Osteoarthritis
Pannus
Polymyositis
Rheumatoid arthritis
Rheumatoid factor
Scleroderma
Sjögren's syndrome
Tenosynovitis

Eva, a 50-year-old grocery store cashier, mother of two teenage children, woke again with severe pain and stiffness as she had every morning for the past few months. Her hands and elbows were swollen and warm to the touch. She had to get up and go to work. She knew her family counted on her income so there was no way that she could call in sick again. Besides, she would feel better in the afternoon like she usually did. Her husband convinced her to see a doctor for an evaluation. She did, and was eventually diagnosed with rheumatoid arthritis.

INTRODUCTION

A. J. Landnia-Beauvais is given credit for the earliest description of rheumatoid arthritis (RA) in his Paris thesis of 1800, although analysis of pictorial art of the late Renaissance has provided some evidence of RA in earlier times. However, it was not until 1858 that A. B. Garrod coined the actual phrase "rheumatoid arthritis" and not until 1941 that the American Rheumatism Association adopted the terminology (1).

There are more than 100 different forms of arthritis. Arthritis is divided into eight major categories, and RA is included under the synovitis category. Although less common than other forms of the disease, such as osteoarthritis, it is more serious.

Data indicate that the economic costs linked with RA are on a level with those of coronary heart disease. In the United States, the direct medical care of RA is typically three times the cost of medical care of a person of the same age and sex who does not have RA. Annually, the per-person medical costs have been estimated at $5400 (in 1994 figures). The indirect costs for RA, principally from lost wages, exceed medical costs by three to four times (2, 3).

ANATOMY

It is important to have an accurate concept of the joint anatomy and its related structures (Fig. 14.1) before discussing the etiology, signs and symptoms, and course of RA. The word "arthritis" comes from the Greek words "anthron" (meaning joint) and "itis" (meaning inflammation or infection). Therefore, the word is defined as "inflammation or infection of the joint" (4). In addition, the base word "rheum" in rheumatoid refers to the stiffness, general aching, weakness, and fatigue that is experienced throughout the body.

The anatomy of a healthy joint (Fig. 14.1) should be kept in mind when, later in the chapter, the disease process and its effect on the joint

are discussed. Refer to the glossary for specific anatomical definitions.

ETIOLOGY

Despite intensive research over many decades, the cause of RA and juvenile rheumatoid arthritis (JRA) are unknown. Current interrelated research has focused on three areas.

First, it is believed that RA is a chronic multi-system disease associated with a malfunctioning immune system, which results in the immune system attacking healthy joint tissue. In turn, this causes inflammation and subsequent joint damage.

Second, research has found that RA may be caused by a virus or bacterium that causes a release of persistent microbial infection (5, 6). It is also speculated that a high proportion of individuals with RA demonstrate circulating antibodies to an antigen present in the Epstein-Barr (EB) virus (7). The inflammatory problem involves a "triggering" of a chronic inflammation that begins in the synovial membrane of the joints and progresses to erosion of the joint capsule, tendons, ligaments, and eventually cartilage and bone. The inflammation usually spreads to other joints, resulting in further joint damage (8)

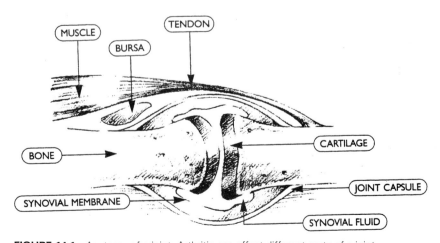

FIGURE 14.1   Anatomy of a joint. Arthritis can affect different parts of a joint.

(Fig. 14.2). Further, because this disease is systemic, chronic involvement includes manifestations that affect the lungs, the cardiovascular system, and the eyes.

Third, genetic factors have been identified as potentially influential in the disease. Rheumatoid arthritis is not inherited; it is not passed directly from parents to children. A susceptibility or tendency to develop RA can be inherited, but not everyone who inherits this susceptibility will have the disease develop.

Leukocytes (white blood cells) have been studied for hereditary factors that predispose a person to RA. One type of leukocyte, the T cell, matures under the influence of the thymus and mediates cellular immunity. This cell-mediated immunity provides the body's main defense against intracellular organisms and involves the identification and removal of foreign substances (antigens) from the body. The entire process depends on the interaction of the antigen with receptors on the surface of the T cell; therefore, T cells are further categorized into genetic classes containing human leukocyte antigen (HLA) receptors. A large accumulation of data links specific HLA antigens with particular disease states in the human (7).

The T cell has a binding cleft (receptor site) with specific sensitivity to certain antigens and is complementary to the structures found in antibodies. One particular class, the HLA-DR4 type, does not distinguish between antigens and healthy tissue and is associated with a susceptibility to RA. As a result, substances that facilitate inflammation of the synovial lining are released.

The following description helps to provide an understanding of the molecular process. Initially, an antigen such as the EB virus comes in contact with the T-cell receptor; the T-cell membrane becomes activated and is transformed into a large

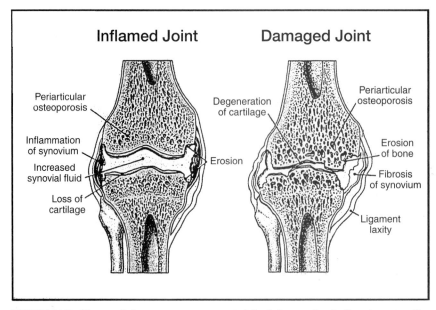

FIGURE 14.2   The postinflammatory response to joint inflammation is fibrosis, not unlike the scarring (fibrosis) that results from a surgical incision. The function of the postinflammatory joint depends on the degree of fibrosis and the destruction that occurred during the inflammatory stage. The damage influences the alignment, angle of tendon pull (joint integrity), range of motion, and stability. (Reprinted with permission from the Arthritis Foundation. The AHPA Arthritis Teaching Slide Collection. 2nd ed. 1988.)

blast cell that then proliferates. The sensitized T cells indirectly stimulate macrophagelike cells of the synovial lining of the joints. During this inflammatory phase, the affected joint demonstrates increased heat, swelling, pain, redness, and decreased range of motion (9).

Later, there is a proliferation of connective tissue and a heavy infiltration by more lymphocytes as well as plasma cells. The activated synovial cells grow out as a malignant pannus (cover) (Fig. 14.3) over the cartilage, leading to cartilage breakdown. This granulation tissue continues to spread, the joint space is slowly effaced by fibrous adhesions, and eventually fibrous ankylosis appears. The byproduct of the synovial lining destruction further stimulates the inflammation process, leading to more tissue damage than tissue repair (10) (Fig. 14.4).

Additional research has demonstrated that individuals who have inherited a specific gene sequence from both parents have a higher risk of developing much more severe RA that could involve internal organs as well as joints. Contin-

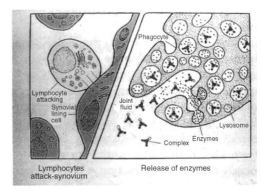

FIGURE 14.4 In the development of inflammatory rheumatic diseases, the normal protective process of inflammation goes awry. Lymphocytes can no longer distinguish between antigens and healthy tissue, and they secrete substances that cause the synovial lining to become inflamed. Phagocytes become overloaded with immune complexes and release lysosomal enzymes into the joint fluid. The enzymes then attack and destroy cells of the joint lining. (Reprinted with permission from the Arthritis Foundation. The AHPA Arthritis Teaching Slide Collection. 2nd ed. 1988.)

ued research on genetic factors could facilitate genetic counseling to identify people at higher risk of developing severe forms of RA or of needing more intensive treatment (11). The North American Rheumatoid Arthritis Consortium (NAARC), consisting of 12 medical centers across the United States, has come together to establish a national registry and repository and repository of families with RA. Researchers will look at clinical data and genetic material from 1000 pairs of siblings, both of whom have RA, and will test about 400 different genetic regions to try to identify specific genes that may play a role in RA (12).

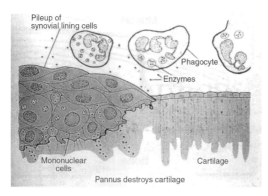

FIGURE 14.3 Synovial lining cells multiply, creating a mass called "pannus." Substances in this mass further damage the underlying cartilage, which softens, weakens, and ultimately is destroyed. The waste products of cartilage cell destruction further stimulate the inflammatory process. New phagocytes rush to the area to clean up the debris. Some lymphocytes and other mononuclear cells are mistakenly rendered capable of attacking cartilage. Lysosomal enzymes and collagenase are released, thus perpetuating the abnormal process. (Reprinted with permission from the Arthritis Foundation. The AHPA Arthritis Teaching Slide Collection. 2nd ed. 1988.)

Juvenile Rheumatoid Arthritis

Juvenile RA is the most prevalent form of arthritis in children age 16 or younger. The diagnostic criteria for JRA are onset at age younger than 16 years, persistent arthritis in 1 or more joints for at least 6 weeks, and exclusion of other types of childhood arthritis (Table 14.1) (13). The three classifications of JRA are summarized in Table 14.2.

TABLE 14.1   Criteria for the Diagnosis of Juvenile Rheumatoid Arthritis

I. General

The JRA Criteria subcommittee in 1982 reviewed the 1977 Criteria (1) and recommended that *juvenile rheumatoid arthritis* be the name for the principal form of chronic arthritic disease in children and that this general class should be classified into three onset subtypes: systemic, polyarticular, and pauciarticular. The onset subtypes may be further subclassified into subsets as indicated below. The following classification enumerates the requirements for the diagnosis of JRA and the three clinical onset subtypes and lists subsets of each subtype that may be useful in further classification.

II. General criteria for the diagnosis of juvenile rheumatoid arthritis:
A. Persistent arthritis of at least six weeks duration in one or more joints
B. Exclusion of other causes of arthritis (see list of exclusions)

III. JRA onset subtypes

The onset subtype is determined by manifestations during the first six months of disease and remains the principal classification, although manifestations more closely resembling another subtype may appear later.
A. Systemic onset JRA: This subtype is defined as JRA with persistent intermittent fever (daily intermittent temperatures to 103° F or higher) with or without rheumatoid rash or other organ involvement. Typical fever and rash will be considered probable systemic onset JRA if not associated with arthritis. Before a definite diagnosis can be made, arthritis, as defined, must be present.
B. Pauciarticular onset JRA: This subtype is defined as JRA with arthritis in four or fewer joints during the first six months of disease. Patients with systemic onset JRA are excluded from this onset subtype.
C. Polyarticular JRA: This subtype is defined as JRA with arthritis in five or more joints during the first six months of disease. Patients with systemic JRA onset are excluded from this subtype.
D. The onset subtypes may include the following subsets:
1. Systemic onset
a. Polyarthritis
b. Oligoarthritis

2. Oligoarthritis (pauciarticular onset)
a. Antinuclear antibody (ANA) positive-chronic uveitis
b. Rheumatoid factor (RF) positive
c. Seronegative, B27 positive
d. Not otherwise classified
3. Polyarthritis
a. RF positivity
b. Not otherwise classified

IV. Exclusions
A. Other rheumatic diseases
1. Rheumatic fever
2. Systemic lupus erythematosus
3. Ankylosing spondylitis
4. Polymyositis or dermatomyositis
5. Vasculitic syndromes
6. Scleroderma
7. Psoriatic arthritis
8. Reiter's syndrome
9. Sjögren's syndrome
10. Mixed connective tissue disease
11. Behçet's syndrome
B. Infectious arthritis
C. Inflammatory bowel disease
D. Neoplastic diseases including leukemia
E. Nonrheumatic conditions of bones and joints
F. Hematologic diseases
G. Psychogenic arthralgia
H. Miscellaneous
1. Sarcoidosis
2. Hypertrophic osteoarthropathy
3. Villonodular synovitis
4. Chronic active hepatitis
5. Familial Mediterranean fever

V. Other proposed terminology

Juvenile chronic arthritis (JCA) and juvenile arthritis (JA) are new diagnostic terms currently in use in some places for the arthritides of childhood. The diagnoses of JCA and JA are not equivalent to each other, nor to the older diagnosis of juvenile rheumatoid arthritis or Still's disease. Hence reports of studies of JCA or JA cannot be directly compared with one another nor to reports of JRA or Still's disease. Juvenile chronic arthritis is described in more detail in a report of the European Conference on the Rheumatic Diseases of Children (2) and juvenile arthritis in the report of the Ross Conference (3).

1. JRA Criteria Subcommittee of the Diagnostic and Therapeutic Criteria Committee of the American Rheumatism Association. Current proposed revisions of the JRA criteria. Arthritis Rheum 1977; 20(Suppl)195–199.
2. Ansell BW. Chronic arthritis in childhood. Ann Rheum Dis 1978; 37:107–120.
3. Fink CW. Keynote address: arthritis in childhood. Report of the 80th Ross Conference in Pediatric Research. Columbus, Ross Laboratories, 1979;1–2.

TABLE 14.2 Juvenile Rheumatoid Arthritis IRA Subtype Characteristics	SYSTEMIC	POLYARTICULAR	PAUCIARTICULAR
Frequency of cases	10%	40%	50%
Number of joints with arthritis at onset	Variable	≥ 5	≤ 4
Sex ratio (F:M)	1:1	3:1	5:1
Frequency of uveitis	1%	5%	20%
Frequency of rheumatoid factor positivity	< 2%	5–10%	< 2%
Frequency of ANA positivity	5–10%	40–50%	75–85%
Frequency of ≥ 5 joints involved any time during course of JRA	50–60%	100%	40%
Frequency of active disease > 10 years follow-up	42%	45%	41%
Frequency of erosions or joint space narrowing on radiographs	45%	54%	28%
Median time to develop erosions or joint space narrowing on radiographs (years after disease onset)	2.2	2.4	5.4
Frequency of adult height < 5th percentile	50%	16%	11%

Abbreviations: ANA, antinuclear antibody.

Systemic JRA (sJRA) affects 10% of children with JRA. It is characterized by intermittent fever spikes of more than 101°. Children with systemic JRA often experience a rash with the high fever; the rash may be present only when temperature is elevated and is most commonly seen on the trunk. Systemic JRA usually affects multiple joints and may facilitate other problems, such as pericarditis, pleuritis, stomach pain, anemia, and an increase in white blood cells (11, 12). General feelings of fatigue, weakness, and weight loss may be experienced as well. The prognosis is decided by the severity of the arthritis that usually develops with the fever and rash. Onset of JRA may begin at any age; however, the peak of onset is 1 to 6 years old. Boys and girls are equally affected (14).

Polyarticular JRA (poJRA) affects approximately 40% of children with JRA and is initiated in several joints at once (five or more). The course usually involves the small joints of the hands and fingers but can also affect the weight-bearing joints. The joints are typically affected symmetrically and fevers may be present. Juvenile RA is subdivided into two groups and identified most readily by the absence and presence of rheumatoid factor (RF). The prognosis for those with an RF-positive factor is that they are at higher risk for erosions, nodules, growth retardation, lack of adequate bone mineralization, anemia, and poor functional status.

Pauciarticular arthritis (paJRA), or oligoarthritis, accounts for 50% of those with JRA. This type of JRA characteristically affects the large joints such as the knees, ankles, or elbows and engages only a few joints (four or fewer) at a time. Pauciarticular JRA is divided into two groups: late onset and early onset. Those with late onset RA are usually girls (outnumbering boys 4 to 1) who are very young (1 to 5 years old), have a 30 to 50% chance of developing chronic eye inflammation with complications, and have the best articular outcome. Late onset JRA affects boys who are HLA-B27 positive, have tendinitis, with the large joints (hip and low back) of the body being the most affected (14).

INCIDENCE AND PREVALENCE

In 1997, there were an estimated 40 million Americans with arthritis, according to the National Health Interview Survey (HIS) (15). One in seven people in the general population is affected, and women are affected three times more often than men (4).

The prevalence of JRA is approximately 1/1000 of the childhood population, with girls being affected 7 times more often than boys (16, 17). The prevalence increases with age until about the seventh decade (18). Eighty percent of all patients who develop RA are between 35 and 50. Sex differences diminish in the older age group (5).

Racial factors also appear relevant in RA. American blacks have a lower occurrence of RA than whites (19). North American Indians have a higher prevalence of RA, whereas native Japanese and Chinese may have a lower prevalence than whites (20). Reasons for these variations are unknown and may be attributed to both genetic and environmental factors. Epidemiological studies in Africa indicate that climate and urbanization have a major impact on incidence and severity of RA in groups with similar genetic backgrounds (21). Long-term studies from the Mayo Clinic, Great Britain, and a population of PIMA Indians suggest that the incidence of RA has declined from 20 to 50% (22–25). Although good evidence supports this decline, several studies have not done so (26). Explanations for the declining incidence include a possible change in a casual infectious agent, the increased use of oral contraceptives that may protect against the disease in some way, or a general improvement in living standards, which may affect disease occurrence and severity. The incidence in other diseases, such as coronary artery disease, seems to be declining at the same time as the incidence of RA.

SIGNS AND SYMPTOMS

Onset of symptoms may be sudden and may vary in degree. Rheumatoid arthritis is frequently characterized by exacerbations (flare-ups) and remissions, in which the disease appears to be quiet and nonexistent. Even though RA is destructive, the course of the disease is variable from person to person. Some individuals experience only a mild, brief monoarticular involvement and minimal joint damage, whereas others will have an ongoing progressive arthritis with significant joint deformity. Most often, RA affects more than one joint at once. In two-thirds of patients, an exacerbation is initiated by feelings of fatigue, generalized weakness, weight loss, malaise, and vague musculoskeletal symptoms until synovitis becomes more obvious. Although joint involvement is generally symmetrical, some patients may experience an asymmetrical pattern (21).

A discussion of joint involvement can be divided into two sections: stages of inflammatory joint disease as experienced overall and specific manifestations to particular joints.

Articular and Periarticular Involvement

Stages

Table 14.3 presents the stages of the inflammatory process: a) acute, b) subacute, c) chronic-active, and d) chronic-inactive.

As mentioned earlier, onset may be sudden, with inflammation occurring in many joints at once. In the acute and subacute phases, fatigue may be extensive enough to cause disability from disuse of joint motion and loss of strength before joint changes actually occur. Various degrees of general soreness and aching are experienced. These are usually followed by progressive, localized symptoms of pain, inflammation, warmth, and tenderness in a joint or multiple joints.

Symmetrical involvement of small hand joints, feet, wrists, elbows, and ankles is typical, but initial manifestations may occur in any joint.

Pain originates primarily from the joint capsule, which is abundantly supplied with pain fibers and is highly sensitive to stretching and distention.

Joint swelling results from the accumulation of synovial fluid, hypertrophy of the synovium,

TABLE 14.3 Stages of Inflammatory Joint Disease		
STAGES	**OBJECTIVE SIGNS**	**SUBJECTIVE SYMPTOMS**
Acute	Limited range of motion Fever Decreased muscle strength Possible cold, sweaty hands Overall stiffness Gel phenomenon most prominent Weight loss Decreased appetite	Pain at rest and movement most severe Inflammation most severe Hot, red joints Decreased function Tingling and numbness in hands and feet
Subacute	Decreased range of motion Poor endurance Mild fever Decreased muscle strength Morning stiffness Gel phenomenon Weight loss Decreased appetite	Pain and tenderness at rest and movement decreases Joints warm and pink Inflammation subsiding Decreased function Tingling and numbness in hands and feet
Chronic-active	Decreased range of motion Fever has subsided Muscle strength decreased Endurance low	Pain and tenderness at rest minimal Pain on motion decreases Inflammation low-grade Increased activity noted, owing to adjustment to pain

Chronic-inactive	Limited range of motion
	
	Muscle atrophy
	Decreased endurance from limited
	  activity in previous stages
	Residuals seen from above stages
	Potential contracture
		Pain at motion caused by stiffness from
		  disuse during pervious stages and
		  instability of joint
		No inflammation
		Residuals seen from above stages
		Functioning may be decreased due to pain

and thickening of the joint capsule. Synovial thickening, the most specific physical finding, eventually occurs in most active joints.

Various degrees of generalized stiffness occur, including the "gel phenomenon," which is the inability to move joints after prolonged rest. Morning stiffness that lasts longer than 1 hour is an almost universal feature of inflammatory arthritis, which distinguishes it from noninflammatory disorders. The length and intensity of the stiffness can be used as a gross assessment of disease activity (21).

In JRA, morning stiffness, gelling after inactivity, and night pain are encountered as frequently as in adult disease. However, children may not discuss these symptoms with anyone so their presence is detected only by caregiver observation. Initial presentation may be detected by the child's increased irritability, joint guarding, or refusal to walk (13).

Also, adults and children with RA have decreased joint motion, decreased muscle strength and endurance, and a loss of appetite and weight. Patients frequently experience chills in their hands and feet, as well as numbness and tingling. As motion is limited by pain, the inflamed joint is usually held in flexion to maximize joint volume and minimize distention of the capsule.

Once the acute and subacute stages have subsided, limited joint range of motion causes contractures to form. Contractures are the result of adhesions that form when the patient avoids movement during the acute, painful phase. Limitations in range of motion result from ankylosis, subluxation, or dislocation. Also, muscle atrophy in chronic stages results from disuse in the earlier, more acute stages.

SPECIFIC JOINT MANIFESTATIONS

Hand

Of all the extremities, the hands are by far the most severely affected by RA (27). Joints with the highest synovium-to-cartilage ratio are those most frequently affected by the disease.

Fusiform or spindle-shaped fingers, a typical sign of RA, result from swelling in the proximal interphalangeal (PIP) joints (Fig. 14.5). This is usually related to bilateral and symmetrical swelling of the metacarpophalangeal (MCP) joints. Pressure on these joints causes tenderness. Distal interphalangeal (DIP) joints are rarely involved, which discriminates RA from osteoarthritis and psoriatic arthritis (4).

Boutonniere and swan-neck deformities are two other common hand disfigurements that result from RA. A boutonniere deformity is a combination of PIP joint flexion and DIP joint hyperextension (Fig. 14.6). More descriptively, it is flexion of the PIP joint through the detached central slip of the extensor tendon, which serves as a "button-hole" through which the joint can pop. The DIP joint is then forced into hyperextension.

Swan-neck deformities result from contractures of the interosseus and flexor muscles and tendons, which in turn produce a flexure contracture of the MCP joint, compensatory hyperextension of the PIP joint, and flexion of the DIP joint (Fig. 14.7).

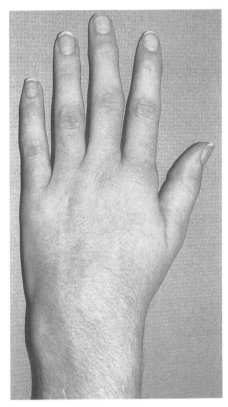

FIGURE 14.5 Fusiform swelling and erythema about the PIP joints, most significant in the long finger. Swelling at the MCP joints has caused loss of definition of joint margins. The extensor carpi ulnaris tendon sheath (sixth dorsal compartment of the wrist) has synovial thickening and swelling.

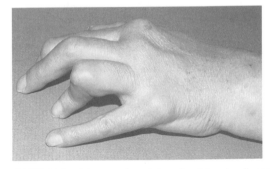

FIGURE 14.6 A boutonniere deformity of the ring finger, flexion deformity of the long finger PIP joint, and mild swan-neck deformity of the index finger. Extensive synovitis at the MCP joints obscures the usual definition of joint margins.

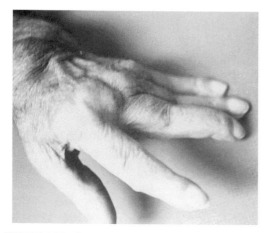

FIGURE 14.7 Swan-neck deformities of long, ring, and little fingers, with concomitant subluxation of the MCP joints.

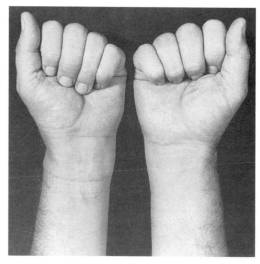

FIGURE 14.8 Flexor tendinitis at the wrist and in the palm leading to decreased flexion of the fingers of the left hand.

Thumb deformities associated with RA have been classified into three categories by E. A. Nalebuff. In type I, MCP inflammation leads to stretching of the joint capsule and boutonnierelike deformity. In type II, edema of the carpometacarpal (CMC) joint leads to volar subluxation during ankylosis of the adductor pollicis. In type III, after sustained disease of both MCP joints, exaggerated adduction of the first metacarpus, flexion of the MCP joint, and hyperextension of the DIP joint result from the patient's need to establish a compensatory method to pinch (28, 29).

Flexor tenosynovitis was seen in 55% of patients with RA in a study done by Gray and Gottlieb (30). Stiffness and crepitary inflammation along the tendon sheath with limitations of flexion and extension were exhibited (Fig. 14.8). Finger "triggering" occurs when thickening or nodule formation of the tendon interplays with the tenosynovial inflammation, trapping the tendon in a flexed position. Tendon rupture most frequently occurs in the abductors of the thumb and extensor carpi ulnaris of the fourth and fifth fingers. Rupture of the latter is usually caused by a combination of synovitis in the tendon sheaths and mechanical irritation from an eroded and subluxed distal ulna (31).

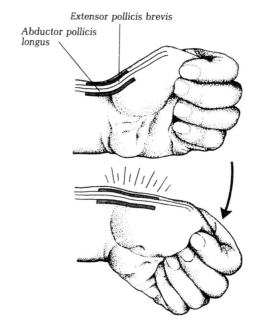

FIGURE 14.9 Finkelstein's test for de Quervain's disease.

de Quervain's tenosynovitis, which involves extensors at the thumb, causes severe pain and discomfort, resulting in a decrease in hand function and the ability to grip (Fig. 14.9).

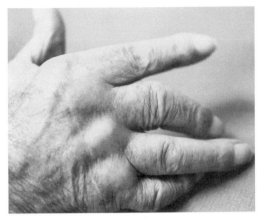

FIGURE 14.10 Arthritis mutilans. The long PIP joint has been destroyed by RA. Deflection of the distal portion of the phalanx is caused by the pull of gravity.

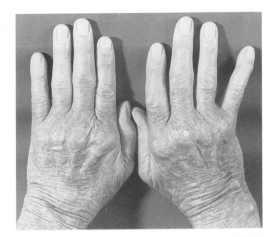

FIGURE 14.11 Subcutaneous tissue atrophy, MCP joint proliferation synovitis with loss of joint definition, and mild PIP joint enlargement. There is slight volar subluxation of the MCP joints and mild ulnar deviation at the MCP joints of the right hand. Involvement of the dominant (right) hand is more pronounced.

Mutilans deformity (opera glass hand) causes transverse folds of the skin of the thumb and fingers, resembling a folded telescope. Pulling on the fingers during examination may lengthen the digit much like opening opera glasses, or the joint may bend in unusual directions just by the pull of gravity. X-rays of the fingers and thumb identify severe bone resorption, erosions, shortening of MCP, PIP, radiocarpal, and radioulnar joints (30) (Fig. 14.10). The grossly unstable thumbs and severely deformed phalanges negatively affect hand function and the ability to complete daily living activities.

Wrist

Ulnar deviations and volar subluxation at the MCP joints or radiocarpal deviation are characteristic signs of RA at the wrist (Fig. 14.11). These problems result from severe tenosynovitis and inflammation where the ligaments surround the joint and eventually lead to edema, joint laxity, erosion of the tendons and ligaments, and muscle imbalance. When ulnar deviation of the MCP is present with radial deviation at the radiocarpal joint, a "zig-zag" presentation of the hand is seen (Figs. 14.12 and 14.13). Dorsiflexion of the wrist often is one of the first movements to be

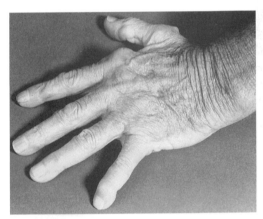

FIGURE 14.12 "Zig-zag" deformity with ulnar deviation of the fingers at the MCP joints and clockwise rotation of carpus on the distal radius.

limited. Carpal tunnel syndrome is commonly diagnosed, resulting from synovial proliferations on the volar aspect of the wrist, which then impinge upon the median nerve (4). This causes paresthesia of the palmar aspect of the thumb, the second and third digits, and the radial aspect of the fourth digit (Fig. 14.14).

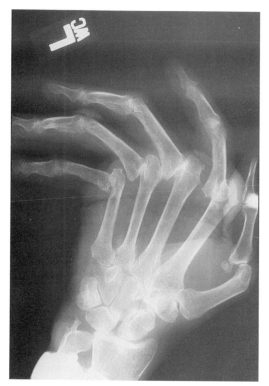

FIGURE 14.13 Severe MCP joint subluxations in the volar and ulnar directions. There is concomitant clockwise rotation of the carpus on the distal radius ("zig-zag deformity"). Erosions of the ulnar styloid and metacarpal heads are evident.

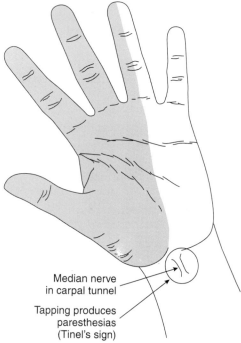

FIGURE 14.14 Distribution of pain or paresthesias (*shaded area*) when the median nerve is compressed by swelling in the wrist (carpal tunnel).

Elbow

Loss of motion due to flexion contractures in addition to inflammation are the most prevalent problems with elbow involvement. Synovial swelling and thickening may be observed in the lateral area between the radial head and the olecranon. A bulge will be seen. Synovitis in the radiohumeral joint can result in decreased motion during pronation and supination of the forearm. Lateral epicondylitis, more often referred to as tennis elbow, is reported as sharply painful when firm pressure is placed on this specific area. Other symptoms include paresthesia over the fourth and fifth fingers and weakness in the flexor muscle of the little finger.

Shoulder

Shoulder involvement is common and can be complicated as RA progresses. The glenohumeral, acromioclavicular, and thoracoscapular joints are the most susceptible. Because the shoulder capsule lies beneath the muscular rotator cuff, inflammation is difficult to detect during physical assessment. Difficulty with shoulder movement and with completing daily living activities is usually the chief complaint, followed by pain and tenderness (32). Because the shoulder relies on extensive coordinated movement, when any one of these joints becomes affected, dysfunction in activities of daily living will be seen.

Localized pain and tenderness, resulting from tendinitis in the glenohumeral area where the supraspinatus muscle or the long head of the biceps tendon inserts, are frequently seen. Rotator cuff tears are likely where the rotator cuff tendon inserts into the greater tuberosity. Erosion is triggered by the proliferative synovitis that develops there (Fig. 14.15) (33). Tendinitis, capsulitis, and bursitis (grouped under the "local conditions" of arthritis categories) are causes of shoulder pain diagnosed more frequently than synovitis.

Synovitis of the glenohumeral area is seen occasionally in those with RA and is observed as a bulge in the anterior or lateral superior area of the shoulder.

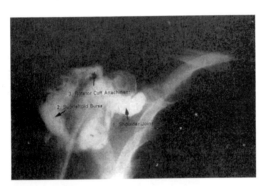

FIGURE 14.15 The supraspinatus, infraspinatus, and teres minor tendons make up a tendinous envelope commonly called the rotator cuff. This structure aids in the rotation of the humeral head and approximates the head to the glenoid fossa, permitting the deltoid to abduct and forward flex the arm. The rotator cuff can undergo degenerative changes. Under conditions of trauma or repetitive stress, it may rupture. In incomplete tears, the patient may have only mild pain, atrophy of muscles in the shoulder region, and slight weakness on abduction. When the rupture is complete, the patient is unable to abduct the arm from 0 to 90 degrees but can hold the arm above that level by deltoid muscle action. This contrast arthrogram shows abnormal communication between the shoulder joint space (*1*) and the subdeltoid bursae (*2*). The rotator cuff (*3*) usually prevents the contrast media, injected into the shoulder joint itself, from entering the bursal space. Presence of contrast in the bursa confirms partial or complete tear. (Reprinted with permission from the Arthritis Foundation. The AHPA Arthritis Teaching Slide Collection. 2nd ed. 1988.)

Loss of motion is a complication of shoulder synovitis, which is seen in progressed cases and is known as a "frozen shoulder."

Head, Neck, and Cervical Spine

The cervical spine is often involved in RA (34, 35). Involvement of C1 and C2 may produce life-threatening situations. Neck pain on motion and occipatal headaches are common symptoms of cervical spine involvement and occur in those individuals who have had RA longer than 10 years (36). Patients with severe deformities in their hands, as in mutilans deformity, are very likely to have had significant amounts of corticosteroids for RA management (37).

During radiological examination of this area in advanced cases of RA, the lower cervical and odontoid processes often appear eroded, as do the cervical apophyseal and intervertebral joints. The first to the fourth cervical joints are those most commonly affected by inflammation and pain (Figs. 14.16 and 14.17). Involvement of the upper cervical spine in advanced cases leads to subluxation, whereas lower cervical spine involvement produces symptoms of cord–root compression. For example, with a C5 root compression, problems are a) sensation on the radial aspect of the forearm, b) muscle weakness with abduction of the shoulder and flexion of the elbow, and c) decreased biceps jerk reflex. Subluxation also can cause twisting and compression of the vertebral arteries, which leads to vertebrobasilar insufficiency. This may be facilitated by syncope on a downward gaze. Flexion and extension of the cervical spine are usually less affected.

The temporomandibular joints (TMJ) have varied involvement in RA, ranging from 1 to 60%. Women are affected three times more often than men. Both TMJs are usually involved (38). Involvement of this synovial joint results in the inability to open the mouth fully because of side-to-side gliding and protrusion. After persistent inflammation, normal approximation of the upper and lower teeth may be affected.

Hoarseness occurs in up to 30% of patients with RA. This stems from inflamed cricoarytenoid

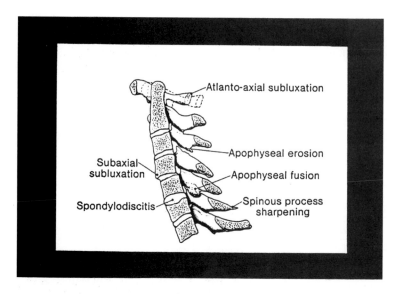

FIGURE 14.16 Neck abnormalities in RA. The neck is usually involved in adult and juvenile RA. The most common disorder is subluxation of the atlantoaxial joint, which occurs particularly on flexion of the neck. C1 moves forward on C2, and the odontoid process can actually cause pressure on the spinal cord posteriorly. Other findings include erosions at the apophyseal joints, fusion of the apophyseal joint, which occurs particularly in JRA , and subluxation at other levels. Disc involvement also may occur, and erosive changes and resorption can cause sharpening of the spinous process. (Reprinted with permission from the Arthritis Foundation. The AHPA Arthritis Teaching Slide Collection. 2nd ed. 1988.)

joints, which rotate with the vocal cords as they abduct and adduct to vary pitch and tone of the voice. If joint motion becomes too severely restricted, tracheostomy may be required (39, 40).

Hip

Approximately one-half of patients diagnosed with RA have radiographic evidence of hip disease (Fig. 14.18). Although hip involvement is common, early manifestations of hip disease are typically not apparent because the location of the joint is deep within the pelvis. Early hip disease might be seen in range of motion (41). In more progressive hip involvement, an abnormal gait pattern, possibly a limp, may be observed. This can result from a variety of factors, including pain, flexion contractures, muscle weakness, or hip instability. Fibrous contractures in flexion or external rotation are standard if restriction of motion is prolonged. Because the hip joint capsule is limited in its ability to stretch, severe RA involvement followed by swelling and massive effusion of synovium into the joint capsule may be extremely painful. Also, hip involvement will result in discomfort and pain in the groin and the medial side of the knee.

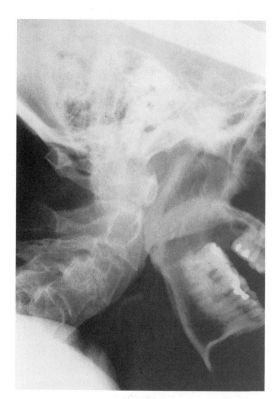

FIGURE 14.17 A lateral radiograph of a patient with RA who is experiencing severe upper extremity neurological decline owing to C2–C3 and C3 and C4 anterior subluxations. The odontoid is not visible because of severe erosion.

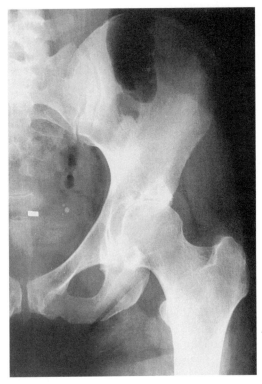

FIGURE 14.18 Hip radiograph of a patient with RA. There is diffuse joint space narrowing, small cysts in the femoral head and acetabulum, and little reparative bony change.

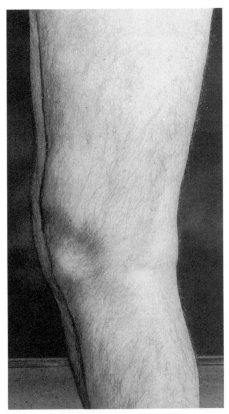

FIGURE 14.19 Lateral view of a patient with RA affecting the knees. There is quadriceps atrophy, significant synovial proliferation with joint effusion in the suprapatellar pouch, and fullness in the popliteal space because of a small synovial (Baker's) cyst.

As involvement increases (e.g., increased flexion contractures), more functional problems will be experienced in activities such as donning pants, sitting in a chair comfortably, walking upstairs, and positioning during sexual relations.

Knee

Hypertrophy and effusion of large amounts of synovium into the joint capsule are common in the knee joint and are more readily demonstrated in the knee than in the hip (Fig. 14.19). More than 5 mL of synovial fluid in the knee may be observed as a "bulge" sign; bulges occur behind the patella when fluid is pushed into the suprapatellar pouch and then back into the joint. Swelling, quadriceps muscle atrophy, ligamentous laxity, and joint instability may be more obvious when the patient stands or walks. Pain and swelling on the posterior knee may be caused by significant increases in intra-articular pressure during flexion, which produces an out-pouching, or Baker's cyst. Popliteal cysts, such as these, may impede superior venous flow in the thigh, producing a dilation of veins and edema (42). When the joint capsule is stretched, a reflex spasm triggers in the hamstring muscles. To relieve joint pain and tension, patients will hold their hips and knees in a flexion position that facilitates contractures. These contractures will cause difficulty in all weightbearing activities (26).

Ankle and Foot

True rheumatic disease is less common in the ankle than in other areas of the body and usually is not seen without concurrent midfoot or metatarsophalangeal (MTP) involvement (43). Tibiotalar swelling and loss of subtalar motion can develop. Ankle synovitis can be palpated in front of, behind, and below the malleoli. The ankle is often very tender and sensitive.

Symptomatic involvement of the feet is reported by 30 to 90% of those who have RA (44). Rheumatoid arthritis of the toes involving the MTP joints results in changes similar to those in the hands. When the MTP joints are affected, normal gait is disrupted. Problems will be observed during the push-off phase of ambulation, causing compensatory action with other weightbearing joints.

Characteristic manifestations of the feet include claw toes, hammer toes, cock-up toes, and hallux valgus. Claw toes result from the hyperextension of the MTP joints and the flexion of the PIP and DIP joints. Hammer toes differ from claw toes in that the DIP joint is hyperextended (Fig. 14.20). Cocking up of the toes may be associated with subluxation of the metatarsal heads and, finally, a clawlike appearance with an elevation of the tip of the toe above the surface on which the foot is resting. Hallux valgus is a common event in which fibular deviation of the first through the fourth toes occurs. This is similar to ulnar deviation of the hands (Figs. 14.21 and 14.22).

Rheumatoid nodules develop over bony prominences that bear more than normal pressure. For individuals affected by painful forefoot weightbearing, rheumatoid nodules can occur on the heels because of increased weightbearing there.

Tarsal joint involvement does not occur as often as in the forefoot; however, it can be detrimental to

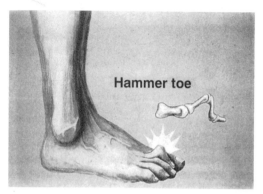

FIGURE 14.20 In this diagram, the second toe has a cockup deformity, which is similar to the boutonniere abnormality of the hand. Often this deformity is associated with subluxation of the corresponding MTP joints. This deformity may be hastened in a patient who wears shoes that are too small. Rubbing of the PIP joints on the shoe causes pain, callus formation, and possibly ulceration. This abnormality is not restricted to patients with RA. (Reprinted with permission from the Arthritis Foundation. The AHPA Arthritis Teaching Slide Collection. 2nd ed. 1988.)

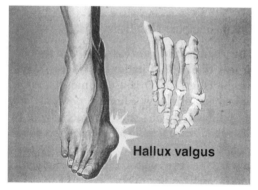

FIGURE 14.21 An anatomical and clinical diagram of hallux valgus. Pes planus and ligamentous laxity lead to lateral deviation of the great toe with a resultant hallux valgus. This deformity can be hastened by the wearing of narrow-toed shoes. Rubbing of the bunion on the shoe surface produces pain, and the lateral deviation of the great toe may impinge on other digits of the foot. This abnormality is not restricted to patients with RA. (Reprinted with permission from the Arthritis Foundation. The AHPA Arthritis Teaching Slide Collection. 2nd ed. 1988.)

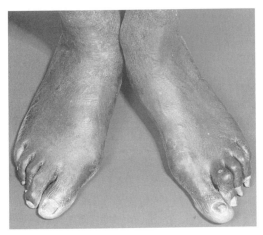

FIGURE 14.22 Mild hallux valgus, with dorsal subluxation of the MTP joints and resultant "hammer toe" deformities of second through fifth toes. Midfoot instability has lead to eversion, with concomitant flattening of the feet.

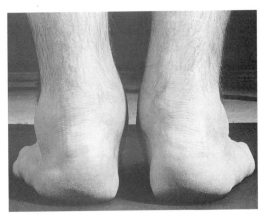

FIGURE 14.23 Significant ankle and midfoot synovitis. Loss of definition of the arch and eversion at the subtalar joint also are evident.

a person's ability to ambulate. As the longitudinal arch in the foot flattens and hindfoot valgus occurs, weightbearing pressure tends to shift medially (Fig. 14.23). This, in turn, facilitates the possible development of callositas and more rheumatoid nodule formations (45).

Muscle Involvement

Most patients with RA have muscle involvement, including muscle weakness. Recent studies suggest at least five stages of muscle disease in the RA process (46):

1. Reduction of muscle bulk associated with muscle atrophy that accompanies the inflammatory process as a result of disuse, bed rest, vascular events, and drug effects (47). A muscle can lose 30% of its bulk in 1 week (48). Loss of muscle bulk is associated with functional decrease (49).

2. Peripheral neuromyopathy, usually owing to mononeuritis multiplex, which is frequently associated with rheumatoid vasculitis involving localized sensory loss (a complication of RA).

3. Steroid myopathy.

4. Active myositis and muscle necrosis (or muscle fiber inflammation resulting in destruction of the muscle fibers).

5. Chronic myopathy resembling a dystrophic process.

Tendon

Tendon damage may result from inflammation of the synovial lining of the tendon sheath (tenosynovitis) and interferes with smooth gliding of the tendon. A lag phenomenon may be seen in patients with tendon damage or muscle weakening, displaying a significant difference between passive and active range of motion.

EXTRA-ARTICULAR SYSTEMIC MANIFESTATIONS

As previously described, RA affects the joint and is systemic. The number and the severity of extra-articular features vary with the duration and extent of the disease and tend to occur in individuals with higher levels of RF in their blood. The following are additional manifestations that may exist in those with RF.

Rheumatoid or Subcutaneous Nodules

Rheumatoid nodule formation is one of the most common extra-articular manifestations of RA and occurs in up to 50% of individuals at some point during the disease course (5, 50). Periarticular structures, extensor surfaces, and areas subject to pressure such as the olecranon (Fig. 14.24), the proximal ulna, the Achilles tendon, the occiput, and the sacrum are primary sites for those growths. Most can develop insidiously and regress at any time.

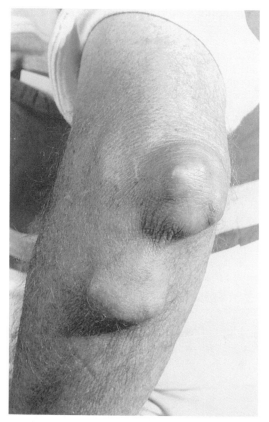

FIGURE 14.24 Large rheumatoid nodules in the ole-cranon bursa and along the extensor surface of the proximal ulna. Each mass is a collection of multiple smaller nodules. A small effusion is present in the ole-cranon bursa.

Pulmonary Manifestations

Pleuritis, interstitial fibrosis, pulmonary nodules, pneumonitis, and other forms of pulmonary obstructive disease occur more frequently in those with RA than in the normal population (51, 52). Evidence of pleuritis is usually found at autopsy, because the disease is usually asymptomatic during life. In a few cases, upper airway obstruction from cricoarytenoid arthritis or laryngeal nodules may develop. Others believe that small-airway dysfunction is related to factors other than RA.

Felty's Syndrome

The condition of leukopenia associated with collagen–vascular disorders, called "Felty's syndrome," occurs in less than 1% of patients with RA (53). This syndrome is usually found in those who have progressed and have chronic RA, as well as those who have high levels of RF (5). Splenomegaly, leukopenia, anemia, neutropenia, thrombocytopenia, and granulocytopenia also are features of this syndrome. Although hypersplenism is proposed as one of the causes of the leukopenia, splenectomies do not correct the abnormality in many patients.

Cardiac Manifestations

Asymptomatic pericarditis is found in nearly 50% of autopsied cases (54). Most pericardial disease develops with synovitis several years into the course of RA. Manifestations may vary from mild to being the cause of death.

Other forms of cardiac disease in RA include rheumatoid carditis, endocardial (valve) inflammation, conduction defects, coronary arteritis, and granulomatous aortitis (55).

Nervous System Manifestations

Neurological manifestations may be caused by cervical spine subluxation. As briefly described in the neck, cervical spine, and wrist sections above,

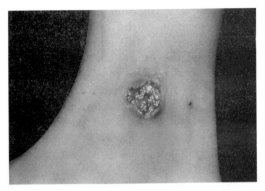

FIGURE 14.25 Vasculitis, defined as inflammation of the small vessels, is common in RA. The most common vascular abnormality in patients with RA is leg ulceration, which may be indolent and difficult to heal. Ulcers are not usually associated with either arterial or venous insufficiency. Other vasculitis problems among patients with RA include benign digital (fingertip) ulceration and severe systemic vasculitis similar to polyarteritis nodosa. (Reprinted with permission from the Arthritis Foundation. The AHPA Arthritis Teaching Slide Collection. 2nd ed. 1988.)

nerve entrapment that is the result of proliferative synovitis or joint deformities may facilitate neuropathies of the median, ulnar, radial, or anterior tibial nerves. In aggressive forms of vasculitis (Fig. 14.25), polyneuropathy and mononeuritis multiplex may result (5). Central nervous system involvement does not appear to occur directly, but vasculitis (as discussed above) and rheumatoid nodulelike granulomas can occur irregularly in the meninges.

Ophthalmological Manifestations

The rheumatoid process involves the eye in less than 1% of patients. Sjögren's syndrome (Fig. 14.26) is a chronic disease of unknown etiology causing corneal and conjunctival lesions and characterized by dry eyes and mouth. Eye discomfort includes the inability to cry and a sandy feeling when blinking. Scleritis, which involves the deeper coats of the eye, may cause pain and visual impairment. Episcleritis is a less serious inflammatory condition and is usually temporary.

Eye involvement occurs in 30 to 50% of early onset JRA patients (Fig. 14.27). In 80% of those

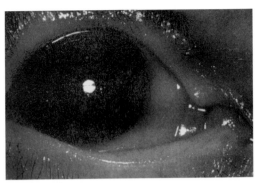

FIGURE 14.26 Patients with RA may also have Sjögren's syndrome. Sjögren's syndrome is a chronic inflammatory disorder characterized by diminished lacrimal and salivary gland secretions (sicca complex), resulting in keratoconjunctivitis sicca and xerostomia. Patients may complain that the eyes feel "as if they have sand in them." The syndrome also may include decreased vaginal lubrication. Keratoconjunctivitis sicca is demonstrated here by flecks of reddish-purple discoloration in the lower portion of the cornea and conjunctiva, which were stained with rose bengal dye. One-half of all patients with Sjögren's syndrome have RA or some other connective tissue disease, particularly systemic lupus erythematosus or systemic sclerosis. More than 90% of these patients are women, with a mean age of 50 years at the time of diagnosis. Keratoconjunctivitis sicca develops in 10 to 15% of all patients with RA. (Reprinted with permission from the Arthritis Foundation. The AHPA Arthritis Teaching Slide Collection. 2nd ed. 1988.)

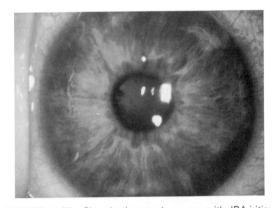

FIGURE 14.27 Chronic changes in an eye with JRA iritis: posterior synechiae (iris-lens adhesions at pupil margin); iris bombe (shallowing of the anterior chamber caused by blockage of aqueous flow from posterior chamber through pupil); secondary cataract. (Reprinted with permission from Hiles DA. Slide atlas of pediatric physical diagnosis. In: Zitelli BJ, Davis HW, eds. Pediatric Ophthalmology. New York: Gower Medical Publishing, 1987;17:15.)

TABLE 14.4   American Academy of Pediatrics Guidelines for Frequency of Screening Eye Examinations in JRA Patients

JRA ONSET SUBTYPE	Age at Onset	
	7 YEARS	≥ 7 YEARS
Systemic	Annual	Annual
Polyarticular		
ANA positive	Every 3–4 months × 4 years, then every 6 months × 3 years, then yearly	Every 6 months × 4 years, then yearly
ANA negative	Every 6 months × 4 years, then yearly	Every 6 months × 4 years, then yearly
Pauciarticular		
ANA positive	Every 3–4 months × 4 years, then every 6 months × 3 years, then yearly	Every 6 months × 4 years, then yearly
ANA negative	Every 6 months × 4 years, then yearly	Every 6 months × 4 years, then yearly

Abbreviation: ANA, antinuclear antibody. Adapted with permission from Yancey and Gross (8).

children who experience eye involvement, the inflammation process primarily involves the anterior chamber of the eye with minimal to no symptoms. However, severe, irreversible eye changes can occur including corneal clouding, cataracts, glaucoma, and partial or total visual loss. Children with JRA should be screened at regular intervals and treated by eye specialists (56) (Table 14.4).

Depression

Depression has been identified as a significant problem for those with arthritis. Research completed at the University of California, San Francisco between 1989 and 1991, found that the greater the negative impact on an individual's ability to accomplish daily living activities, the greater the likelihood that he or she would develop symptoms of depression (57).

Body Composition

Researchers at the USDA Human Nutrition Center on Aging at Tufts University and New England Medical Center found that among persons with RA, changes in their immune system and the substance it produces resulted in higher metabolism, loss of lean body mass, and loss of appetite. This,

in turn, suggests that the use of measures for lean mass in those with RA might identify high risk individuals who could then be identified for interventions, such as nutritional counseling, to improve body composition (58).

COURSE AND PROGNOSIS

The course of RA tends be uncertain because its effects differ significantly from person to person. Onset of the disease is usually gradual or insidious, although it may be abrupt. Because of the cyclical nature of the RA process, an individual's ability to function can fluctuate according to the stage and severity of the disease. Approximately 20% of patients will improve spontaneously, or even achieve remission, especially in the first year of the disease; however, chronic disease progression and functional deterioration occur in the majority. Long-term studies have shown that patients with RA have 6 times the probability of restrictions in daily activities, 4 times as many restricted activity days, and 10 times the work disability rate as the general population (4).

In children with JRA, 70 to 90% make a satisfactory recovery from their disease without serious disability. A small percentage will have a recurrence as adults (13).

After diagnosis, it is helpful to monitor the patient carefully during the next 3 months to predict the course of the disease, if evidence of progressive disease is not apparent at initial presentation.

Studies have found that some patients do experience spontaneous remission. Short et al. found that only 10% of patients see clinical remission during more than a decade of follow-up (60). Other research completed by Ragan concurred with those findings but also concluded that those patients who experienced remission did so in the first 2 years of disease onset (61) (Table 14.5).

Features that appear to have prognostic importance are: a) number and length of remissions (62), b) levels of RF, c) presence of subcutaneous nodules, d) extent of bone erosion seen radiographically at initial evaluation, and e) sustained disease activity for more than 1 year. In addition, it has been discovered that in patients younger than age 50, women tend to have a worse prognosis with regard to persistence and severity (63).

Classification and prognosis of RA also can be assessed by functional analysis (Table 14.6). The functional capacity of an individual declines as the disease becomes more prevalent. Studies have established both an immediate and long-term relationship between arthritis and limitations in function (64). Self-reported functional status and the physical demands of work are the best pre-

---

TABLE 14.5 Proposed Criteria for Clinical Remission in Rheumatoid Arthritis[a]

Five or more of the following requirements must be fulfilled for at least 2 consecutive months:
1. Duration of morning stiffness not exceeding 15 minutes
2. No fatigue
3. No joint pain (by history)
4. No joint tenderness or pain on motion
5. No soft tissue swelling in joints of tendon sheaths
6. Erythrocyte sedimentation rate (Westergren method) less than 30 mm/hr for a female or 20 mm/hr for a male

---

[a]These criteria are intended to describe either spontaneous remission or drug-induced disease suppression, which simulates spontaneous remission. To be considered for this designation, a patient must have met the American Rheumatism Association criteria for definite or classic rheumatoid arthritis at some time in the past. No alternative explanation may be invoked to account for the failure to meet a particular requirement. For instance, in the presence of knee pain that might be related to degenerative arthritis, a point for "no joint pain" may not be awarded.
Exclusions: Clinical manifestations of active vasculitis, pericarditis pleuritis, or myositis, and unexplained recent weight loss or fever attributed to RA will prohibit a designation of complete clinical remission.

TABLE 14.6 Classification of Functional Capacity in Rheumatoid Arthritis

Class I: Complete functional capacity with the ability to carry on all usual duties without handicaps
Class II. Functional capacity adequate to conduct normal activities despite handicap of discomfort or limited mobility of one or more joints
Class III: Functional capacity adequate to perform only a few or none of the duties of usual occupation or self-care
Class IV: Largely or wholly incapacitated, with patient bedridden or confined to wheelchair, permitting little or no self-care

dictors of disability. Lack of autonomy over the work schedule, the pace of the work, and the nature of the job all increase the likelihood of becoming disabled (65, 66). Early mortality has been linked closely to functional disability (67).

Although there is no cure for RA, treatment methods continue to improve. Data suggest that individuals currently admitted to the hospital for RA are likely to have a decreased number of contractures and less fusion of peripheral joints at admission than did patients 20 years ago (27). The median life expectancy of individuals with RA is shortened by 3 to 7 years (21). Upon completion of a thorough evaluation by a physician, early diagnosis can assist with developing a treatment approach to diminish joint pain, impede the disease process, and decrease joint deformity. Early classification of the disease facilitates earlier intervention and, possibly, a "retarding" of the disease progress.

Emotional and financial support for treatment both contribute to the prognostic outcome and performance of children and adults. Studies have demonstrated a high incidence of depression, decreased self-esteem, and social withdrawal. In those with a progressed case of RA, the type of treatment prescribed plays a key part in life expectancy. For example, drug therapy, especially the more aggressive, systematic corticosteroid drugs, may play a role in increased mortality rates.

DIAGNOSIS

Individuals with joint disease delay seeking medical care an average of 2 to 4 years (5). It is much more difficult to establish a diagnosis of RA in the early development of the disease than in the more progressed, later stages. Several visits to a physician for evaluation and testing may be needed before a diagnosis can be confirmed. The American College of Rheumatology (ACR), formerly the Rheumatism Association (ARA), first developed diagnostic criteria for the classification of RA in 1958, with revisions in 1987 (Tables 14.7 and 14.8). Originally, these criteria were guidelines for classification of

---

TABLE 14.7   Classification of Progression of Rheumatoid Arthritis[a]

Stage I—Early
*1. No destructive changes on roentgenographic examination
 2. Roentgenological evidence of osteoporosis may be present

Stage II—Moderate
*1. Roentgenological evidence of osteoporosis with or without slight subchondral bone destruction; slight cartilage destruction may be present
*2. No joint deformities, although limitation of joint mobility may be present
 3. Extensive muscle atrophy
 4. Extra-articular soft tissue lesions, such as nodules and tenosynovitis, may be present

Stage III—Severe
*1. Roentgenological evidence of cartilage and bone destruction in addition to osteoporosis
*2. Joint deformity such as subluxation, ulnar deviation, or hyperextension, without fibrous or bony ankylosis
 3. Extensive muscle atrophy
 4. Extra-articular soft tissue lesions, such as nodules and tenosynovitis, may be present

Stage IV—Terminal
*1. Fibrous or bone ankylosis
 2. Same criteria of stage III

---

[a]An asterisk marks criteria required for classification in the particular stage. See Table 14.5 for clinical remission criteria.

TABLE 14.8   1987 ARA Revised Criteria for the Classification of Rheumatoid Arthritis[a]

CRITERION	DEFINITION
1. Morning stiffness	Morning stiffness in and around the joints lasting at least 1 hour before maximal improvement
2. Arthritis of three or more joint areas	At least 3 joint areas at the same time have had soft tissue swelling or fluid observed by a physician. The 14 possible areas are right or left PIP, MCP, wrist, elbow, knee, ankle, and MTP joints.
3. Arthritis of hand joints	At least one area swollen in a wrist, MCP, or PIP joint
4. Symmetric arthritis	Simultaneous involvement of the same joint areas on both sides of the body (bilateral involvement of PIPs, MCPs, or MTPs is acceptable without absolute symmetry)
5. Rheumatoid nodules	Subcutaneous nodules over bony prominences or extensor surfaces or in juxta-articular regions, observed by a physician
6. Serum rheumatoid factor	Demonstration of abnormal amounts of serum RF by any method for which the result has been positive in 5% of normal subjects
7. Radiographic changes	Radiographic changes typical of RA on posteroanterior hand and wrist X-rays, which must include erosions or unequivocal bony decalcification localized in (or most significant adjacent to) the involved joints.

[a]A person is to be diagnosed with RA if he or she has met at least four of seven of the established criteria. The criteria of morning stiffness, arthritis of three or more joint areas, at least one area swollen in the hand joints, and presence of symmetrical involvement must be present for at least 6 weeks to establish a diagnosis of RA as well. Note that failure to meet these criteria, especially in the early stages, does not exclude the diagnosis. Patients with two clinical diagnoses are not excluded. Designation as classic, definite, or probable RA is not to be made.

disease syndromes to allow a correct diagnosis in individuals taking part in clinical research investigations. However, the criteria have also been used as guidelines for the specific diagnosis of individuals in general (1). The ACR continues to monitor the criteria for accuracy and validity. When diagnosis is still in doubt, further biopsies should be completed, if possible, on subcutaneous nodules to differentiate them from gouty tophi and amyloid and other types of nodules. Even though RA shares many characteristics of other collagen diseases, particularly systemic lupus erythematosus, the latter can usually be identified by the characteristic skin lesions on the light-exposed areas, temporal frontal hair loss, oral and nasal mucosal lesions, and in joint fluid with a white blood count seen as "overlap syndrome" (5).

Diagnosis of JRA may be a long, drawn out process. The diagnosis depends on symptoms experienced in the first 6 months of the illness. The primary steps include many of those taken to diagnose RA in an adult. These include:

• A comprehensive health history to help determine the length of time symptoms have been present
• A physical examination to look for joint inflammation, rashes, nodules, and eye problems
• Laboratory tests to rule out other diseases
• X-ray examinations of joints to identify other possible conditions
• Tests of fluids from joints and tissues to check for infections or inflammation

MEDICAL/SURGICAL MANAGEMENT

The goals of medical management of RA and JRA are: 1) relief of pain and stiffness, 2) reduction of inflammation, 3) preservation of muscle strength and joint function, 4) minimizing drug side effects, 5) maintenance of as much of a normal lifestyle as possible and, for children, 6) promotion of normal growth and development. Another objective is to attempt to resolve or modify disease progress through early, aggressive drug therapies advocated because of the diagnosis, prognosis, and reversible damage in the articular cartilage within the first 2 years of the disease (4).

Because the etiology of RA is unknown and the mechanisms of therapeutic interventions uncertain, therapy remains experimental. None of the interventions are curative; therefore, all must be viewed as palliative, aimed at relieving the signs and symptoms of the disease.

A comprehensive therapeutic management program for those with JRA and RA include a) physical management (includes occupational and physical therapy), b) psychosocial care (includes self-image, pain management work, and school participation, leisure, family functioning, family education, and financial aspects), c) nutritional aspects, d) pharmacological management, and e) other medical aspects.

An interdisciplinary approach that focuses on physical, functional, and psychosocial issues is common with RA patients. Physical and occupational therapy interventions, including exercise and rest strategies, physical agent modalities (i.e. heat, ultrasound, etc.), and splinting to allow proper alignment of deformed joints, have all assisted with managing symptoms.

Patient and family education that centers on self-help and self-management of RA have demonstrated positive results. Review of medical and patient education outcomes research shows that medications offer a 20 to 50% improvement in arthritis symptoms for most patients and that patient education interventions, such as the Arthritis Self Help Courses, offered through the Arthritis Foundation, can reduce symptoms an additional 15 to 30% (68, 69).

DRUG THERAPY

Many different drugs are used in the medical management of RA. Five different types of drugs are important: analgesic drugs, nonsteroidal anti-inflammatory drugs, including salicylates, corticosteroids, disease modifying antirheumatic drugs (DMARDs), which are considered second-line drugs, and cytotoxics, which are considered third-line drugs.

Treatment is focused on anti-inflammatory and immunosuppressive effects to both prevent destruction of the joint and give pain control. However, as mentioned above, treatment should not be limited to drug therapy.

As seen in the pyramid approach (Fig. 14.28), which was the key philosophy during the 1980s,

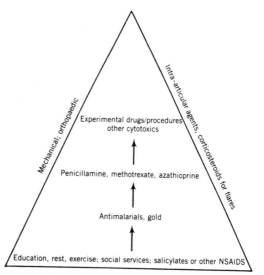

FIGURE 14.28 Treatment pyramid for RA. (Reprinted with permission from The Arthritis Foundation. The Primer on the Rheumatic Diseases. 9th ed. 1988.)

medical management began with the most conservative method and then assumed a more aggressive approach as the disease progressed. This thought process began to change somewhat when methotrexate, a cytotoxic drug, demonstrated that it could control RA with minimal toxicity compared with other second-line DMARDs. In the 1990s, the pyramid approach has been used less frequently. Instead, more aggressive therapy consisting of immunosuppressives (including cytotoxic drugs) is implemented as the first part of treatment and combined with DMARDs to obtain disease control before severe joint destruction occurs (68).

Salicylates (e.g., aspirin) or the newer nonsteroidal anti-inflammatory drugs (NSAIDs) are the primary, and less toxic drugs, available for RA treatment. They provide relief from pain, reduce inflammation, and are fairly inexpensive.

SURGERY

Surgery plays a role in the management of RA in severely damaged joints. Hip and knee arthroplasties and total joint replacements have offered the most success, even though these procedures are completed on a number of joints. The goals of surgery are 1) pain reduction, 2) correction of deformity, and 3) functional improvement. As with any major surgery, there are inherent risks that must be carefully weighed. The patient must prepare for the surgery and expect to be an active participant in rehabilitation (70).

IMPACT ON OCCUPATIONAL PERFORMANCE

Effects on occupational performance for individuals with RA are usually disruptive but not life threatening. A person with RA will experience varying degrees of improvement, depending on the progression of the disease, anatomical structures involved, systemic problems experienced, financial support available, and psychological outlook (Table 14.9).

Trombley calls identifying occupational performance problems as the first step in assessment a more "top down" approach (as opposed to the "bottom up" approach of evaluating performance components like joint range of motion and muscle strength). Taking the top down approach also gives a better understanding of the context within which the person functions and the priorities he or she believes are key (71, 72). A variety of tools are available to assess performance problems and performance components. These evaluations include both health status questionnaires (i.e., Arthritis Impact Measurement Scale 2 [AIMS2] [73] and Juvenile Arthritis Functional Assessment Report [JAFASR] [74]) and functional status assessments (Canadian Occupational Performance Measure [COPM] [75]). It is important to focus on the context in which the individual must perform daily activities, as this will determine the feasibility and appropriateness of intervention.

Sensory Integration

Sensory processing may be affected, specifically tactile, proprioceptive, visual, and auditory. Nerve impingement from the loss of soft tissue integrity can affect both tactile and proprioceptive processing throughout both proximal and peripheral joints. Visual changes occur in 1% of the population, resulting from iridocyclitis (described above). Auditory changes can result from inflammation of the inner ear bone joints.

NEUROMUSCULAR

The most prominent deficit in the neuromuscular component is decreased range of motion in the major joints, with subsequent muscle weakness. Joint deformities are common, especially in the direction of flexion. The inflammation of RA causes joint swelling. Joint stiffness, especially in the morning, is a common complaint. The cumulative effects of immobility, stiffness, and pain result in generalized fatigue that exacerbates the

TABLE 14.9   Occupational Performance Profile

I. PERFORMANCE AREAS	II. PERFORMANCE COMPONENTS	III. PERFORMANCE CONTEXTS
A. Activities of Daily Living	**A. Sensorimotor Component**	A. Temporal Aspects
1. Grooming	**1. Sensory**	1. Chronological
2. Oral Hygiene	a. Sensory Awareness	2. Developmental
3. Bathing/Showering	**b. Sensory Processing**	3. Lifecycle
4. Toilet Hygiene	**(1) Tactile**	4. Disability Status
5. Personal Device Care	**(2) Proprioceptive**	B. Environment
6. Dressing	(3) Vestibular	1. Physical
7. Feeding and Eating	**(4) Visual (only 1%)**	2. Social
8. Medication Routine	**(5) Auditory**	3. Cultural
9. Health Maintenance	(6) Gustatory	
10. Socialization	(7) Olfactory	
11. Functional Communication	c. Perceptual Processing	
12. Functional Mobility	**(1) Stereognosis**	
13. Community Mobility	**(2) Kinesthesia**	
14. Emergency Response	**(3) Pain Response**	
15. Sexual Expression	(4) Body Scheme	
B. Work and Productive Activities	(5) Right–Left Discrimination	
1. Home Management	(6) Form Constancy	
a. Clothing Care	(7) Position in Space	
b. Cleaning	(8) Visual–Closure	
c. Meal Preparation/ Cleanup	(9) Figure Ground	
d. Shopping	(10) Depth Perception	
e. Money Management	(11) Spatial Relations	
f. Household Maintenance	(12) Topographical Orientation	
g. Safety Procedures	2. Neuromusculoskeletal	
2. Care of Others	**a. Reflex**	
3. Educational Activities	**b. Range of Motion**	
4. Vocational Activities	**c. Muscle Tone**	
a. Vocational Exploration	**d. Strength**	
b. Job Acquisition	**e. Endurance**	
c. Work or Job Performance	**f. Postural Control**	
d. Retirement Planning	**g. Postural Alignment**	
e. Volunteer Participation	**h. Soft Tissue Integrity**	
C. Play or Leisure Activities	3. Motor	
1. Play or Leisure Exploration	**a. Gross Coordination**	
2. Play or Leisure Performance	b. Crossing the Midline	
	c. Laterality	
	d. Bilateral Integration	
	e. Motor Control	
	f. Praxis	
	g. Fine Coordination/Dexterity	
	h. Visual–Motor Control	
	i. Oral–Motor Control	

(continued)

TABLE 14.9 Occupational Performance Profile (Continued)		
I. PERFORMANCE AREAS	**II. PERFORMANCE COMPONENTS**	**III. PERFORMANCE CONTEXTS**

	B. Cognitive Integration and Cognitive Components
	 1. Level of Arousal
	 2. Orientation
	 3. Recognition
	 4. Attention Span
	 5. Initiation of Activity
	 6. Termination of Activity
	 7. Memory
	 8. Sequencing
	 9. Categorization
	 10. Concept Formation
	 11. Spatial Operations
	 12. Problem Solving
	 13. Learning
	 14. Generalization
	C. Psychosocial Skills and Psychological Components
	 1. Psychological
	  a. Values
	  b. Interests
	  c. Self-Concept
	 2. Social
	  a. Role Performance
	  b. Social Conduct
	  c. Interpersonal Skills
	  d. Self-Expression
	 3. Self-Management
	  a. Coping Skills
	  b. Time Management
	  c. Self-Control	

mobility impairment. Decreased strength may be seen in patients during functional strength testing. A patient may demonstrate good strength in a pain-free portion of joint range and unmeasurable strength in painful areas of joint range. Strength also may vary during times of the day when joint stiffness is decreased.

Motor

The most likely motor impairment will be depressed activity tolerance due to the decreased neuromuscular status. Fatigue should be carefully evaluated during a 24-hour period, as well as over several days or weeks to gain full understanding of patterns and impact on function over time. Heart rate, respiratory rate, and blood pressure should all be measured during functional activities. Although a passive and active range-of-motion and strength assessment is useful, if joint pain or poor activity tolerance prohibit measurement of range of motion, consideration should be given to completing a functional range of motion test to see the range of motion available for performing functional activities. Documenting time of day can assist with identifying cycles of stiffness. Joint instability may be a significant deterrent to completing daily living activities. Areas of impact that require assessment include mobility and gait, as well as gross and fine coordination.

Cognitive

Rheumatoid arthritis has no direct cognitive effects. However, difficulty with attention span, short-term memory, sequencing, and problem solving may be caused by depression.

Psychosocial Skills and Psychological Components

It is not unusual for an individual with RA to have disease exacerbation as the result of major psychological stressors (76). The breakdown in coping mechanisms may lead to feelings of hopelessness and helplessness, which creates a reduction in self-management and self-concept. Depression and anxiety are other potential problems. It has been found that 43 to 52% of patients with RA report dysfunction in the areas of social interaction, communication with others, and emotional behavior (77). The individual with RA or JRA must routinely implement a series of changes in daily life with respect to medications, exercise, and self-care. Failure to comply with professional recommendations is often interpreted as a rejection of the caregiver's assistance or maladaptive behavior. The caregiver must allow the individual some control and autonomy to set the direction of the treatment and identify personal goals for the best outcome.

CASE STUDIES

CASE 1

M. C. is a 37-year-old housewife and mother of an energetic 10-year-old son and an 8-year-old daughter. She was diagnosed with RA 5 years ago and has,

until her most recent flare-ups, been able to take care of her home and her own self-care responsibilities.

Before this exacerbation, M. C. had always been very involved with her children and their activities. In addition, she did volunteer secretarial work at the local Arthritis Foundation and taught Sunday school. M. C. enjoyed doing needlework and went golfing with a friend. M. C. did most of the household maintenance because her husband is a salesman who travels and works long hours.

Since her last flare-up, M. C.'s lifestyle has been dramatically affected in all occupational performance areas. She displays moderate involvement in the neuromuscular and motor areas. Range of motion and muscle strength are affected in all movement of extension in her elbows, wrists, and hands. A slight ulnar drift is noted at the MP joints. Prehension skills are within normal limits, but grip strength is below normal. Endurance has declined to 1.5 hours of light activities before fatigue sets in. Because of pain and stiffness in the small joints of the hands, fine coordination has become significantly slowed. M. C. has left most of the housekeeping chores (e.g., laundry, vacuuming, and lawn cutting) to her husband, children, and supportive sister because she has lessened activity tolerance and pain. She has been able to continue her own self-care, simple meal preparation (using many convenience items), light housework with several rest breaks, and teaching Sunday school. She has completely discontinued her volunteer activities, her needlework, and her golfing.

Owing to the effects of her neuromuscular and motor problems, M. C. is having difficulty adjusting psychologically and socially. Previously, she exhibited a high level of self-esteem for her flexibility, planning skills, and ability to cope with the unexpected events that occur in raising a family. Now she has difficulty concentrating for long periods and has a poor appetite. She feels guilty and angry about no longer being the "supermom" she once thought herself to be. She feels that she is a burden to others, especially to her husband who must now add most of the household chores to his already busy and tiring schedule. She also is very frustrated by the fact that she was once a great source of support and motivation for others with arthritis and is now "letting them down."

CASE 2

M. S. was a fairly normal 9-year-old fourth grader who enjoyed swimming, soccer, collecting baseball cards, and science class. He is the third of four children (two boys and two girls). M. S.'s mother is a part-time teacher and his father is a banker.

Three months ago, M. S. was diagnosed with JRA of the pauciarticular type (four or fewer joints involved). The diagnosis was made after a series of laboratory tests, x-rays, and physical examinations by his pediatrician. Before the diagnosis, M. S. had been complaining of intermittent mild pain and stiffness in his lower back and hips for approximately 2 months.

Play, activities of daily living, and education are the areas primarily affected. The intensity of his symptoms fluctuates significantly.

Involved neuromuscular components include hip and trunk range of motion, lower extremity muscle strength, endurance, and, occasionally, postural control. Hip range of motion is limited, and muscles appear "stiff" in the last quarter of the range early in the morning, after sitting for more than 45 minutes, and before going to bed. Muscle strength is measured as fair/fair+ on hip flexion and extension, and fair+ for trunk extension. At the highest degree of hip and trunk stiffness, his postural control is compromised and he cannot react quickly during play. His musculoskeletal endurance decreases in the afternoon, especially after a morning of school activities.

M. S.'s gross motor coordination (and activity tolerance) declines on "bad days," which significantly affects his ability to play on the school soccer team. M. S.'s parents have met with his teachers to explain his special needs so he can function at his optimal level. The teachers must allow M. S. to walk around the classroom from time to time to prevent stiffness and rest more frequently if he is doing a great deal of walking on a field trip.

On a functional level, M. S. can dress and bathe independently; however, some days it takes him much longer because of the stiffness. Feeding and grooming present no problems at this point. Functional mobility is affected after M. S. has been sitting for a time. He experiences increased stiffness and even walks with a limp when his back pain increases.

For the most part, M. S. has been able to maintain most of his leisure interests except soccer. His regular swim session at the local Y.M.C.A. helps to decrease pain and stiffness in his hips and back. The whole family has become involved at the open swim night, which has helped promote good family fun and relations.

Psychosocially, M. S. has had some difficulty adjusting to limitations, even though his parents have been very supportive. To maintain his role within the family, M. S.'s parents have attempted to treat him as they do their other children so he is not perceived as the "special" or "sick" child. M. S.'s self-esteem fluctuates, depending on his ability to participate in activities with his friends. M. S. has not told his friends that he has JRA. He fears that they will not want to play with him, will avoid him because he has a contagious disease, or will make fun of him. The time that he was devoting to soccer he now spends with the science club at school, at his mother's insistence. M. S. has periodic temper tantrums and displays anger about JRA and sometimes refuses to take his medications. M. S. and his parents attend a family support group for children with JRA, where the whole family has met new friends and has been able to share their feelings in a nonthreatening environment.

CONCLUSION

During the last decade, the health care environment has and will continue to be stressed in regards to reimbursement and funding for assessment and treatment of those with RA and JRA. Managed care is still growing across the country, which will have a significant impact on where the treatment of those with arthritis will take place. The "gate-keeper" will be the primary care physician who will determine the need for referral to specialists, including rheumatologists. Because positive results have been found with the initiation of early, aggressive intervention, primary care physicians will need to be proactively educated with appropriate protocols and treatment regimens.

Clinicians will have increased demands for outcomes research to demonstrate the positive effects of their interventions. Client-centered treatment, including self-help, self-management, and education, will continue to be advocated, along with the clinicians' responsibility to facilitate realistic goal setting and provide patients with encouragement, optimism, and hope for the future.

Growth of resources, including community based and those found on the Internet, can foster an individual's quality of life. As researchers continue to seek the cause of, and a cure for RA, the challenge for physicians and allied health professionals, including occupational and physical therapists, will be to assist those with RA to "take charge" of their lives and to learn to live as comfortably, productively, and independently as possible.

Acknowledgments

In writing this chapter, I have renewed my great respect for all those individuals who have JRA and RA and have learned positive coping and management strategies in their daily lives.

I am also extremely proud to be a part of, and very encouraged by, the progress that the medical community has made in the area of research, gaining understanding of the etiology and comprehensive management of RA and JRA. Even with the challenges ahead, there are optimistic expectations of disease regression and cure in the near future.

I also would like to express my thanks to my fiancé, family, colleagues, and the Arthritis Foundation, National Office and Michigan Chapter, for their assistance and support during the work on this chapter.

POINTS FOR REVIEW

1. List the various anatomical aspects of a joint.

2. What is the cause of arthritis?

3. Describe the current focus in research regarding the etiology of RA.

4. What are the three major criteria for diagnosis of JRA?

5. What is the peak onset age for JRA? Is there a difference in incidence between gender groups?

6. When someone with RA is in an exacerbated state of the disease, what characteristics may be observed?

7. Describe the three stages of the inflammatory process.

8. Of all the extremities, which are most affected by RA?

9. Describe conditions of the hand associated with RA.

10. Describe conditions of the shoulder associated with RA.

11. Why does hoarseness of the voice occur in 30% of persons with RA?

12. Describe the five stages of muscle disease in RA.

13. What systems, other than joint structures, are involved?

14. Why should children with JRA be screened by an ophthalmologist?

15. Describe the functional capacity indicators used to classify RA.

16. What is the focus of medical management for persons with RA?

17. What areas of the occupational performance components would need to be evaluated?

REFERENCES

1. Benedict T. History of the rheumatic disease. In: Klippel JH, Weyland CM, Wortman RL, eds. Primer on the Rheumatic Diseases. 11th ed. Atlanta: Arthritis Foundation, 1997.

2. Schned ES, Reinertsen JL. The social and economic consequences of rheumatic disease. In: Klippel HJ, Weyland CM, Wortman RL, eds. Primer on the Rheumatic Diseases. 11th ed. Atlanta: Arthritis Foundation, 1997.

3. Yelin E, Callahan LF. The economic and social and psychological impact of musculoskeletal conditions. Arthritis Rheum 1995;38:1351–1362.

4. Arnett F. Rheumatoid arthritis. In: Bennett JC, Plum F, eds. Cecil's Textbook of Medicine, Volume 2. 20th edition. Philadelphia: WB Saunders Co., 1996.

5. Berkow R, Fletcher AJ, eds. Rheumatoid arthritis. In: The Merck Manual. 16th ed. Whitehouse Station, NJ: Merck and Co. Inc, 1992.

6. Winchester R. Studying genetic susceptibility to rheumatoid arthritis. Joint Movement 1989;1:4.

7. Roitt I. Essential Immunology. 4th ed. Boston: Blackwell Scientific Publications, 1980:85, 287, 321.

8. Anonymous. The immune system. Joint Movement 1989;1:4.

9. Anonymous. Inflammation. Joint Movement 1989; 1:2.

10. Silverman EH. Rheumatic diseases: evaluation and treatment. In: Logigian MK, ed. Adult Rehabilitation: A Team Approach for Therapists. Boston: Little, Brown & Co., 1981:111–115.

11. Arthritis Foundation. Gene may predict severity in rheumatoid arthritis. In: New Arthritis Research pg 1. (http://www.arthritis.org/news/nmr/pimemos/93_06.html)

12. Briley M. Why me? Arthritis Today 1998;12:1:31–32.

13. Cassidy J. Juvenile rheumatoid arthritis. In: Kelley WN, Ruddy S, Harris ED, et al, eds. Textbook of Rheumatology. 5th ed. Philadelphia: WB Saunders Co., 1997.

14. Lovell DJ. Pediatric rheumatic diseases: juvenile rheumatic diseases and juvenile spondyloarthritis. In: Klippel JH, Weyand CM, Wortman RL, eds. Primer on the Rheumatic Diseases. 11th ed. Atlanta: Arthritis Foundation, 1997.

15. Arthritis Foundation. Demographic and economic information, 1998. (http://www.arthritis.org/offices/al/about/demecoinfo.html)

16. Lawrence RC, Hunchberg MC, Kelsey JL, et al. Estimates of the prevalence of selected arthritis and musculoskeletal diseases in the United States. J Rheumatol 1989;16:427–441.

17. Arthritis Foundation. Status of pediatric rheumatology, part 1, 1997. (http://www.arthritis.org/ajao/arhreya_part_1.html)

18. Silman AJ, Hockberg MC. Epidemiology of the Rheumatic Diseases. Oxford University Press, 1993.

19. Cunningham LS, Keesley JL. Epidemiology of musculoskeletal impairments and associated disability. Am J Public Health 1984;74:574–579.

20. Beasley RP, Bennett PH, Len CC. Low prevalence of rheumatoid arthritis in Chinese: prevalence survey in a rural community. J Rheumatoid Arthritis 1983; 10:11–15.

21. Lipsky P. Rheumatoid arthritis. In: Harrison TR, Isselbacher KJ, Braunwald E, et al, eds. Harrison's Principles of Internal Medicine, Vol. 2. 13th ed. New York: McGraw-Hill, 1994.

22. Felson DT. Etiology of the rheumatic disease. In: Koopman WJ, ed. Arthritis and Allied Conditions: A Textbook of Rheumatology, Vol. 1. 13th ed. Baltimore: Williams & Wilkins, 1997.

23. Linos A, Worthington JW, O'Fallon WM, et al. The epidemiology of rheumatoid arthritis in Rochester, Minnnesota: a study of incidence, prevelance and mortality. Am J Epidemiol 1980;111:97–98.

24. Hochberg MC. Changes in the incidence and prevalence of rheumatoid arthritis in England and Wales, 1970–1982. Semin Arthritis Rheum 1990: 294–302.

25. Jacobson LTH, Hanson RL, Knowler WC, et al. Decreasing incidence and prevelance of rheumatoid arthritis in PIMA Indians over a 25 year period. Arthritis Rheum 1994;33:735–739.

26. Silman AJ. Trends in the incidence and severity of rheumatoid arthritis. J Rheum 1992;19(32):71–73.

27. Fallahi S, Halla JT, Hardin JG. Clinical Research 1983;31:650.

28. Melvin JL. Rheumatic Disease: Occupational Therapy and Rehabilitation. 2nd ed. Philadelphia: FA Davis, 1982.

29. Nalebuff EA. Diagnosis, classification and management of rheumatoid thumb deformities. Bull Hosp Jt Dis 1968;24:119.

30. Gray RG, Gottlieb NL. Hand flexor tenosynovitis in rheumatoid arthritis. Arthritis Rheum 1977;20: 1003–1007.

31. Fuchs HA, Sergent JS. Rheumatoid arthritis: the clinical picture. In: Koopman WJ. Arthritis and Allied Conditions, Vol. 1. 13th ed. Baltimore: Williams & Wilkins, 1997.

32. Anderson RJ. Rheumatoid arthritis: clinical and laboratory features. In: Klippel JH, Weyand CM, Wortmann RL, eds. Primer on the Rheumatic Diseases. 11th ed. Atlanta: Arthritis Foundation, 1997.

33. Post M. The Shoulder: Surgical and Non-surgical Treatment. Philadelphia: Lea and Febiger, 1978.

34. Moncur C, Williams HJ. Cervical spine management in patients with rheumatoid arthritis. Phys Ther 1988;68:508.

35. Kramer J, Jolesz F, Kleefield J. Rheumatoid arthritis of the cervical spine. Semin Arthritis Rheum 1985;14:187–195.

36. Komusi T, Jolesz F, Kleefield J. Rheumatoid arthritis of the cervical spine. Rheum Dis Clin North Am 1991;17:757.

37. Rasker JJ, Cosh JA. Radiological study of the cervical spine and hand patients with rheumatoid arthritis of 15 years duration: an assessment of corticosteroid treatment. Ann Rheum Dis 1978;37: 529–535.

38. Ryan D. Painful temporomandibular joint. In: McCarty DJ, ed. Arthritis and Allied Conditions. 11th ed. Philadelphia: Lea and Febiger, 1989.

39. Leicht MJ, Harrington TM, Davis DE. Cricoary-tenoid arthritis: a cause of laryngeal obstruction. Ann Emerg Med 1987;16:885–888.

40. Lawry GV, Finerman ML, Hanaffee WN, et al. Laryngeal involvement in rheumatoid arthritis: a clinical, laryngoscopic and computerized tomographic study. Arthritis Rheum 1984;27:873–882.

41. Anderson RJ. Rheumatoid arthritis: clinical and laboratory features. In: Klippel JH, Weyand CM, Wortmann RL, eds. Primer on the Rheumatic Diseases. 11th ed. Atlanta: Arthritis Foundation, 1997.

42. Bennett JC. Rheumatoid arthritis: clinical features. In: Schumacher HR, Klipper JH, Robinson DR, eds. Primer on Rheumatic Diseases. 9th ed. Atlanta: Arthritis Foundation, 1988.

43. Vidigal E, Jacoby RK, Dixon ASJ, et al. The foot in chronic rheumatoid arthritis. Ann Rheum Dis 1975;34:292–297.

44. Valniok K. The rheumatoid foot, a clinical study with pathological roentgenological comments. Am Clin Gynecol 1956;45:1–5.

45. Frieberg RA, Moncur C. Arthritis of the foot. Bull Rheum Dis 1991;40:1.

46. Pearson CM. Polymyositis and dermatomyositis. In: McCarthy DJ, ed. Arthritis and Allied Conditions. 9th ed. Philadelphia: Lea and Febiger, 1978.

47. Mullen EA. Influence of training and activity on muscle strength. Arch Phys Med Rehabil 1990;51:449–469.

48. Kottle F. The effects of limitation of activity on the human body. JAMA 1966;196:825–830.

49. Harris E. Rheumatic arthritis: the clinical spectrum. In: Kelly WH, ed. Textbook of Rheumatology. Philadelphia: WB Saunders, 1981.

50. Moore CP, Wilkens RF. The subcutaneous nodule: its significance in the diagnosis of rheumatic disease. Semin Arthritis Rheum 1977;7:63–79.

51. Jurik AG, Davison D, Graudal H. Prevalence of pulmonary involvement in rheumatoid arthritis and its relationship to some characteristics of the patients. Scand J Rheumatol 1982;11:217–224.

52. Hunninghald GW, Fauci HS. Pulmonary involvement in the collagen vascular diseases. Am Rev Resp Dis 1979;119:471–503.

53. Rosenstein ED, Kramer N. Felty's and Felty's syndrome. Semin Arthritis Rheum 1991;21:129–142.

54. Berkow R, Talbott JH. Merck Manual. 13th ed. Rahway, NJ: Merck, 1977:1312, 1331, 1656–1675.

55. Robert WC, Kehoe JA, Carpenter DF. Cardiac valvular lesion in rheumatoid arthritis. Arch Intern Med 1968;122:141–146.

56. Arthritis Foundation. Treatment for juvenile arthritis eye care, 1997. (http://www.arthritis.org/ajao/tellmemore/treatments.html)

57. Arthritis Foundation. Depression in arthritis. In: New Arthritis Research, 1990. (http://www.arthritis.org/news/nmr/pimemos/93_06.html)

58. Arthritis Foundation. Body composition and rheumatoid arthritis. In: New Arthritis Research, 1990. (http://www.arthritis.org/news/nmr/pimemos/93_06.html)

59. Pincus T. Rheumatoid Arthritis. In: Wegener ST, Belza BL, Gall EP. Clinical Care in the Rheumatic Diseases. Atlanta: American College of Rheumatology, 1996;26:151–152.

60. Short CL, Bauer W, Reynolds WE. Rheumatoid Arthritis. Cambridge: Harvard University Press, 1957.

61. Ragan C, Farrington E. The clinical features of rheumatoid arthritis. Prognostic indices. JAMA 1959;2:16.

62. Pinals RS, Masi AT, Larsen RA, et al. Preliminary criteria for clinical remission in rheumatoid arthritis. Arthritis Rheum 1981;24:1308–1315.

63. Masi AT, Maldonado-Cocco JA, Kaplan SB, et al. Prospective study of the early course of rheumatoid arthritis in young adults: comparison of patients with and without rheumatoid factor positivity at entry and identification of variables correlating with outcome. Semin Arthritis Rheum 1976;5:299–326.

64. Guccione AA. Arthritis and the process of disablement. Phys Ther 1994;74:408–414.

65. Eberrhardt K, Larsson BM, Nived K. Early rheumatoid arthritis—some social, economical and psychological aspects. Scand J Rheumatol 1993;22:119–123.

66. Yelin E, Henke C, Epstein W. The work dynamics of the person with rheumatoid arthritis. Arthritis Rheum 1987;30:507–512.

67. Pincus T, Callahan L. Taking mortality in rheumatoid arthritis seriously. Predictive markers, socioeconomic status and comorbidity. J Rheumatol 1986;13:841–845.

68. Melvin J. Issues and trends in rheumatologic rehabilitation. In: Melvin JL, Jensen G. Rheumatologic rehabilitation series: assessment and management, part 1. Bethesda, MD: American Occupational Therapy Association, 1998.

69. Hirano PC, Laurent DD, Lorig K. Arthritis patient education studies, 1987–1991: a review of the literature. Patient Education Counseling 1994;24(1):9–54.

70. Ganz SB, Viellion G. Pre and post surgical management of the hip and knee. In: Wegener ST, Belza BL, Gall EP. Clinical Care in the Rheumatic Diseases. Atlanta: American College of Rheumatology 1996; 17:103–106.

71. Trombley CA. Theoretical foundations for practice. In: Trombley CA, ed. Occupational Therapy for Physical Dysfunction. 4th ed. Baltimore: Williams & Wilkins, 1995:15–27.

72. Backman C, Functional assessment. In: Melvin JL, Jensen G. Rheumatologic rehabilitation series: assessment and management, part 1. Bethesda, MD: American Occupational Therapy Association, 1998.

73. Meenan RF, Mason JH, Anderson JJ, et al. AIMS2: The content and properties of a revised and expanded Arthritis Impact Measurement Scales Health Status questionnaire. Arthritis Rheum 1992;35:1–10.

74. Howe S, Levinson J, Shear E, et al. Development of a disability measurement tool for juvenile rheumatoid arthritis: the juvenile arthritis functional assessment report for children and their parents. Arthritis Rheum 1991;34:873–880.

75. Law M, Baptiste S, Carswell A, et al. Canadian Occupational Performance Measure. 2nd ed. Toronto, Ontario: CAOT Publications, 1994.

76. Affleck G, Tennen H, Pfeiffer C, et al. Appraisals of control and predictability in adapting to a chronic disease. J Pers Soc Psychol 1987;53:273–279.

77. Deyo RA, Inui TS, Leininger J, et al. Physical and psychosocial function in rheumatoid arthritis: clinical use of a self-administered health status instrument. Arch Intern Med 1982;142:879–882.

SUGGESTED READINGS

Brattstorm M. Joint Protection and Rehabilitation in Chronic Rheumatic Disorders. Rockville, MD: Aspen, 1987.

Canthum CJ, Clawson DL, Decker JL. Functional assessment of the rheumatoid hand. Am J Occup Ther 1969;23:122.

Dequeker J. An Atlas of Radiology of Rheumatic Disorders. New York: Wolfe Medical Publications Ltd., 1982.

Dunkin MA. Drug guide. Arthritis Today 1997:44:26–46.

Ehrlich GE, ed. Rehabilitation Management of Rheumatic Conditions. 2nd ed. Baltimore: Williams & Wilkins, 1986.

Gall EP, Gibofsky A, eds. Rheumatoid Arthritis: Clinical Tools for Outcome Assessment. Atlanta: Arthritis Foundation, 1994.

Gerber LH. Rehabilitative therapies for patients with rheumatic disease. In: Schumacher HR, Wippel JH, Robertson DR, eds. Primer on the Rheumatic Diseases. 9th ed. Atlanta: Arthritis Foundation, 1988.

Gibofsky A, Gall EP, et al. Early Diagnosis and Treatment of Rheumatoid Arthritis: The Changing Role of the Family Practice Physician. Atlanta: Arthritis Foundation, 1996.

Kate WA. Diagnosis and Management of Rheumatic Diseases. 2nd ed. Philadelphia: JB Lippincott, 1988.

Klippel JH, ed. Primer on the Rheumatic Diseases. Atlanta: Arthritis Foundation, 1997.

Koopman WJ. Arthritis and Allied Conditions: a Textbook of Rheumatology, Vols. 1 and 2. 13th ed. Baltimore: Williams & Wilkins, 1997.

McCarty DJ, ed. Arthritis and Allied Conditions. 11th ed. Philadelphia: Lea and Febiger, 1989.

Melvin JL. Rheumatic Disease in the Adult and Child: Occupational Therapy and Rehabilitation. 3rd ed. Philadelphia: FA Davis, 1989.

Melvin JL, Jensen GM, eds. Rheumatologic Rehabilitation Series, Vol. 1: Assessment and Management. Bethesda, MD: American Occupational Therapy Association Inc., 1998.

O'Sullivan SB, Schmitz TJ. Physical Rehabilitation: Assessment and Treatment. 3rd ed. Philadelphia: F.A. Davis Co., 1994.

Peck JR, Smith TW, Ward JR, et al. Disability and depression in rheumatoid arthritis. Arthritis Rheum 1989;32(9):1100–1106.

Riggs GK, Gall EP, eds. Rheumatic Disease: Rehabilitation and Management. Boston: Butterworth, 1984.

Schumacher HR, Gall EP. Rheumatoid Arthritis: An Illustrated Guide to Pathology, Diagnosis and Management. New York: Gower Medical Publishing, 1988.

Sculo TD. Surgical treatment of rheumatoid. St.Louis: Mosby and Year Book, Inc., 1992.

Wegener S, Belza BL, Gall EP. Clinical Care in the Rheumatic Diseases. Atlanta: American College of Rheumatology, 1996.

RESOURCES

CONSUMER AND PROFESSIONAL RESOURCES
Health Organizations

Arthritis Foundation (AF)
1330 West Peachtree Street
Atlanta, GA 30309

404-872-7100
800-283-7800
404-872-0457 (fax)
http://www.arthritis.org

American Juvenile Arthritis Organization (AJAO)
Same as above for AF

Arthritis Society (Canada)
250 Bloor Street East
Suite 901
Toronto, Ontario, M4W3P2
416-979-3760

HEALTH (Higher Education and Adult Training for People with Handicaps)
11 Dupont Circle
Suite 700
Washington, DC 20036-1193

International League Against Rheumatism
c/o Charles M. Plotz
SUNY Downstate Medical Center
450 Clarkston Avenue
Brooklyn, NY 11203

National Chronic Pain Outreach
4922 Hampden Lane
Bethesda, MD 20814
301-652-4948

Rheumatism Disease Foundation
5106 Old Harding Road
Franklin, TN 37064
615-646-1030
615-646-1030 (fax)

Support Groups
Contact the Arthritis Foundation for local groups across the United States.

Professional Organizations

American College of Rheumatology (ACR)/Arthritis Health Professionals Assocation (AHPA)
1800 Century Place
Suite 250
Atlanta, GA 30345
404-633-3777
404-633-1870 (fax)
acr@rheumatology.org (email)
http://www.rheumatology.org
http://www.rheumatology.org/arhp/about.html

For JRA Information
http://www.rheumatology.org/patient/jra.htm

American Occupational Therapy Association (AOTA)
4720 Montgomery Lane
PO Box 31220
Bethesda, MD 20824-1220
800-SAY-AOTA
301-652-7711
301-652-7711 (fax)
800-377-8555 (TDD)
http://www.aota.org

American Physical Therapy Association (APTA)
111 N. Fairfax Street
Alexandria, VA 22314
800-999-2782
703-684-7343 (fax)
703-683-6748 (TDD)
http:www.apta.org

Journals and Newsletters

Arthritis and Rheumatism
Published by American College of Rheumatology
1800 Century Place
Suite 250
Atlanta, GA 30345
404-633-3777

AJAO Newsletter
Published by Arthritis Foundation
1330 West Peachtree Street
Atlanta, GA 30309
404-872-7100

Arthritis, Rheumatic Diseases and Related Disorders
Annual Report
Published by National Arthritis and Musculoskeletal
    and Skin Diseases
Information Clearinghouse
9000 Rockville Pike
PO Box AMS
Bethesda, MD 20892-2903
301-495-4484

Arthritis Today
Published by Arthritis Foundation
1330 West Peachtree Street
Atlanta, GA 30309
800-933-0032
http://www.arthritis.org/at/

Arthritis Today Newsletter (free)
Published by University of Alabama at Birmingham
Multipurpose Arthritis Center

108 Basic Health Science Building
Birmingham, AL 35294
205-934-0542

Bulletin on the Rheumatic Diseases (free)
Published by Arthritis Foundation
PO Box 6996
Alpharetta, GA 30009-6996
800-207-8633

Current Opinion in Rheumatology
Published by Current Science Ltd.
20 N. Third Street
Philadelphia, PA 19106-2199
800-552-5866

Research Alert: Arthritis
Published by Institute for Scientific Information
3501 Market Street
Philadelphia, PA 19104
800-523-1850

Rheumatic Disease Clinics of North America
Published by W. B. Saunders Co.
6277 Sea Harbor Drive
Orlando, FL 32887-4800
800-654-2452

The Journal of Rheumatology
Published by The Journal of Rheumatology Publishing
    Co. Ltd.
920 Young Street
Suite 115
Toronto, ON M4W3C7
416-967-5155

**Research Centers, Institutes,
    and Clearinghouses**

Arthritis Center
Boston University
Conte Building
5th Floor
71 E. Newton Street
Boston, MA 02118
617-534-5154

Arthritis Center
University of Missouri-Columbia
MA427 Health Sciences Center
1 Hospital Drive
Columbia, MO 65212
314-882-8738

Arthritis Clinical and Research Center
Medical University of South Carolina
171 Ashley Avenue
Charleston, SC 29425
803-792-2000

Arthritis Research Institute of America
300 S. Duncan Avenue
Suite 240
Clearwater, FL 34615
813-461-4054

Multipurpose Arthritis Center
University of Connecticut
School of Medicine
Division of Rheumatic Diseases
Farmington, CT 06030
203-679-2160

Multipurpose Arthritis Center
University of Michigan
3918 Taubman Center
Ann Arbor, MI 48109-0358
313-936-9539

**National Arthritis and Musculoskeletal
    and Skin Diseases**
Information Clearinghouse (NAMSIC)
9000 Rockville Pike
PO Box AMS
Bethesda, MD 20892
301-495-4484

Northeast Ohio Multipurpose Arthritis Center
Case Western Reserve University
University Hospitals of Cleveland
2074 Abington Road
Cleveland, OH 44106
216-844-3168

Adaptive Aids
These companies have catalogs that contain resources
    for those with arthritis.

Aids for Arthritis, Inc.
3 Little Knoll Court
Medford, NJ 08055

Adapt Ability
PO Box 513
Colchester, CT 06415-0515
800-288-9941

AliMed Rehabilitation Products, Inc.
297 High Street
Dedham, MA 02026-9135
800-255-2160

Amigo Mobility International, Inc.
6693 Dixie Highway
Bridgeport, MI 48722
800-248-9131

Back Saver
53 Jeffrey Avenue
Department 50
Holliston, MA 01746
800-251-2225

Bruce Medical Supply
411 Waverly Oaks Road
PO Box 9166
Waltham, MA 02254
800-255-8446

Cleo, Inc.
PO Box 1076
White Plains, NY 10602
800-435-8573

College Video Specialists
Complete Guide to Exercise Videos
5390 Main Street, N.E.
Minneapolis, MN 55421
800-433-6769

DeRoyal/LMB, Inc.
PO Box 1181
San Luis Obispo, CA 93406
800-541-3992

Electronic Cart and Wheelchair Company
415 North Mulberry Street
Elizabethtown, KY 42701
800-227-1919

Endless Pools
200 E. Dutton Mill Road
Department A12
Aston, PA 19014
800-732-8660

Enrichments
PO Box 5071
Bolingbrook, IL 60440-5071
800-435-8573

Exer-Spa
Department AR9813
4216 6th Avenue South
Seattle, WA 98108
http://www.exerspa.com

Futuro, Inc.
5405 Dupont Circle
Suite A
Milford, OH 45150-2735
513-272-5000

Hoveround Corporation
2151 Whitfield Industrial Way
Sarasota, FL 34243
800-771-6565

Independent Living Aids, Inc.
27 East Mall
Plainview, NY 11803
800-537-2118

Invacare Corporation
899 Cleveland Street
Elyria, OH 44036
800-333-6900

Lumex Medical Products
100 Spence Street
Bay Shore, NY 11706-2290
800-645-5272

Maddak, Inc.
PO Box 384
Penquannock, NY 07440-1993
800-443-4926

North Coast Medical, Inc.
187 Stauffer Boulevard
San Jose, CA 95125-1042
800-821-9319

S & S AdaptAbility
PO Box 513
Colchester, CT 06415-0515
800-266-8856

Sammons Preston
PO Box 5071
Bolingbrook, IL 60440-5071
800-323-5547

Sears Health Care
9804 Chartwell Drive
Dallas, Texas 75243
800-326-1750

Select Comfort Direct Corporation
6105 Trenton Lane North
Minneapolis, MN 55442
800-831-1211 ext. 8089

SelfCare
Products for Healthy Living
104 Challenger Drive
Portland, TN 37148-1716
800-520-9924

Smith and Nephew, Inc.
Rehabilitation Division
PO Box 1005
One Quality Drive
Germantown, WI 53022-8205

Thera-Kinetics
55 Carnegie Plaza
Cherry Hill, NJ 08003
800-800-4276

**Patient and Professional Resources from
    the Arthritis Foundation**
To Order:
Arthritis Foundation
PO Box 6996
Alpharetta, GA 30009-6996
800-207-8633

CONSUMER INFORMATION BOOKLETS

Understanding Arthritis
Back Pain
Bursitis, Tendonitis and Other Soft Tissue
Rheumatic Syndromes
Carpal Tunnel Syndrome
Rheumatic Arthritis
Sjögren's Syndrome

Self Management for Healthier Living
Arthritis in the Work Place
Diet and Arthritis
Exercise and Your Arthritis
Managing Your Fatigue
Managing Your Health Care
Managing Your Pain
Managing Your Stress

General Information
Arthritis Answers
Arthritis and Pregnancy
Choosing a Health Plan
Guide to Lab Tests
Surgery: Information to Consider
Understanding Arthritis in African-Americans

Understanding Medications
Aspirin and Other NSAIDs
Corticosteroids
The Drug Guide
Gold Treatment
Hydrochloroquine
Medications: Using Them Wisely
Methotrexate
Penicillamine
Sulfasalazine

Tips for Active Living
Gardening and Arthritis
Gold and Arthritis
Walking and Arthritis

Help for Juvenile Arthritis
Arthritis in Children
Decision Making with Teenagers with Arthritis
When Your Student Has Arthritis: A Guide for Teachers

Consumer Books
Arthritis 101: Questions You Have, Answers You Need
250 Tips for Making Life with Arthritis Easier
Health Organizer: A Personal Health Care Record
Help Yourself: Recipes from the Arthritis Foundation

Self-Help Programs
Participant and Trainer Information Available
Bone Up on Arthritis: Arthritis Self Care Information
Pathways to Better Living with Arthritis
PACE (People with Arthritis Can Exercise)
Pool Exercise Program (PEP)

ADDITIONAL WEB SITES WITH ARTHRITIS INFORMATION

http://www.ama-assn.org
    This American Medical Association site has several
    medical and health resources, a nationwide
    physician directory, and reports on medical research.
http://www.arcade.uiowa.edu/hardin-www/md.html
    This site links you with the Hardin Meta Directory
    of Internet Health Sources—a link to access more

sites on specific medical topics, including rheumatology.

http://www.arthritis.org

The official Arthritis Foundation website includes the latest news and research on arthritis and arthritis-related diseases, local offices, and Arthritis Foundation print materials and products. This is a comprehensive resource room and link to other sites with arthritis information.

http://www.drweil.com

An interactive medical clinic where a doctor answers questions online daily. The site also has access to a referral directory and treatment database.

http://www.duq.edu/PT/RA/PreventionOfDisability.html

Discusses the approaches used to reduce and prevent disability from becoming worse for people with rheumatoid arthritis.

http://www.healthfinder.gov

A website from the federal government offering easy-to-read information prepared by health agencies and other reliable sources. It offers links to more than 500 other sites, online documents, and databases.

http://www.hsc.missouri.edu/arthritis/handtips.html

Arthritis Wise; Tips for Living Well with Arthritis. Information about joint protection, especially the hands.

http://www.medicinenet.com

An electronic database that includes a forum where users can ask doctors specific disease- and health-related questions.

http://www.merck.com/!!rGBNN2da4/pubs/manual/html/sectoc.htm

A definitive source of information about disease. Very technical.

http://www.plsgroup.com/arthritis.htm

A doctor's guide to the internet on arthritis. Medical news and alerts about arthritis. Includes an overview of arthritis and a study of rheumatoid arthritis.

Provides links to discussion groups and newsgroups and other sites that have arthritis-related information.

misc.health.arthritis

This newsgroup focuses on discussions on arthritis and related topics.

alt.support.arthritis

This site functions as a support group for people with arthritis.

http://www.nih.gov

National Institute of Health (NIH)

http://www.nih.gov/niams

National Institute of Arthritis, Musculoskeletal and Skin Diseases (NIAMS)

http://www.cdc.gov

National Centers for Disease Control and Prevention (CDC)

Other Juvenile Arthritis Web Sites

http://www.wp.com/pedsrheum

The Pediatric Rheumatology Home Page by Thomas Lehman

This site contains information for patients from physicians from the Hospital for Special Surgery in New York.

http://www.mc.vanderbilt.edu/peds/pidl/rheum/jra_pauc.html

Pauciarticular Juvenile Rheumatoid Arthritis

http://www.vanderbilt.edu/peds/pidl/rheum/jra.html

Juvenile Rheumatoid Arthritis (Systemic Onset)

http://proteus.mig.missouri.edu/som/mmr/1995fall/arthrit.html

Reaching Out to Children with Arthritis

http://www.immunology.meei.harvard.edu/review4.htm

Questions for Juvenile Rheumatoid Arthritis

http://www.mcg.edu/news/95features/arthritis.html/cc16550

Arthritis Can Strike Children As Well As Adults

CHAPTER 15

ORTHOPAEDICS

Joanne Phillips Estes

CRITICAL TERMS

Anti-inflammatory
Certified hand therapist
Closed fracture
Colles' fracture
Comminuted fracture
Compartment syndrome
Compound fracture
Delayed union
Disuse phenomenon

Fibrosis
Inflammatory phase
Malunion
Nonunion
Open fracture
Open reduction internal
 fixation
Orthostatic hypotension

Osteodystrophy
Osteomyelitis
Osteoporosis
Pathological fracture
Reflex sympathetic dystrophy
Remodeling phase
Reparative phase
Total hip arthroplasty

Ellie is a healthy, 82-year-old widow of 17 years, who lives alone in the same small house she's lived in for the past 63 years. She is rarely home because of her many activities. These include yoga, line dancing, golf, bridge, sewing club, occasional babysitting, travel, and socializing. Ellie is described by others as happy, cheerful, and energetic.

On March 13, 1997, as she was hurrying out the door for exercise class, Ellie slipped on a small patch of ice on her porch. She experienced excruciating pain and was unable to get up or bear weight on her right leg. At the emergency room, she was diagnosed as having a right intertrochanteric femur fracture (Fig. 15.1). This isolated incident may be the most significant event of her life in terms of its impact on her ability to function at the high level she's enjoyed.

INTRODUCTION

Ellie's experience is not unusual. The National Center for Health Statistics (1980) reports that "33 percent of healthy community-dwelling elders (older than age 65) fall annually" (1). Furthermore, 85% of these falls occur in homes among people who live independently (2). The most common fractures that result from falls are humeral, wrist, pelvic, and hip (1).

A fracture is simply a break in the continuity of bone that is usually caused by external force. Soft tissue surrounding the fracture site is typically damaged. Falling is a common cause of fractures,

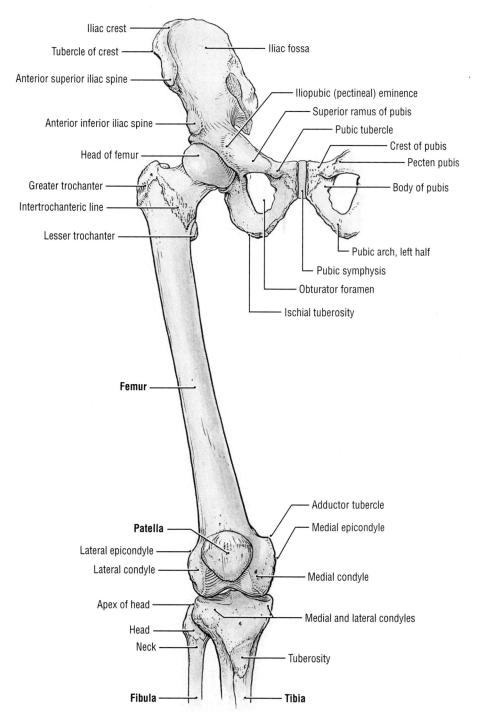

FIGURE 15.1 Lower extremity, anterior view. (Reprinted with permission from Agur AMR. Grant's Atlas of Anatomy, 9th ed. Baltimore: Williams & Wilkins, 1991:256.)

especially for elderly individuals. The elderly are more prone to falls, their bones are more likely to break during a fall, and the course of healing is likely to be more complicated than for younger people. Accidental falls and resultant fractures among elderly people are significant problems in health care today.

ETIOLOGY

Fractures occur when physical force is applied that is greater than the bone can withstand. They occur in healthy bone and in bone structurally compromised by disease. Diseased bone is more vulnerable to fracture. Spontaneous fractures (i.e., those resulting from normal, everyday movement, such as rolling over in bed) occur in bone weakened by pathological conditions such as tumors or osteomyelitis. Direct trauma from an external force, however, is the most common cause. Bones weakened from other diseases (such as osteoporosis or osteoarthritis) are more easily fractured by trauma.

Osteoporosis is a "disease characterized by low bone mass, microarchitectural deterioration of bone, and susceptibility to fracture" (3). It is particularly common in postmenopausal women, and more than half of these women will develop a spontaneous fracture because of it (3). Furthermore, 1.5 million osteoporosis-related fractures occur annually in the United States; approximately 70% of fractures in persons older than age 45 are related to osteoporosis (3). The most common sites of osteoporosis-related fractures are the neck of the femur, humerus, and distal radius (4).

Most fractures from trauma are the result of auto accidents, sports injuries, direct hit with a blunt object, and accidental falls. Accidental falls are common in older people and are reported by one-fourth of people ages 65 to 74 and one-third of the people older than age 75 (5). A variety of factors place older adults at higher risk for falls. These include normal physiological degenerative changes associated with aging, underlying diseases, side effects of medication, and environmental hazards.

Most organ systems undergo degenerative change with aging. This can impede an older per-

son's ability to safely interact with his or her environment. Examples of sensorimotor components that may be compromised are balance, visual acuity, focus, and resistance to glare (6). Neuromusculoskeletal components include decreased strength and endurance (owing to decreased cardiac output and blood flow) and postural instability (6). Decline in motor functioning includes impaired motor control due to stiffened joints, decreased return of equilibrium after exertion, and decreased speed of response (6).

Several disorders that are common to elderly people can exaggerate dysfunction because of degenerative changes (1). These include neurological conditions such as cerebral vascular accident (CVA), peripheral neuropathies, and Parkinson's disease. Cardiovascular (myocardial infarction, orthostatic hypotension), gastrointestinal (bleeding, diarrhea, or defecation syncope), metabolic (hypothyroidism, anemia, dehydration, or hypoglycemia), and genitourinary (incontinence, nocturia) disorders also can increase the risk of falling. Finally, musculoskeletal (arthritis, deconditioning) and psychological (depression, anxiety) disorders may increase risk as well.

Medications taken for the above disorders have side effects that can further impair ability to safely navigate through one's environment. Common types of medications associated with falls in older persons include: diuretics, narcotics, phenothiazines, select antihypertensives, tricyclic antidepressants, and benzodiazepines (7); the risk of hip fractures from falls *doubles* with the use of certain anti-psychotic and long-acting benzodiazepines" (1). Potentially dangerous side effects include blurred vision, dizziness, fatigue, or disorientation.

Finally, characteristics of the physical environment can increase the risk of falls. These include poor lighting, unstable (or no) grab bars or hand rails, slippery or uneven floor surfaces, throw rugs, electrical cords, or furniture arranged without adequate clearance. Each of these individual factors (normal changes in aging, underlying disorders, medication side effects, or environmental hazards) will increase an elderly person's risk of falling and sustaining a fracture. In reality, it is more typical that several of these factors are operating simultaneously.

INCIDENCE AND PREVALENCE

The most common sites in the skeletal system for fractures are the metacarpal and phalanges (8). The scaphoid is the most common wrist bone to be fractured (8). Fracture of the distal radius (known as Colles' fracture) is the most common site for forearm fracture (9); it is also the most common fracture site in adults older than age 50 (8). Colles' fractures typically are the result of falls onto an extended upper extremity. Women are more likely to sustain this injury than men owing to weakened, osteoporotic bones (8, 10).

Men ages 30 to 40 are more likely to sustain a fracture from job-related injuries (9). Accidental falls, however, are the major cause of fractures. Rothstein cites the following (1):

- "Until age 75 years falls occur more frequently in women. The frequency is the same for both genders between ages 75 and 85 years, and after 85 years, white men have the highest death rate from falls.
- Thirty-three percent of healthy community dwelling elders (older than 65 years) fall annually.
- Sixty-seven percent of nursing home residents fall annually.
- Falls contribute to 40% of admissions to nursing homes.
- Five percent of falls among older people will result in fractures.
- The most serious fracture (i.e., with the greatest likelihood of morbidity and mortality) after falls in the elderly are hip fractures (greater than 250,000 per year in people older than 65 years)."

SIGNS AND SYMPTOMS

Fractures have two symptoms. The patient will complain of localized tenderness at the fracture site and experience a sharp pain in the area of the fractured bone. With hip fracture, pain may occur in the knee rather than the hip (referred pain).

Clinical signs of fracture are structural breaks in bone as shown in radiographic (x-ray) studies. There is also swelling in the involved limb. Examination of a Colles' fracture will reveal gross angular or rotational deformities of the fractured bone. These deformities of the radius are "displacement backwards, tilt backward, and tilt in a radial direction" (11). They give the appearance of an upside down dinner fork. Thus, it is called a dinner fork deformity (Fig. 15.2) (12). If there is a break in the skin at the fracture site, it is termed an open fracture. If not, it is a closed fracture.

The examiner of a hip fracture will observe external rotation and shortening of the involved lower extremity (LE). X-rays will show a fracture line at the head or neck of the femur. The types of neck fractures are subcapital (where the head meets the neck) or transcervical. Femur head fractures are either intertrochanteric or subtrochanteric (below the trochanteric region) (Fig. 15.1).

COURSE AND PROGNOSIS

Functional outcomes for fractures are influenced by the quality of the healing process that begins immediately after the fracture occurs. Time required to heal depends on age of patient, site and type of break, initial displacement of bone, and blood supply to fragments (4). In adults, union of upper extremity (UE) fractures takes 6 to 12 weeks; LE fractures take 12 to 30 weeks. Factors that can impede the healing process (and ultimately the prognosis) include type, severity, and location of injury, premorbid state of health, whether the patient smokes, and complications during healing.

Abnormal healing is one complication. There are three types: malunion, delayed union, and nonunion. In a malunion, fracture healing has occurred at the normal time but in an unsatisfactory position. A delayed union fracture eventually heals but takes considerably longer to do so. A nonunion occurs when the fracture fails to completely heal by bony union. Causes of abnormal

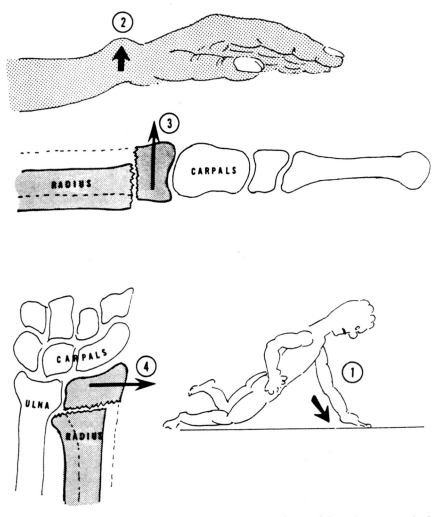

FIGURE 15.2 Colles' fracture. *1,* Fracture usually occurs from a fall on the outstretched hand. *2,* The typical "dinner fork" deformity is noted. *3,* The distal fragment is displaced backward (dorsally) and *4,* outward (radially) (Reprinted with permission from Caillet R. Hand Pain and Impairment, 3rd ed. Philadelphia, FA Davis, 1982, p138.)

healing include open fractures, fractures separated by soft tissue interposition, poor blood supply, or iatrogenic interference (8). Additional complications are infection (osteomyelitis), phlebitis, vascular damage, neurological damage, or compartment syndrome.

During healing of a Colles' fracture, patients experience decreased functional use of the involved extremity. Specifically, edema and decreased range of motion (ROM) (especially in the wrist and forearm), strength, and grip are noted. Not using the UE for these reasons can result in "disuse phenomena" of the entire upper quadrant. Twenty percent of patients with a Colles' fracture have residual symptoms, and 10% have significant functional impairment (13).

Sudeck's atrophy or osteodystrophy is a late-occurring complication found particularly after a

Colles' fracture. The cause and nature of this condition are not understood, and incidence is low (14). Reflex sympathetic dystrophy (RSD), another potentially disabling complication, causes eventual atrophy of tissues with joint contracture, chronic edema, and fibrosis (15).

Surgery is usually indicated after a hip fracture (15). Elderly patients do not physically tolerate periods of confinement. They should be out of bed and ambulating after surgery, usually the next day. Mental deterioration occurs in 90% of older patients after surgery; it "usually subsides but may persist due to preexisting arteriosclerosis" (15). Patients must avoid external rotation and flexion of more than 90° in the involved hip for at least 6 weeks postoperatively to allow bony union.

Estimates of functional outcomes after a hip fracture vary. Dambro states "65% of patients (with hip fractures) can be expected to return to their former state of health" (15). Others report "50% of elderly who can walk before a hip fracture cannot do so after the fracture, and 50% are unable to live independently after a hip fracture" (1). Favorable prognostic indicators for return home after hip fracture are the patient's general medical condition, that he or she lives with someone else, and has a pattern of social contacts outside the home (16).

DIAGNOSIS

To diagnose a fracture, physicians obtain a detailed history, perform a systematic physical evaluation, and view x-rays. The patient's history provides clues about causes and underlying factors contributing to the injury. Physical examination for swelling, tenderness, and the ability to move fracture fragments is done. Radiographic studies show the actual break in continuity of bone (fracture line). Computed tomography (CT) or magnetic resonance imaging (MRI) scans are not usually necessary, as diagnosis is obvious from x-rays (15).

Physical examination and x-rays are also used to determine state of fracture healing. If there is neither movement nor pain during physical examination, the fracture is "clinically" united. At that time, x-rays will show bony callus formation and a still-visible fracture line. "Clinical" union precedes "radiographic" union by months (8).

Imaging for hip fractures includes the pelvis to rule out the possibility of pelvic fracture and to give information about the noninvolved side for comparison (15). Views should include the entire femur to the knee. X-rays of all painful areas should be taken. Other fracture sites are common and may be overlooked because of the pain from a hip fracture (15).

MEDICAL/SURGICAL MANAGEMENT

Medical/surgical intervention is individualized to each patient. Four goals of fracture management are to relieve pain, realign fractured bones, help bony union, and restore functional use of the limb. A variety of methods are used to achieve these goals.

Common to all fractures is realignment (known as reduction) of bones to allow healing. Closed fractures are usually manually reduced and immobilized by plaster cast. Open reduction and internal fixation (ORIF) is indicated with closed comminuted fractures or open fractures. Internal fixation can be established by orthopaedic nail, pin, screw, rod, wire, or plate (4).

External skeletal fixation may be used to maintain the reduction by insertion of pins, through the skin, proximal and distal to fracture site. The pins are held together by a rigid external bar. This is used primarily with Colles' fractures and open fractures with soft tissue loss (8).

Open reduction and internal fixation is usually done with intertrochanteric and subtrochanteric fractures (17). Some fractures of the neck and head of the femur require partial joint replacement. The head and neck are replaced with a metal prosthesis. A total hip arthroplasty (THA) is indicated if there are destructive changes in both the femur and acetabulum.

Medications

After a fracture, medication is primarily for pain relief. This can consist of nonprescription analgesics such as aspirin or Tylenol. Prescribed narcotic pain relievers may be given for relief of more severe pain. Common narcotic pain relievers are oral opioids or morphine (14). "Dosage should be lower in older people to avoid respiratory problems" (14). (See Appendix II for listing of pain-relief medications).

IMPACT ON OCCUPATIONAL PERFORMANCE

The function of several performance components may be compromised by fracture (Table 15.1). The degree of the patient's impairment depends on the severity of injury, other anatomical structures injured, and premorbid condition. Sensorimotor is the major performance component compromised. In all fractures, neuromusculoskeletal and motor components are the primary areas affected. Diminished function in these areas could be the direct result of the injury. Impaired neuromuscular and motor function of noninvolved structures also could result from disuse of that extremity.

One's psychosocial skill and psychological components may be affected by a UE or LE fracture. Injury may change the appearance of the hand and result in diminished function, which can impair one's self concept. Self-expression may be compromised if one cannot use his or her hands for nonverbal expression. Finally, a patient may be unable to implement previous coping skills or develop new ones, especially if physical activity has been used as a coping technique.

TABLE 15.1   Occupational Performance Profile

I. PERFORMANCE AREAS	II. PERFORMANCE COMPONENTS	III. PERFORMANCE CONTEXTS

A. Activities of Daily Living
  1. Grooming
  2. Oral Hygiene
  3. Bathing/Showering
  4. Toilet Hygiene
  5. Personal Device Care
  6. Dressing
  7. Feeding and Eating
  8. Medication Routine
  9. Health Maintenance
  10. Socialization
  11. Functional Communication
  12. Functional Mobility
  13. Community Mobility
  14. Emergency Response
  15. Sexual Expression
	A. Sensorimotor Component
	  1. Sensory
	   a. Sensory Awareness
	   b. Sensory Processing
	    (1) Tactile
	    (2) Proprioceptive
	    (3) Vestibular
	    (4) Visual
	    (5) Auditory
	    (6) Gustatory
	    (7) Olfactory
	   c. Perceptual Processing
	    (1) Stereognosis
	    (2) Kinesthesia
	    (3) Pain Response
	    (4) Body Scheme
	    (5) Right–Left Discrimination
	    (6) Form Constancy
	    (7) Position in Space
	    (8) Visual–Closure
	    (9) Figure Ground
	    (10) Depth Perception
	    (11) Spatial Relations
	    (12) Topographical Orientation
		A. Temporal Aspects
		  1. Chronological
		  2. Developmental
		  3. Lifecycle
		  4. Disability Status
		B. Environment
		  1. Physical
		  2. Social
		  3. Cultural

(continued)

TABLE 15.1 Occupational Performance Profile (Continued)

I. PERFORMANCE AREAS	II. PERFORMANCE COMPONENTS	III. PERFORMANCE CONTEXTS

B. Work and Productive Activities
1. **Home Management**
   a. **Clothing Care**
   b. **Cleaning**
   c. **Meal Preparation/ Cleanup**
   d. **Shopping**
   e. Money Management
   f. **Household Maintenance**
   g. **Safety Procedures**
2. **Care of Others**
3. **Educational Activities**
4. **Vocational Activities**
   a. Vocational Exploration
   b. Job Acquisition
   c. **Work or Job Performance**
   d. **Retirement Planning**
   e. Volunteer Participation
C. Play or Leisure Activities
1. **Play or Leisure Exploration**
2. **Play or Leisure Performance**

2. **Neuromusculoskeletal**
   a. Reflex
   b. **Range of Motion**
   c. **Muscle Tone**
   d. **Strength**
   e. **Endurance**
   f. **Postural Control**
   g. **Postural Alignment**
   h. **Soft Tissue Integrity**
3. **Motor**
   a. **Gross Coordination**
   b. Crossing the Midline
   c. Laterality
   d. **Bilateral Integration**
   e. Motor Control
   f. Praxis
   g. **Fine Coordination/Dexterity**
   h. Visual–Motor Control
   i. Oral–Motor Control
B. Cognitive Integration and Cognitive Components
1. Level of Arousal
2. Orientation
3. Recognition
4. **Attention Span**
5. Initiation of Activity
6. Termination of Activity
7. **Memory**
8. Sequencing
9. Categorization
10. Concept Formation
11. Spatial Operations
12. Problem Solving
13. Learning
14. Generalization
C. Psychosocial Skills and Psychological Components
1. Psychological
   a. Values
   b. Interests
   c. Self-Concept
2. **Social**
   a. **Role Performance**
   b. **Social Conduct**
   c. **Interpersonal Skills**
   d. **Self-Expression**
3. **Self-Management**
   a. **Coping Skills**
   b. **Time Management**
   c. **Self-Control**

Fractures can potentially influence function of all performance areas. The extent of impact depends on the type and severity of the injury. This is further influenced by contexts in which the individual must perform. Age, premorbid health status, and environmental supports/barriers are all factors that can contribute to increased or decreased abilities.

CASE STUDIES

CASE 1

Colles' Fracture

Jim, a 41-y.o.-white male, sustained a fracture of his left (nondominant) distal radius on 3/17/97. Injury occurred when he was atop an 8-foot ladder at the top of a staircase, wiping walls. The ladder became unsteady and Jim jumped off to avoid tumbling down the steps. He extended his left upper extremity (LUE) to break the fall and sustained a Colles' fracture. At the emergency room, an orthopaedic surgeon manually reduced the fracture and placed a cast on Jim's wrist and forearm (Fig. 15.3). Two days later, Jim sought the opinion of a second orthopaedic surgeon. On 3/25/97, this surgeon openly reduced the fracture and placed an external fixator on for 6 weeks.

When the fixator was removed there was severe pain and edema in Jim's distal LUE and he said, "My hand looked like a softball with sausages for fingers." Jim was sent to a physical therapist who placed the LUE in a sling for 1 week, then advised him to begin using his hand. Jim reports he used his LUE functionally "almost constantly."

Jim returned to the surgeon 4 weeks after fixator removal, complaining of severe edema, lack of

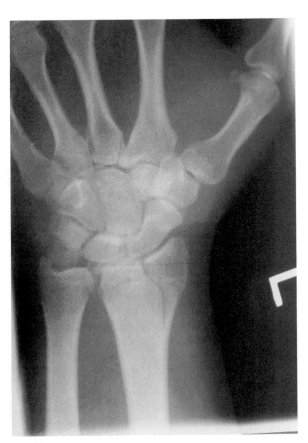

FIGURE 15.3 Radiographic study of Jim's Colles' fracture, dorsal view. The fracture site is indicated by a "vertical line" denoting the break in continuity of bone near the radial styloid.

movement and function, and pain in his LUE. The physician accused him of "not doing the home exercise program." Jim became upset and reports that he "semidiscreetly" corrected the physician. The surgeon again sent him to a physical therapist who applied heat and forcefully snapped his wrist into extension. Jim found this "extremely painful" but managed to maintain small ROM gains for a few weeks.

Still dissatisfied with the lack of functional use of his LUE, Jim sought the opinion of yet another orthopaedic surgeon in August 1997. This physician referred him to a hand therapy clinic, where Jim began treatment with an occupational therapist who is a certified hand therapist (CHT). Jim states, "when you grow up poor, you learn to keep fighting for what you need until you get it."

Past medical history is significant for alcohol abuse ("dry" for 14 years) and migraine headaches since 1989. Jim lives with his wife and two children (son and daughter ages 8 and 6 years) in a two-story home. He has a bachelor of science degree in elementary education, along with graduate credit in learning disabled (LD) education. Jim works as an LD tutor and maintenance man at a local elementary school and does maintenance work on the side for extra income. His wife worked full time but lost her job in June 1997. She currently receives unemployment benefits. Jim's hobbies include coaching kids' sports teams, socializing with friends, maintenance work, and woodworking.

Several occupational performance components are affected by Jim's injury. His deficits are primarily in the neuromusculoskeletal and motor components. Pain, swelling, and stiffness limit the function of his LUE.

Jim also has difficulties in psychosocial skills and psychological components. He reports having "periods of blues" throughout his recovery. This was especially true initially when he was unable to coach kids' baseball. In addition, he reports a significant depression since June when his wife lost her job. He has difficulty coping with the stress of lost income and is particularly frustrated with his inability to generate income from side maintenance work. This has led to a strained relationship with his wife.

Jim manages most occupational performance area tasks using his right upper extremity (RUE) dominantly and his LUE assistively. He is unable to button, tie shoes, or bathe his RUE. Turning door knobs with his LUE is painful and difficult.

Jim is unable to carry groceries with his LUE or any load larger than 30 lb using both UEs. He currently does not attempt woodworking projects and is unable to get his camper on and off the hitch.

Jim has missed only 2 days of work from this injury. He continues his full-time job as LD tutor and does light maintenance tasks at school. His employer is understanding of his limitations and accommodates accordingly. Jim reports a lack of confidence in doing certain maintenance tasks, like installing ceiling fans. He has a fear of further injury from not having normal strength and movement in his LUE.

Being a husband and father of young children places Jim in a position of responsibility for the care of others. This injury has interfered with his being able to do this in a satisfying way. His environment, however, provides supports to maximize his functional capabilities.

CASE 2

Hip Fracture

Ellie, introduced in the opening vignette, underwent surgical repair of the fracture later that day. Open reduction internal fixation (using a nail and femoral plate) was done. Ellie had postoperative confusion and memory loss. She was unable to follow postoperative restrictions to allow healing. These restrictions were to a) avoid hip flexion beyond 90°, b) no hip rotation, c) no crossing of involved leg, and d) no adduction of the operated leg (16). This necessitated minimum to moderate physical assistance to complete lower extremity bathing and dressing tasks.

On 3/24/97 Ellie was admitted to a nursing facility. Her choice was to return to her home, but she was unable to manage daily activities within the above restrictions. Ellie's son, daughter, and grandchildren (ages 12 to 21) all live in nearby states. Her family visited during the acute care hospital stay but had to return to work and school after 1 week. They were devastated by having to place Ellie at the nursing facility. They felt they were putting her away and grieved at her loss of independence and freedom to do her activities. However, they realized that there was no other option as no one was available to care for her at her home. They hoped that the nursing home placement would be transitional until Ellie could tolerate subacute or rehabilitation center levels of services.

Upon admission to the nursing facility, Ellie displayed significant signs of depression (flat affect, avoidance of eye contact). She rarely interacted or socialized with others and typically refused to participate in organized activities. Nursing staff often observed her crying in bed during the day. When approached by nursing, Ellie discussed fears of becoming a burden to her family. She expressed sadness at her inability to participate in previous activities that were so important to her identity. These impairments in psychosocial skills and psychological components slowed her recovery and affected her functional independence.

Sensorimotor components were also affected. Neuromusculoskeletal abilities in ROM were moderately deficient in the noninvolved extremities because of disuse during the past week. Strength, endurance, and postural alignment were similarly compromised.

She continued to display mild confusion and moderate memory deficits. This further impeded function of cognitive integration and cognitive components. Decreased attention span and problem-solving abilities were noted.

Her fracture resulted in impaired function of all occupational performance areas. She continued to be dependent in LE bathing and dressing because of her postsurgical restrictions. Ellie required physical assistance with toilet hygiene, functional mobility, and medication routine. She no longer socialized, participated in her previous leisure activities (cards, yoga, sewing), or was willing to explore new leisure activities.

POINTS FOR REVIEW

1. What causes a bone fracture?

2. What is ORIF and when is it used?

3. When narcotic pain relievers are prescribed to older adults, what is the one precaution that physicians must keep in mind?

4. Why is the context particularly important when determining the risks of falls (and fractures) for older adults?

REFERENCES

1. Rothstein J, Roy S, Wolf S. The Rehabilitation Specialist's Handbook. Philadelphia: F. A. Davis, 1997:723–733.

2. Hettinger J. Encouraging activity in older adults. OT Week, 2-8-96:15–16.

3. National Fund for Medical Education. Working with Patients to Prevent, Treat, and Manage Osteoporosis: A Curriculum Guide for the Health Professional, 1996:1.

4. Daniels M, Strickland R. Occupational Therapy Management in Adult Physical Dysfunction. Gaithersburg, MD: Aspen Publishers, Inc., 1992:149–154.

5. Hettinger J. Falling down. OT Week 9-14-95:18–19.

6. Davis L, Kirkland M. Role of Occupational Therapy with the Elderly. Rockville, MD: The American Occupational Therapy Association, Inc., 1988:41–67.

7. Abrams SW, Beers M, Berkaw R. The Merck Manual of Geriatrics. 2nd ed. New Jersey: Merck Research Laboratories, 1995:68.

8. Smigielski M. Lecture: Upper Extremity Orthopaedics. Ypsilanti, MI, February 4, 1986.

9. Reed C. Quick Reference to Occupational Therapy. Gaithersburg, MD: Aspen Publishers, 1991:247–251.

10. Jebson P. Occupational hand fractures and dislocations. In: Kasden M, ed. Occupational Hand and Upper Extremity Injuries and Diseases. Philadelphia: Hanley and Belfus, Inc., 1997:213–231.

11. Lamb DW, Hooper G. Hand Conditions. New York: Churchill-Livingstone, 1984:17.

12. Calliet R. Hand Pain and Impairment. Philadelphia: FA Davis, 1983:138.

13. Lidstrom A. Fractures of the distal end of the radius: a clinical and statistical study of end results. Acta Orthop Scand 1959:41.

14. Adams JC. Outline of Fractures. New York: Churchill-Livingstone, 1983:12, 71, 161.

15. Dambro M. Griffith's Five Minute Clinical Consult. Baltimore: Williams & Wilkins, 1997:484–485.

16. Bear J. Orthopaedic conditions. In: Trombly C, ed. Occupational Therapy for Physical Dysfunction. 4th ed. Baltimore: Williams & Wilkins, 1995:753–754, 761–762.

17. Platt J. Occupational Therapy Practice Guidelines for Adults with Hip Fracture/Replacement. Baltimore: The American Occupational Therapy Association, Inc., 1996:3–7.

CHAPTER 16

CHRONIC PAIN

Catherine Heck Edwards

CRITICAL TERMS

Analgesic
Catabolites
Causalgia
Crepitus
Dermatome
Fibrositis

Malingerer
Muscle loading
Myofascial pain
Neuralgia
Neuritis

Neuroma
Nociceptors
Projected pain
Radiculopathy
Referred pain

Valerie has worked at the hospital for the past 8 years. She had started as a dishwasher and worked her way up to being a food server on the tray line, then to salad and dessert preparation, and is now a cook. She enjoys her job and hopes her next promotion will be to kitchen supervisor.

Six months ago, Valerie gained custody of her 4-year-old nephew who has cerebral palsy. Her own son, who is 17, has been watching the young nephew after school until Valerie gets home from work. In 2 months, however, her son will be going away to college on a scholarship, and Valerie has been concerned about the after-school child care costs that she'll incur when her son leaves.

During a busy morning rush, Valerie slipped on a wet floor and fell, straining her back. She has tried returning to her job several times, but each time has experienced an increase in back pain after 2 or 3 days back at work. Her job requires standing for 7 hours a day, as well as frequent lifting, carrying, and bending. Recovery also has been hampered by the custodial needs of her nephew, whom she needs to lift and carry frequently. Valerie's accident occurred more than a month ago, and the concerns around her son's departure, combined with her back pain, are weighing heavily on her.

INTRODUCTION

Pain is best described as a subjective response to distress that cannot be quantitatively measured. There are three components to pain: physiological, pathological, and psychological. Pain may result from one or any combination of the three components. The degree to which each component contributes to the individual's experience of pain is difficult to assess. However, to provide effective treatment, every attempt must be made to evaluate all three accurately, keeping in mind that no matter what the cause, the effects can be equally disabling.

There are three types of pain: acute, chronic, and that associated with malignancy. The emphasis of this chapter is on chronic pain, particularly pain associated with soft tissue injuries. Individuals with this complaint are being seen more frequently in occupational therapy settings.

Chronic pain is defined as pain that lasts 6 months or longer or 3 to 4 weeks after "normal" healing should have occurred, in the absence of any objective pathological findings. Early identification and treatment of this problem increases the likelihood that the person can either overcome or learn to manage the pain effectively, thus minimizing the chance of prolonged disability.

ETIOLOGY

The literature on chronic pain is extensive, complicated, and often conflicting. Scientists and researchers have yet to determine how the human body and mind communicate, interpret, and respond to pain. As a consequence, there are numerous theories about the etiology of pain in general and, specifically, about the true nature of chronic pain.

This section of the chapter contains a review of some possible causes of pain that are specifically related to human anatomy and physiology. The major emphasis is on the transmission of acute pain. This is followed by a description of some of the major pathological and psychological factors in chronic pain. These theories provide a framework for understanding the general characteristics of chronic pain. (For more detailed information, see the references and recommended readings at the end of the chapter.)

Anatomy and Physiology of Acute Pain

The exact pathways by which pain is transmitted have not been clearly identified, nor is there any clear correlation between amount of tissue damage and the degree of pain and disability. A recently developed theory about the physiology and anatomy of pain poses the following explanation (1). At the time of injury, the peripheral nerves respond to the noxious or nociceptive (painful) stimulus. When the peripheral, somatic nerve endings receive a painful impulse, an afferent cue is transmitted through specific nerve fibers and pathways. The small-diameter nerve fibers appear to be the primary transmitters of pain, and they are able to respond selectively to either high-intensity or low-intensity pain stimuli. Also, certain nociceptors may play a role in further differentiating the intensity and the type of stimulus (e.g., heat).

With the onset of acute pain, the type of noxious stimulus (e.g., electrical shock, pin prick, laceration, or contusion) is usually obvious. Once the pain threshold has been reached, a pain signal is sent to warn the individual that tissue damage is occurring. Tissue damage usually begins at the same time the pain threshold is reached. Because of the tissue damage, acute pain is often accompanied by inflammation.

When nerve endings receive a painful stimulus, amines and peptides such as prostaglandin (1, 2) and substance P (1–4), among others, are released by the nerve cells. These neurotransmitters trigger the firing of an electrical impulse by the nerves. This impulse travels through designated pathways in the central nervous system (CNS). The dorsal horn, spinothalamic tract (1–5), and spinoreticular tract (1, 3) are commonly identified as the primary conduits for pain transmission in the spinal column. As the fibers enter the brain and divide, information is sent to different areas. The first supraspinal receptors of pain seem to be the reticular formation (1, 3, 4) and the thalamus (1–4). The thalamus interprets the signal as pain and relays messages to the limbic system, where an immediate emotional awareness is generated. Impulses are also sent to the somatosensory cortex (1–4), which consciously evaluates and locates the pain. The final transmission is to the frontal cortex (3), where emotional and physical responses are organized and carried out.

Descending analgesic pathways suppress the pain sensations through a linking mechanism in the brain that activates the body's natural defenses against pain. Studies using electrical stimulation reveal that descending pathways transmit analgesics (1, 2) produced at the midbrain level (2–4). Specifically, the periaqueductal, periventricular gray matter in the midbrain has been identified as having a large concentration of opiate receptor cells, thus playing a key role in producing analgesia (5). Some research suggests that the body's natural analgesic abilities are enhanced as the descending messages pass through opiate neurotransmitters in the spinal column, which in turn block ascending pain messages (1). At the spinal cord level, the substantia gelatinosa, with a high concentration of opiate receptors, assists in the modulation of pain (1, 2, 5). The fact that pain pathways seem capable of self-activating their own modulatory systems (1) may yet lead researchers to more effective means of controlling pain.

Another conceptualization of pain transmission is the "gate theory" of Melzack and Wall (6). Although subsequent research has disproven parts of the theory, the concept of "gating" is still considered valid (1). Although a painful stimulus triggers the small fibers to fire, Melzack and Wall believe that nonpainful stimuli trigger the firing of large nerve fibers. Thus, the perception of pain depends on the balance between the transmissions by the two types of fibers. The final effect is based on the networking of these different sensory nerves (large and small) converging in the substantia gelatinosa of the dorsal horn in the spinal cord (5, 7). If more large than small fibers are firing, the gate is closed and there is no pain perception. Facilitating a dominance of large fibers is done by either decreasing the noxious stimulus or applying a nonnoxious stimulus. The old remedy of rubbing a bump or bruise to make it feel better is a good illustration of increasing nonnoxious stimuli to decrease pain. Similarly, the basis for the use of transcutaneous electrical nerve stimulation (TENS) is that it induces competitive inhibition by stimulating the large nerve fibers.

A further review of current literature suggests that multiple sites and mechanisms affect both the transmission and modulation of pain and that these mechanisms may have either selective or multiple functions. The individual's response will differ, depending on the type or intensity of the pain. It is clear from this brief discussion that much is still unknown about how the body and the brain receive, analyze, and respond to pain.

Pathology of Chronic Pain

The models that have been developed to describe chronic pain are fewer and generally less advanced that those for acute pain. Chronic pain is often explained by the pathological changes in the nervous or musculoskeletal system, including prolonged muscle spasm, trigger points, radiculopathy, peripheral neuropathy, and causalgia.

One theory (1) proposes that in the absence of a tissue-damaging stimulus, neuronal elements may cause inappropriate firing of the nerve fibers. For example, a damaged nociceptive terminal may produce chemicals that lower the threshold of other nociceptive fibers (1, 2). This causes typically nonnoxious stimuli to be interpreted as painful. A second hypothesis suggests that damaged axons may regenerate by forming abnormal nerve sprouts (1, 2), which may fire in the absence of any stimuli or may be hypersensitive. The CNS is then inappropriately signaled that tissue damage is occurring. A third is the theory of dysfunctional gating (1). For some reason the CNS becomes unable to differentiate the sensory information from nerves. Signals become garbled like a poor telephone connection and result in an erroneous pain message being sent. This may happen without any stimulus being applied or may cause the sensation of pain in locations distant from the stimulus.

Pathology of Soft Tissue Pain

One of the leading scholars in this field, Rene Cailliet, believes that the primary causes of soft tissue pain are muscle spasm and decreased circulation. He believes that prolonged muscle contraction or spasm may result from an imbalance of the agonist–antagonist muscles, nerve malfunction, or internal changes in the muscle (8). These spasms cause catabolites to accumulate in the muscle, producing pain. Catabolites are the byproducts of muscle metabolism and are normally removed from the muscle by capillary action. With a prolonged contraction, however, the catabolites build up. Once this happens, it is difficult to remove them. Even after the muscle contraction has stopped, an accompanying reflexive vasospasm still exists. The presence of concentrated catabolites, combined with a lack of efficient capillary action, affects the proximal nociceptors and triggers a pain signal. A cyclical response may begin with the prolonged muscle contraction, a buildup of catabolites, pain signal, emotional tension, and further muscle contraction.

Ischemia may also be a cause of soft tissue pain (8). Changes in arterial pressure may quicken the onset of pain and cause it to be more severe (8). An example is shoulder or upper back pain caused by activity that requires reaching overhead for extended periods, as when painting a ceiling.

Another explanation used by Dr. Cailliet and others is called myofascial pain, myalgia, or myofascitis. One of the primary concepts of myofascial pain is the trigger point, a hypersensitive point within a muscle or its fascia (8, 9), which may be accompanied by inflammation. A trigger point is speculated to be caused or perpetuated by muscle loading or emotional stress (8, 9). It is very painful when pressure is applied (9). The location of these trigger points is similar from individual to individual. Each trigger point has an area of referred pain that is also generally consistent from person to person (9). Pressure on the trigger point reproduces pain in the referred pain area. Researchers have been able to draw a map of common trigger points and their associated areas of referred pain.

A spasm in a segment of the muscle with a trigger point is another identifying trait. When palpated or "strummed," a localized twitch response is seen. There may also be a palpable "ropy" feeling to the muscle, as when you roll a thick cord back and forth between your index finger and thumb. The muscle may feel locally "hard," and there is always extreme local tenderness when deep pressure is applied to the trigger point. Relief may be achieved through injection of the trigger point with a local anesthetic or a steroid. The effects may not be permanent, however (8, 9).

Psychology of Chronic Pain

A third component of chronic pain is psychological. Emotional distress such as anxiety, depression, or hysteria can intensify pain (7, 10). Ultimately, there is a psychogenic component to all chronic pain—if not as a primary cause, then as a result of the pain's duration and debilitating effects. If a patient experiences a muscle spasm after an injury, there may be an unconscious increase in muscle tension. This increase in muscle tension produces a state of emotional tension that further aggravates the spasm and pain (Fig. 16.1). Thus, a psychophysiological cycle is established that perpetuates the pain. This is commonly seen in muscles of the spine, especially the neck and trunk, where a flexion/extension injury has occurred (7).

However, psychological distress alone can heighten the perception of pain. This can occur in the absence of a painful stimulus or can cause nerve signals to be misinterpreted. Pain tolerance

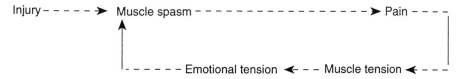

FIGURE 16.1   Cycle of psychophysical response to pain.

can be influenced by psychological factors such as emotional tension, stress, or fatigue. A person with chronic pain is likely to have a lowered pain tolerance and, as a result, functions less effectively (7).

Significant, predisposing factors for persons with chronic pain are associated with their childhood experiences. Often they have been verbally or physically abused as a child, had a family member with a physically debilitating condition, or were unable to deal with significant losses, such as death of a family member, in a normal and timely manner (11). Other common characteristics include previous psychiatric illness; psychosocial problems, such as a poor work history or family problems; or a history of frequent medical problems that the person perceives as having responded poorly to medical care (12).

Examples of psychological disturbances that may precede or follow chronic pain include depression, anxiety disorder, hypochondriasis, hysterical neurosis, somatization disorder, malingering, and substance abuse disorder (7, 10, 12). These disturbances may exist prior to chronic pain or may develop as its result. Regardless of their etiology, such disorders will certainly affect the pain the individual experiences and his or her response to treatment.

Organic complaints sometimes accompany psychological problems. Such complaints may be a result of treatment, such as failed surgery or postsurgical scar tissue. Other problems may be caused by medications. Common side effects of medication include gastrointestinal distress, loss of appetite, swelling, and drowsiness, among others. It is important to differentiate psychological issues and organic causes of pain to provide effective treatment.

Beliefs about health and illness also can play a role in the perpetuation of chronic pain. In our society, the expectation is that most illnesses and injuries can be cured. On the other hand, a sick person is expected to be dependent and exempt from certain social responsibilities (7, 11). The intertwining of these perceptions can lead to the following expectations:

"If I have pain, I must be sick; the pain will go away when I am better."

"Too much activity will only make me sicker."

"I need to rest if I am going to heal."

"I am in pain; therefore, something is wrong."

With medical and pharmacological advances, society has come to expect a "cure" for most ailments. Within this context it is not surprising that many people with chronic pain view themselves as disabled.

Most individuals with chronic pain are earnestly seeking relief. A small minority, however, complain of chronic pain to receive unwarranted financial remuneration through workers' compensation or Social Security benefits. These individuals are labeled as malingerers. They will exaggerate their pain and are often very dramatic in their verbal and nonverbal communication about their pain. However, it is important to remember that persons who have genuinely high levels of emotional distress will often respond in a similar fashion. Along with an incongruence between the malingerers' complaints and medical findings, they also have normal physical abilities. Experienced clinicians estimate that only 2 to 5% of persons with chronic pain are malingerers (Jerome J. Unpublished data. Lansing: MI, Ingham Medical Center).

Another challenge in working with individuals with chronic pain are patients who achieve secondary gains from their disability. Secondary gains are events or responses that result from the pain/disability and serve to reinforce the problem's existence. These gains may be subtle or obvious. An example of secondary gain is the individual who initially injures himself at his factory job and, during the course of his recovery, is able to devote more time to his college studies and get better grades. Another example is a mother with young children who no longer has to struggle with the conflict of spending too much time away from home, working to supplement the family income. Secondary gains are the "silver lining" to the "cloud" of pain. As time progresses, the individual may become consciously aware of the secondary gains and try to either eliminate or perpetuate them.

Conclusion

As mentioned earlier, there are differences between acute and chronic pain. A common medical management problem is that individuals with chronic pain are treated the same as those with acute pain. It is important to distinguish the cause(s) of the pain, as well as whether it is acute or chronic, inasmuch as chronic pain does not respond to conventional acute pain treatments. Refer to Table 16.1 for a summary of some of the major differences between acute and chronic pain.

INCIDENCE AND PREVALENCE

Chronic pain and related illness and injury are major health problems in this country and have a significant impact on health costs. Recent estimates indicate that at least $75 billion are spent each year on these conditions, in both direct medical expenses and indirect costs associated with lost productivity. When other expenses, such as retraining, medical disability, early retirement, and others are considered, the cost is estimated to be $100 billion. Each year, at least 1400 days of work are missed per 1000 workers because of back pain alone (13).

There are no precise statistics, however, on the actual prevalence and costs associated with

TABLE 16.1 Overview of Differences Between Acute and Chronic Pain

ACUTE	CHRONIC
Provides warning of tissue damage occurrence	Has no known function
Fast, sudden, sharp, followed by dull ache	Ache, cramp, or burn; constant or intermittent
Initially discrete, well localized, then more diffuse	Generally more diffuse and may have radiating component
Usually has identifiable cause such as injury, pathology, or disease	May or may not have associated injury, pathology, or disease
Pain pattern follows known dermatomes and nerve distribution	May stray from known dermatomes and nerve distributions
Usually accompanied by objective findings	May or may not be accompanied by objective findings
Responds to analgesics or narcotics	Analgesics have little or no effect; narcotics become addictive

chronic pain, because there is no systematic record-keeping or data collection.

It is important to note that of those aged 60 years and older, the number diagnosed with chronic pain (250/1000) is double that of those younger than age 60. Eighty-five percent of older adults have at least one chronic condition that may result in pain. In fact, pain is the most frequently reported symptom when a physician is contacted for consultation (14).

It is hard to obtain precise data on the numbers of individuals with chronic pain for three main reasons. One is the lack of a common pool of data because information is not shared among medical providers, insurance carriers, and governmental agencies. The second is the way the data are collected. Existing data are organized according to the type of problem and body part affected (e.g., low back pain) and do not indicate the degree of chronicity. Third, much of the data details on-the-job injuries only and disregards injuries, for example, that happen at home.

Difficulty in determining the exact cost of chronic pain can be largely attributed to the inability to estimate indirect costs such as lost productivity, hiring and training replacement employees, and increased insurance premiums. Ultimately, these increased costs are passed on to the consumer and the public.

The remainder of this chapter focuses on two conditions that are commonly associated with chronic pain: lower back pain and cumulative trauma disorder. Both are seen frequently in occupational therapy settings.

Lower back pain is a pervasive disability. It is estimated in the literature that 80% of the population in the United States will experience back pain at some time during their lives. Low back pain is ranked as the second leading cause of all visits to a physician in the United States. It is the most frequent cause of activity limitations in people younger than age 45 (15).

One study suggests that 5% of the U.S. population has experienced chronic low back symptoms that have permanently disabled 2.6 million individuals and temporarily disabled another 2.6 million (16). A second study (17) reports that chronic back problems will disable 1% of Americans on a total and permanent basis and partially disable many more. A third study reported that approximately 74% of workers with back injuries return to work within a month, whereas 7% are unable to return for more than 6 months (18). This latter group incurs more than 75% of medical costs and overall compensation for low back injuries (18). The likelihood of these individuals returning to work after a 6-month absence is 50%. After 1 year, the rate of return is reduced to 25%, and those absent for more than 2 years never return to gainful employment (16). The estimated costs for those with back pain range from $5 billion per year for medical costs (19) to $56 billion when compensation costs are included (20).

The other primary type of soft tissue disability associated with chronic pain is cumulative trauma disorder. In 1989, 147,000 cases of cumulative trauma disorder were reported to the Bureau of Labor Statistics, making them the leading cause of increases in job-related occupational illnesses (21).

The American Academy of Orthopedic Surgeons has estimated that national costs for cumulative trauma disorders, including medical care and lost wages, are approximately $27 billion per year (22). Carpal tunnel syndrome, one type of cumulative trauma disorder, occurs at the average rate of 0.8 cases/1000 workers in general industry (21). These figures are as high as 15 to 20% for workers in high-risk occupations (21).

A company at high risk for cumulative trauma injuries will spend an estimated $250,000 per year/100 employees for costs associated with the problem (23). To illustrate, only 5% of individuals who are diagnosed with carpal tunnel require surgery. In a study of meatcutters, however, of those who had surgery, 50% had not returned to their original jobs 1 year later (24).

Data seem to indicate that cumulative trauma disorders occur more frequently in certain occupations and that in severe cases (i.e., those not responding to conservative treatment), a high percentage of individuals are unable to return to work because of chronic pain.

SIGNS AND SYMPTOMS

It is important to reiterate that, at the present time, there is no objective way to measure pain. Pain is a subjective response that can be substantiated through observation and possibly by the results of clinical tests/assessments. The signs and symptoms of chronic pain vary, depending on such factors as the presence or absence of an underlying pathology, the type and location of pathology, physical fitness, and psychological state. Table 16.2 lists some common signs and symptoms associated with soft tissue chronic pain of the upper extremity and lower back. Signs and symptoms listed in the table may be present because of pathology, a psychological problem, or a combination of the two. The only universally recognized measure of chronic pain is its presence over time.

The individual's personal and medical histories are often good predictors of dysfunction from chronic pain and should be given careful consideration. The person's psychosocial history (refer to the previous section on the psychology of pain) and the course of previous events and treatment for the condition are important aspects of the total clinical picture.

Many individuals share a common experience or series of events that led to their disability. Frequently he or she has undergone a significant amount of testing to rule out various disorders and pathologies. There is a history of unsuccessful treatments, surgeries, and medications with poor pain control. The person may

---

TABLE 16.2 Signs and Symptoms of Chronic Pain

SIGNS
A. Objective
Asymmetry—structural or postural
Atrophy
Autonomic discharge—sweating, flushing, tachycardia, elevated blood pressure
Crepitus
Edema
Erythema
Incoordination
Inflammation
Muscle spasm, tightness, hardness, ropiness, or twitch response
Reflex exaggerated, diminished, or absent
Skin temperature increased or decreased
Spinal irregularities—misalignment, flattening, general asymmetry
Vascular abnormalities—discoloration, diminished or absent hair growth or pulses, ulcerations

B. Objective but requiring accurate patient report or cooperation
Balance
Gait abnormalities
Fluidity of motion
Muscle cramps or weakness
Numbness
Pain usually poorly localized

Paresthesias (tingling)
Projected pain
Radiculopathy
Range of motion limitation, passive or active
Sensory impairment
Sudden motor loss (e.g., dropping things or falling without warning)
Trigger points

SYMPTOMS
Antalgic movement and postures
Eating pattern changed—increased or decreased
Emotional distress—anger, irritability, depression, anxiety, emotional lability, etc.
Fatigue
Functional capacity diminished
Glove anesthesia
Muscle weakness observed as a sudden, giving way to applied resistance
Pain behaviors—guarding, grimacing, sighing, holding or rubbing body parts, etc.
Preoccupation with pain
Referred pain
Tenderness
Tolerance to pain diminished
Sexual activity diminished
Sleeping disturbances
Social withdrawal

have consulted a number of physicians and therapists, seeking alternative methods of treatment for relief. This is sometimes referred to as "doctor shopping" and can significantly inflate the costs of medical care. Having seen a variety of medical providers, the patient is often confused about the cause of the pain, the diagnosis, appropriate treatments, and safe activity level. With contradictory advice, it is not surprising that the patient becomes confused, suspicious, or defensive.

As pain persists, the person becomes more and more distressed, especially when no medical cause is found for the continuing pain. The distress may manifest itself in a number of ways, depending on such factors as premorbid personality, cultural influences, and financial incentives or disincentives. Distress may result in anger directed at self or others, depression, anxiety, and guilt. These responses can heighten emotional tension and, thus, the perception of pain.

Drug dependency can be another result of frequently changed or mismanaged care (7). The patient finds that narcotic medication helps "take the edge off," even though it doesn't cure the pain. In extreme situations, the person will change doctors or see several concurrently to maintain drug dependence.

Some individuals find it necessary to "prove" that they have a disability. Insurance carriers/employers often require an independent medical evaluation (IME). The intent is to provide an objective, impartial physician's opinion. This is not unusual when the employee has been unable to return to work and has a history of chronic pain of unknown origin. In some states, if the IME reveals no objective findings to substantiate the patient's continued complaints of pain, it is possible, particularly in workers' compensation cases, that the patient will be asked to return to work or risk losing benefits. In this situation, the person may concentrate on proving that the disability is real.

In summary, some of the precipitating factors leading to the diagnosis of chronic pain are:

1. Pain that extends beyond the normal course of healing
2. Lack of objective physical signs, or fluctuating physical findings
3. Significant functional disability as a result of the pain
4. Psychological dysfunction
5. Multiple failed treatments or surgeries
6. Use of many different medications
7. Inability to be gainfully employed
8. Receiving financial remuneration for disability or involvement in litigation to determine disability

DIAGNOSIS

The diagnosis of chronic pain is made when pain lasts beyond the normal healing period. Underlying pathology and psychological factors may be present or absent. Chronic pain is considered dysfunctional when it interferes with the individual's performance.

Chronic pain can be present in an unlimited number of diagnoses. This section focuses on diagnostic tests done to determine if an underlying pathology can be identified for lower back or upper extremity conditions associated with chronic pain. Positive test results substantiate the likelihood of a pathological condition and associated chronic pain. A negative test result, however, does not rule out the existence of chronic pain. Psychological tests are used to determine whether there is an underlying affective disorder, to gain an understanding of how the patient perceives pain, and how the pain affects the individual both personally and socially.

MEDICAL/SURGICAL MANAGEMENT

The use of medication will vary according to the presence of an underlying organic pathology, the type of pathology, and its stage. If no organic pathology is identified, medications are prescribed according to the duration of the pain. Selection of appropriate medication depends on a specific diagnosis. For example, medications prescribed for an inflammatory flare-up are different than those prescribed to manage ongoing pain.

Information on medications (27–32) is included in the medications appendix at the end of the book. Dosages and daily maximum levels are approximate guidelines. Potential side effects that are common and may affect occupational performance are listed. A word of caution: narcotic analgesics generally are not used for chronic pain because they are addictive. In some situations, they are prescribed on a limited basis for short-term bouts of increased pain.

In addition to the drugs listed in the medications appendix, such medications as Zantac or Cytotec are used to inhibit the secretion of gastric acid and relieve problems of secondary gastrointestinal distress caused by other medications. Antihistamines can be prescribed (50 to 100 mg) to help induce sleep, in place of a sedative with addictive properties.

Diagnostic or therapeutic nerve blocks, which are an injection of local anesthetics, are used to identify or relieve pain in the peripheral nerves, nerve roots, or viscera; decrease trigger point pain; interrupt reflex sympathetic activity; and improve vascular supply (27). Steroid injections are given to reduce inflammation.

IMPACT ON OCCUPATIONAL PERFORMANCE

As previously discussed, chronic pain can be, by itself, a disabling condition, regardless of the etiology. The person who is experiencing chronic pain encounters limitations in a number of performance components and performance areas. These factors may be present or absent for any particular individual or may be experienced to varying degrees by different people.

Performance Components

Sensorimotor

Neuromuscular disruptions are common. There is usually a limitation in active and sometimes passive range of motion. Patients have pain when they attempt to use the muscles, tendons, etc. that have been damaged. For example, in lateral epicondylitis ("tennis elbow"), the patient experiences pain at the muscle's points of origin when attempting to forcefully extend and sometimes supinate the wrist. This condition is caused by forcefully snapping the wrist into extension as with a tennis stroke or by mechanical overload of the muscle(s) through repetitive work. To minimize the pain, the person will avoid wrist extension, especially to maximum range or against force. Initially, passive range of motion is normal; however, it may diminish with prolonged inactivity over time. Pain is reproduced when the involved muscles are put to maximum stretch. In this example, pain may occur when the wrist is passively placed in full flexion. In less severe cases, this may only be referred to as "tightness" by the patient.

Loss of strength and endurance are significant and common problems for chronic pain patients. They often result from prolonged inactivity because of pain avoidance or overuse of orthotic devices. Extended periods of inactivity will cause muscle weakness and atrophy. Generalized deconditioning can also affect activity tolerance.

If the patient avoids using the body part (either actively or passively), the muscles can shorten and the connective tissues lose their "glide" quality. This, in turn, can cause secondary pain. In addition, inflammation and crepitus compromise soft tissue integrity and can cause pain.

In sum, a self-perpetuating cycle is established as a result of initial pain, later sustained by secondary pain (Fig. 16.2). Also, because chronic pain is diffuse and poorly localized, there may be a tendency to protect areas of referred pain. This draws additional soft tissues/muscle groups into the chronic pain syndrome, and there is an addi-

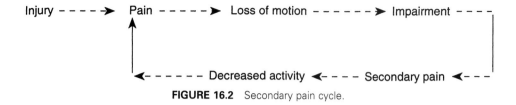

FIGURE 16.2   Secondary pain cycle.

tive effect on limitations in activities as more and more muscles are involved.

Postural control is another potential area of dysfunction. As a guarding mechanism, the patient may hold the body part in a protective, abnormal position. This is particularly common with upper extremity injuries. The extremity is held close to the body with slight elevation of the shoulder. Holding the arm in this position for long periods can cause prolonged static muscle contraction and referred pain in the upper back, particularly the trapezius and levator scapulae. This results in fatigue and loss of symmetry. A person with low back pain can be observed shifting weight to the unaffected side or leaning to the painful side to avoid stretching muscles of the lower back. Greater energy demands are made when maintaining a position against gravity, such as holding the injured arm in slight abduction or laterally flexing the trunk. Unnatural weight distribution can also reduce normal range of motion because of muscle shortening.

Proprioception is associated with postural control. The areas of particular concern are the shoulders, scapulae, and smaller joints of the spine. Normally, a person is aware of the gross position of these structures, but fine positioning, such as slight flexion of C3 or shoulder rounding, is often not perceived. Poor proprioception may play a cumulative role in chronic pain (5).

Finally, sensory awareness and processing may be impaired with chronic pain. This impairment may manifest as tactile hyposensitivity or hypersensitivity to noxious stimuli. For example, pain messages may be sent to the brain when no stimulus is present. Also, the person who has chronic pain may not be able to differentiate various stimuli and may have exaggerated responses.

Cognitive

The individual with chronic pain often becomes very focused on the pain, and as a result, cognitive function may be affected. Perceptions, capacities, and processing are distorted or inhibited because of the emotional stress or fatigue caused by the pain. Some typical changes in cognitive function follow.

Attention span becomes limited. The pain distracts the patient by interrupting concentration. This is seen in tasks that are monotonous or repetitious, in which there is little cognitive challenge or emotional interest. When the perceived pain overrides concentration on the activity, the quality of performance may suffer.

Similarly, increased focus on the pain may decrease the patient's ability to attend to things in the surrounding environment. Therefore, as a result of the attention deficit, short-term or recent memory may be affected. This may be further compounded by depression, which also contributes to poor attention and short-term memory.

Issues of dependency and fear of additional pain or injury can influence problem solving, particularly that related to managing the pain to maintain function. Dependent patients who allow others to do the work until they are "better" may not take the initiative, for example, to analyze everyday activities that are aggravating the pain. This is more common when there is no incentive for the patient to learn to function independently, such as when there is someone else available to perform the task or it is associated with a role that the patient is willing to give up.

Patients often fail to use good problem-solving skills or judgment when they are "having a good day." Often, in this instance, patients will try to do too much. In failing to properly pace activities, they may experience a subsequent increase in pain, which will help perpetuate their misconceptions about their actual abilities and tolerances.

Finally, patients frequently have a hard time learning new strategies to manage their pain. This is especially evident in the psychophysical response to pain, that is, learning to relax muscles when pain occurs instead of increasing muscle tension. It is often difficult for patients to learn to associate relaxation with the pain response.

Psychosocial

Chronic pain often has a strong psychological component that limits functional capacities and perpetuates the pain cycle. The person experiences dramatic changes or even losses of societal roles. Self-concept is inevitably affected, as are values, interests, and social interactions. The loss of familiar roles and activities affects the patient's management of self, because there has been a loss of control over his or her daily life.

A role change or loss may be the single and most apparent effect for the patient to manage. Subsequent psychological components may be directly affected by role interruption. Chronic pain can affect many performance components; therefore, any number of roles can similarly be affected. Because a sense of identity and worth are largely defined by an individual's roles and multiple roles can be affected, there may be substantial feelings of loss, grief, and anger in every aspect of the patient's daily life. In some cases, familiar roles may even be reversed, further complicating the sense of self.

Values may change, as roles and perspectives are modified or reversed. Typically, if a new role is assumed, the person assumes the values associated with that role. A threat to personal or familial security may intensify the focus on some values and diminish it on others. There may be

an increased awareness of mortality, causing patients to reassess what is important.

As a result of changes in performance components over time, patients may experience a change in interests. If there is an activity in which they can no longer participate, there may be a resulting loss of interest. An increase in unstructured time, as a result of limitations in roles, may go unchanneled, demonstrating poor time management skills, or the patient may develop new interests or routines to fill the time.

A change in self-concept almost always follows a significant or long-standing change in roles. As the role definition changes, so does a person's self-concept. These changes may be interpreted by the patient as either good or bad. The interpretation depends on how closely the changes match the patient's long-term goals or motivations. A patient's personal perception may be that he or she is worthless or a failure, or the perception may be one of success in shedding an unwanted role.

Social skills are often affected. A patient's conduct may not be appropriate to the situation when their focus on pain overrides the discussion or issues at hand. Nonverbal communication such as sighing or grimacing may send signals to others about the patient's state of mind. These behaviors can guide or otherwise affect the patient's interpersonal relationships in very significant, but subtle, ways.

As a result of the emotional effects of long-term pain, changes, and loss of control among others, coping skills are invariably affected. In the long run, the effects can be positive or adverse. A formerly shy, introverted patient may learn to express herself openly and assertively. Conversely, others may become withdrawn and dependent. New coping skills are developed in response to the situations in which patients find themselves. Very often, however, feelings of anger, loss, fear, and an inability to sleep soundly impair a person's ability to cope with day-to-day stresses on top of the pain. As a result, sudden, angry outbursts, crying, blaming others, and personal distancing are seen. The patient perceives a loss of control and often demonstrates a personal loss of self-control.

Performance Areas

Work

Because chronic pain primarily affects adults, work is the most commonly affected performance area. Working requires some level of activity tolerance, whether it involves standing for long periods or frequent handling of small objects. The inability to sustain activity over time is why many people with chronic pain conditions are unable to work, particularly outside of the home. In other cases, particular tasks associated with their jobs cause an increase in pain. If the employer can provide work that is within their physical abilities, and the patient feels able to do the job, the patient may be able to continue working. Otherwise, long-term or permanent restrictions may prevent the individual from returning to his or her job. These same restrictions may require the patient to examine alternative or transferrable work skills to find a new job. A role reversal may occur if, for example, a husband is no longer able to work outside of the home. He may stay home with the children while his wife takes a job to ensure an adequate income.

Educational activities may be affected in the same way. In other instances, however, individuals with chronic pain use the change in their work capacity to return to school and obtain new skills. This is particularly common when an individual can no longer perform a manual occupation and must learn job skills that involve higher level cognitive skills.

Work activities that involve home management or caring for others may be limited by physical and emotional tolerances to the pain. A mother may find that she has a shorter temper with her children or she may become more reliant on her children to complete tasks around the house. If there is no one else to assist with the work, patients with chronic pain may find that they do less work or pace themselves so that they can do the essential chores. For example, cleaning may become less important so the patient can save energy for shopping, cooking, and laundry.

Activities of Daily Living

Activities that require either endurance or motion can be affected. Persons with lower back pain may modify the way they dress to avoid the pain associated with bending. Chronic hip pain can be managed by using a tub seat instead of climbing in and out of the tub. A woman with hand pain may be unable to use her curlers or blow dryer without aggravating her pain.

More pervasive, however, are problems encountered with mobility. Lower back pain can impair an individual's ability to walk or ride long distances. Similarly, chronic hand pain can impair tolerance for driving. Limitations in mobility may further affect a person's ability to get to and from work, to get around on the job, to visit friends, or to attend leisure events.

Finally, impaired mobility and flexibility can affect sexual expression. The capacity for sexual interaction may be impaired both physically and psychologically, although adaptation and modification of physical expression can be satisfying.

Leisure Activities

Involvement in leisure activities may change. This can be solely the result of physical limitations (e.g., the father who cannot play football with his son because of chronic back pain) or it can be limited by psychological function (e.g., the depressed individual who has withdrawn from club activities). Finally, increased focus on the pain may draw on the attention span so a person may no longer enjoy former activities (e.g., crocheting or doing crossword puzzles).

A summary of occupational performance components and performance areas commonly seen in chronic pain patients is provided in Table 16.3. From the preceding discussion, it is apparent that each of the three primary performance components and areas can be affected by chronic pain. Although the table provides an overview, the following case studies provide some specific examples of chronic pain and its impact on occupational performance.

TABLE 16.3 Occupational Performance Profile

I. PERFORMANCE AREAS	II. PERFORMANCE COMPONENTS	III. PERFORMANCE CONTEXTS

A. Activities of Daily Living
  1. Grooming
  2. Oral Hygiene
  3. Bathing/Showering
  4. Toilet Hygiene
  5. Personal Device Care
  6. Dressing
  7. Feeding and Eating
  8. Medication Routine
  9. Health Maintenance
  10. Socialization
  11. Functional Communication
  12. Functional Mobility
  13. Community Mobility
  14. Emergency Response
  15. Sexual Expression
B. Work and Productive Activities
  1. Home Management
    a. Clothing Care
    b. Cleaning
    c. Meal Preparation/ Cleanup
    d. Shopping
    e. Money Management
    f. Household Maintenance
    g. Safety Procedures
  2. Care of Others
  3. Educational Activities
  4. Vocational Activities
    a. Vocational Exploration
    b. Job Acquisition
    c. Work or Job Performance
    d. Retirement Planning
    e. Volunteer Participation
C. Play or Leisure Activities
  1. Play or Leisure Exploration
  2. Play or Leisure Performance
	A. Sensorimotor Component
	  1. Sensory
	    a. Sensory Awareness
	    b. Sensory Processing
	      (1) Tactile
	      (2) Proprioceptive
	      (3) Vestibular
	      (4) Visual
	      (5) Auditory
	      (6) Gustatory
	      (7) Olfactory
	    c. Perceptual Processing
	      (1) Stereognosis
	      (2) Kinesthesia
	      (3) Pain Response
	      (4) Body Scheme
	      (5) Right–Left Discrimination
	      (6) Form Constancy
	      (7) Position in Space
	      (8) Visual–Closure
	      (9) Figure Ground
	      (10) Depth Perception
	      (11) Spatial Relations
	      (12) Topographical Orientation
	  2. Neuromusculoskeletal
	    a. Reflex
	    b. Range of Motion
	    c. Muscle Tone
	    d. Strength
	    e. Endurance
	    f. Postural Control
	    g. Postural Alignment
	    h. Soft Tissue Integrity
	  3. Motor
	    a. Gross Coordination
	    b. Crossing the Midline
	    c. Laterality
	    d. Bilateral Integration
	    e. Motor Control
	    f. Praxis
	    g. Fine Coordination/Dexterity
	    h. Visual–Motor Control
	    i. Oral–Motor Control
		A. Temporal Aspects
		  1. Chronological
		  2. Developmental
		  3. Lifecycle
		  4. Disability Status
		B. Environment
		  1. Physical
		  2. Social
		  3. Cultural

(continued)

TABLE 16.3 Occupational Performance Profile (Continued)		
I. PERFORMANCE AREAS	**II. PERFORMANCE COMPONENTS**	**III. PERFORMANCE CONTEXTS**

	B. Cognitive Integration and Cognitive Components
	  1. Level of Arousal
	  2. Orientation
	  3. Recognition
	  4. Attention Span
	  5. Initiation of Activity
	  6. Termination of Activity
	  7. Memory
	  8. Sequencing
	  9. Categorization
	  10. Concept Formation
	  11. Spatial Operations
	  12. Problem Solving
	  13. Learning
	  14. Generalization
	C. Psychosocial Skills and Psychological Components
	  1. Psychological
	    a. Values
	    b. Interests
	    c. Self-Concept
	  2. Social
	    a. Role Performance
	    b. Social Conduct
	    c. Interpersonal Skills
	    d. Self-Expression
	  3. Self-Management
	    a. Coping Skills
	    b. Time Management
	    c. Self-Control	

CASE STUDIES

CASE 1

C. S. is a 43-year-old man employed as a manual laborer at a small chrome plating plant. He has been employed there for 12 years, has a good work record, and is well liked by supervisors and co-workers. He has only one previous workers' compensation claim for an incident 6 years ago when he was exposed to toxic chemical fumes. He is married with three children, ages 7, 9, and 11 and has a good relationship with his wife and children. His wife works as a waitress at a hotel. C. S. is illit-

erate. In his spare time, he enjoys playing basketball and riding motorcycles. He belongs to a motorcycle club and is active in their volunteer work to raise money for a local charity. He also assists with his sons' Little League, driving the team to games, handling the equipment, and cheering the team on. In the winter, he spends a lot of time working on his motorcycle and pickup truck in a neighbor's heated garage.

C. S. injured his lower back while lifting at work. He was taken to the hospital's emergency department; radiographs showed no structural damage, and examination found no neurological deficits. A severe muscle spasm in the right, lower back was the only positive finding. A diagnosis of severe lumbosacral strain was made. He was given prescriptions for anti-inflammatory agents and muscle relaxants and told to go home to bed for 3 days and then follow-up with his family doctor.

After 3 days of bed rest, C. S. still had difficulty getting up and down from a seated position, standing, and walking. His family doctor noted a paravertebral spasm in the right low back. Further examination revealed trunk flexion limited by pain to 30 degrees; full extension was measured at –10 degrees. When he straightened from sitting, C. S. used his hands on his thighs to "walk" himself back up. Side bending was normal on the right but limited by 20 degrees on the left. Rotation was limited in both directions. Straight leg raising was negative on the left and positive at 25 degrees on the right. His stance and gait showed a pain scoliosis on the right. Sensory and reflex testing were normal. Bowel and bladder function were reported to be normal. Muscle strength appeared good, although he had "give away" response (sudden release of a muscle contraction when resistance is applied) in his right hip flexors and extensors. The doctor confirmed the diagnosis of back strain and renewed his prescriptions. He told C. S. to stay home and rest for a week but to gradually begin increasing his activities. The doctor would run some laboratory tests to rule out organic pathologies. The doctor asked him to return in a week.

C. S. again went home and tried to resume some of his activities. He dressed each day but found it very painful to get into his pants, shoes, and socks. He was most comfortable in his recliner chair and spent significant time watching television. His wife and children were very concerned and tried to help him as much as possible.

When he returned to the doctor, C. S. was very concerned about new pain that had developed in his right buttock and anterior thigh. A few of the same tests were quickly repeated, but little change was found. The laboratory results had all been normal. C. S. told the doctor he wasn't ready to go back to work. The following week, when C. S. did feel ready, his employer was unable to offer him restricted work.

C. S. returned to his doctor several times. He was growing restless and bored at home, and the constant pain made him irritable. The doctor, who had observed little improvement, felt there was nothing more he could do. He referred C. S. to an orthopaedic specialist. The orthopaedist reviewed C. S.'s x-ray films and conducted a detailed examination and interviews, including whether C. S. had been experiencing any personal problems at home or at work. C. S. began to wonder if the doctor thought he was faking. During the examination, the doctor repeated many of the tests the family doctor had done. Other tests included standing on one leg, walking on his heels and then his toes, reflex testing, and measuring the lengths and circumferences of his legs. Upon completing his examination, the doctor told C. S. there was nothing structurally wrong. He suggested physical therapy to ease the pain, relax the muscles, and stretch out tightened muscles.

It was now 8 weeks since the injury and C. S.'s discontent and concern were growing. Why wasn't the pain going away? Were the doctors missing something? He was anxious and confused. He continued with the therapy, working hard under his physical therapist's direction. He saw an occupational therapist for several sessions, who showed him how to do things like put on his pants and get out of bed without aggravating the pain. He began to feel that he had some control over the pain and that he was making progress.

C. S. then reinjured his back at home. He returned to the emergency department and was again told there was no structural damage but that he should follow-up with his doctor as soon as possible. The pain was worse than before. He returned to his orthopaedic physician, very upset and agitated. The doctor noted that C. S.'s posture again listed to the right and his trunk range of motion was limited by pain. The muscle spasm was back. C. S. reported that the buttock and thigh pains were worse, going all the way down into his calf. Magnetic resonance imaging results were normal. C. S. asked the doctor what exactly was causing the pain. The doctor again told him it was muscle spasm. C. S. wondered why a back spasm caused leg pain, but he didn't ask the doctor.

Weeks passed and C. S. experienced more and more problems at home. His family was beginning to tire of his short temper and dependency. They were also feeling the financial strain of reduced income. He felt guilty about his wife having to work more and about being so short tempered, but he couldn't help it. This increased his irritability and he felt rejected. He was also frustrated by the limits his back pain had put on his sexual life. As his depression grew, so did his withdrawal from the motorcycle club's activities. He no longer went to his neighbor's, even to talk, because it angered him that he couldn't work on his truck, something that had always helped him relax.

His employers wanted to know when he was coming back to work. They were short of help and needed him. C. S., angry that his boss didn't even ask how he was doing, yelled, "When I'm ready!" and hung up the phone. The employer wondered if C. S. was really trying.

It is now 8 months since the initial injury, and C. S. is still at home. He has good and bad days but is fearful of reinjuring his back. He also doubts his ability to keep up with others at work. The problems he has at home are at least familiar to him; he doesn't know if he can handle returning to work.

CASE 2

B. A. is the single mother of two children, ages 3 and 6. She is 27 years old and was divorced 6 months ago after a difficult marriage to an abusive husband. She lives in a rented trailer.

She works in a large manufacturing plant where plastic components for car dashboards are made. She has worked there for 9 months. Her mother took a medical retirement from the same plant because of carpal tunnel syndrome in both wrists. Her mother had worked there for 17 years.

For the last 3 months, B. A. has been cutting off the "flash" (i.e., seams on plastic that has been hot molded) with a razor knife. She began to notice an aching in her right, dominant forearm at the end of her shift one Friday. By Saturday morning it was gone, and she didn't think twice about it. As the weeks passed, however, the aching developed earlier in her shift and lasted into the next day. Then it became constant. The pain runs from her elbow into the dorsum of her forearm.

She was sent to a doctor frequently used by the company. He asked about the pain: what it felt like, where it was, and what seemed to make it worse. B. A. noted that cutting the plastic flash seemed to bother it the most. The doctor palpated the arm and checked for tender spots. He asked about any numbness or tingling, touched the arm for hot spots, and looked at the color. He noted that B. A. was extremely tender at the lateral epicondyle but less so in her dorsal forearm. He told her she had epicondylitis and gave her a wrist splint to wear at work. She wore the splint at work for a few days, but it interfered with her cutting. She discarded it and the pain persisted.

She then began to have difficulty doing household chores (e.g., cutting food, opening jars, and lifting her toddler). Keeping up with production at work became more and more difficult. B. A. returned to the doctor, and when asked how things were going, she broke into tears and said that the splint hadn't helped, her pain had increased, and she didn't think she could keep on working. He gave her several days off work. Without the rigorous work demands, the pain decreased. She felt more relaxed and enjoyed the time at home with her children.

When she went back to work, the pain quickly returned. At the doctor's suggestion, her supervisor moved her to a job that required removing duct tape from components that had just been painted. This job also bothered her arm.

She asked to see a doctor of her own choice who specialized in industrial injuries. She explained the problem and how it had developed, adding that she now had a generalized numbness and tingling in her fingers. Tearfully, she requested she be given time off work as it had helped before. The doctor agreed after noting a significant amount of crepitus in the common extensor tendon and suggested that B. A. have an electromyelogram (EMG).

Again, with rest, she improved. Her mother was concerned and sympathetic. She warned her daughter not to let "them" ruin her, as she herself had been ruined.

Over the next 6 months, with intermittent therapy, B. A. was on and off work. She found she could tolerate some light-duty jobs, but her employer insisted that she be able to return to her regular job before they could approve her for another job on a permanent basis. Each time she returned to the cutting job, her pain grew worse. Her EMG results were negative.

At this point, B. A. got angry with her employers, blaming them for what had happened to her. She sought out various specialists, received injections, and went to therapy. Nothing seemed to help the pain. Eventually she had surgery to debride the tendon, but the pain did not subside.

B. A. feels she can never go back to work at the plant because the work increases her pain. The employer sent her for an IME, which showed "no objective findings." Her employer maintains that she can return to work and has cut off her workers' compensation benefits. She has filed a dispute and it will be 6 to 8 months before the matter is legally settled. In the meantime, she is handicapped.

CONCLUSION

Pain is a multifaceted phenomenon with many components. We are still learning much about the way pain works. Its presence, over time, affects sensorimotor, physical, cognitive, and psychological performance, yet often no cause is found. Because chronic pain can affect all aspects of a person's life, it can cause the individual to feel "out of control." Occupational therapists can analyze an individual's deficits in specific performance components and determine how these deficits affect the person's occupational performance. The occupational therapist works with patients to improve occupational performance, giving them back a sense of control over both the pain and their lives.

1. Track the transmission of pain from the point of a noxious stimulus to the final transmission to the frontal cortex.

2. Explain the "gate theory" of pain.

3. Describe the three theories that explain the pathology of chronic pain.

4. Explain the relationship between psychological dysfunction and pain.

5. Discuss the incidence and prevalence of chronic pain in the United States.

6. List the objective signs of chronic pain.

7. What signs are objective but require accurate patient report to be deemed reliable?

8. List the symptoms of chronic pain.

9. Profile the effect of chronic pain on occupational performance.

REFERENCES

1. Collins JG. Pain mechanisms. In: Wu W, ed. Pain Management: Assessment and Treatment of Chronic and Acute Syndromes. New York: Human Sciences Press, 1987:23–43.

2. Iggo A. Physiology of pain. In: Burrows GD, Elton D, Stanley GV, eds. Handbook of Chronic Pain Management. New York: Elsevier, 1987:7–18.

3. Smith GC. The anatomy of pain. In: Burrows GD, Elton D, Stanley GV, eds. Handbook of Chronic Pain Management. New York: Elsevier, 1987:1–5.

4. Fessler RG. Physiology, anatomy and pharmacology of pain perception. In: Camic PM, Brown FD, eds. Assessing Chronic Pain: A Multidisciplinary Clinic Handbook. New York: Springer-Verlag, 1989:5–19.

5. Zohn DA. Musculoskeletal pain, diagnosis and physical treatment. 2nd ed. Boston: Little, Brown and Co., 1988.

6. Melzack R, Wall PD. Pain mechanism: a new theory. Science 1965;150:971–979.

7. Gildenberg PL, DeVaul RA. The Chronic Pain Patient: Evaluation and Management. Pain and Headache, vol. 7. New York: Karger, 1985.

8. Cailliet R. Soft Tissue Pain and Disability. Philadelphia: FA Davis, 1977.

9. Travell JG, Simons DG. Myofascial Pain and Dysfunction: The Trigger Point Manual. Baltimore: Williams & Wilkins, 1983.

10. Benca RM. In: Camic PM, Brown FD, eds. Assessing Chronic Pain: A Multidisciplinary Clinic Handbook. New York: Springer-Verlag, 1989:148–160.

11. Grzesiak RC, Perrine KR. In: Wu W, ed. Pain Management: Assessment and Treatment of Chronic and Acute Syndromes. New York: Human Sciences Press, 1987:44–69.

12. Savitz D. Medical evaluation of the chronic pain patient. In: Aranoff GM, ed. Evaluation and Treatment of Chronic Pain. Baltimore: Urban & Schwarzenberg, 1985:39–60.

13. Bonica JJ. Importance of the problem. In: Aranoff GM, ed. Evaluation and Treatment of Chronic Pain. Baltimore: Urban & Schwarzenberg, 1985:xxxi–xliv.

14. Mushinski M. Average hospital charges for medical and surgical treatment of back problems. United States Statistical Bulletin, vol. 76., no.2, Apr–June 1995.

15. Schneider B. Clinical protocol series for care managers in community based long-term care. Philadelphia Corporation for the Aging, 1995.

16. Morrey B. Departments of Labor, Health and Human Services, Education. Appropriations for 1996 Hearing. GPO: Washington, DC, 1996.

17. Frymoyer JW, Gordon SL. Research perspectives in low-back pain. Spine 1989;14:1384–1388.

18. Mayer TG, Gatchel RJ, Mayer H, et al. A prospective two-year study of functional restoration in industrial low back injury. JAMA 1987;258:1763–1767.

19. VanOort G, Frederick M, Pinto D, et al. Back injuries require integration of aggressive and passive treatment. Occup Health Saf 1990;59(1):22–24.

20. Morris A, Randolph JW. Back rehabilitation programs speed recovery of injured workers. Occup Health Saf 1984;53(7):53–68.

21. Bauer WI. Scope of industrial low back pain. In: Wiesel SW, Feffer HL, Rothman RH, eds. Industrial Low Back Pain: A Comprehensive Approach. Charlottesville, VA: The Michie Co, 1985:1–35.

22. AOTA. Repetitive motion disorders lead to increase in job illness. OT Week, 12-13-90:12.

23. Joyce M. Ergonomics will take center stage during 90s and into the new century. Occup Health Saf 1991;60(1):31–37.

24. Barrer S. Gaining the upper hand on carpal tunnel syndrome. Occup Health Saf 1991;60(1):38–43.

25. Field T. A rise in pain from repetitious work. USA Today, 7-23-90:4D.
26. Gourlay GK, Cousins MJ, Cherry DA. Drug therapy. In: Handbook of Chronic Pain Management. New York: Elsevier, 1987:163–192.
27. Fessler RG. Pharmacologic treatment of chronic pain. In: Camic PM, Brown FD, eds. Assessing Chronic Pain: A Multidisciplinary Clinic Handbook. New York: Springer-Verlag, 1989:115–147.
28. Physicians' Desk Reference. 47th ed. Oradell, NJ: Medical Economics Co., 1993.
29. Sunshine A, Olson NZ. Non-narcotic analgesics. In: Wall PD, Melzack R, eds. Textbook of Pain. New York: Churchill-Livingstone, 1984:670–685.
30. Twycross RG, McQuay HF. Opioids. In: Wall PD, Melzack R, ed. Textbook of Pain. New York: Churchill-Livingstone, 1984:686–701.
31. Monks R, Merskey H. Psychotropic drugs. In: Wall PD, Melzack R, ed. Textbook of Pain. New York: Churchill-Livingstone, 1984:702–721.
32. Thomas CL, ed. Taber's Cyclopedic Medical Dictionary. 17th ed. Philadelphia: FA Davis, 1993.

SUGGESTED READINGS

Cromwell FS, ed. Occupational Therapy and the Patient with Pain. New York: Haworth Press, 1984.
Hadler NM. Medical Management of the Regional Musculoskeletal Diseases. Orlando, FL: Grune & Stratton, 1984.
Hendler NH, Long DM, Wise TM, eds. Diagnosis and Treatment of Chronic Pain. Boston: John Wright-PSG, 1982.
Kirkaldy-Willis WH, ed. Managing Low Back Pain. 2nd ed. New York: Churchill-Livingstone, 1988.
Pawl RP. Chronic Pain Primer. Chicago: Year Book Medical Publishers, 1979.
Philips HC. Psychological Management of Chronic Pain: A Treatment Manual. New York: Springer, 1988.
Sternbach RA, ed. The Psychology of Pain. 2nd ed. New York: Raven Press, 1986.
Wall PD, Melzack R, eds. Textbook of Pain. 2nd ed. New York: Churchill Livingstone, 1989.

CHAPTER 17

DIABETES MELLITUS

Joanne Phillips Estes

Insulin-dependent diabetes mellitus

Non–insulin-dependent diabetes mellitus

Polyuria

Polydipsia

Polyphagia

Hypoglycemia or insulin shock

Hyperglycemia

Diabetic ketoacidosis

Diabetic nephropathy

Diabetic neuropathy

INTRODUCTION

Diabetes mellitus (DM) is a condition marked by a deficiency of, or reduced sensitivity to insulin, a hormone produced by the pancreas, whose purpose is to regulate glucose metabolism. Insulin is required for the cellular uptake of glucose, which is required for energy. Without insulin, liver, muscles, and fat tissues cannot take up absorbed nutrients (1). This ultimately leads the body to use its own fat or lipids as an energy source, which produces toxic acid waste products in the blood called ketones. High concentrations of ketones in the blood are lethal. Until insulin was characterized and manufactured in the 1920s, the diagnosis of diabetes often was a death sentence. Although this is no longer so, diabetes does carry a significant risk for individuals to develop major disabling conditions. In the United States, diabetes is the fourth most common reason for physician visits (2). It also is the leading cause of blindness among working-age people, end-stage renal disease (ESRD), and nontraumatic limb amputation (2). Furthermore, diabetes increases

the risk of cardiac, cerebral, and peripheral vascular disease from twofold to sevenfold (2). Few diseases have the same potential for damaging as many organ systems.

Diabetes is classified as either type I or type II. Type I, formerly known as juvenile-onset diabetes mellitus, is referred to as insulin-dependent diabetes mellitus (IDDM) and occurs predominantly in children. Type II, formerly known as adult-onset diabetes mellitus, is called non–insulin-dependent diabetes mellitus (NIDDM) and occurs primarily in adults.

ETIOLOGY

The exact cause of diabetes is unknown. In patients with type I diabetes, an autoimmune response occurs that produces antibodies against and destroys pancreatic beta cells that produce insulin (2). It is thought to involve some type of genetic predisposition along with an environmentally based inciting event. The inciting event may be an acute illness (2) or virus (3), diet (high in fat or nitrosamines), environmental toxins, or emotional or physical stress (3). The pancreas continues to produce insulin in type II diabetes. However, the amount may not be enough to meet bodily demands (4) or there may be desensitization of insulin receptors (2). Genetic factors are thought to be involved, but little is known about specific genetic abnormalities (2). Obesity also is associated with a risk for developing type II diabetes (3), as at least 85% of type II diabetics are obese (2). Finally, aging (40 and older) is believed to contribute to etiology.

INCIDENCE AND PREVALENCE

Type I diabetes occurs at a rate of 15/100,000 per year (3) and accounts for approximately 10% of all diabetic cases (2). The mean age at onset is 8 to 12 years (3). It occurs equally among males and females; however, the mean onset age is 1.5 years earlier in females (3). Prevalence of type I diabetes is associated with ethnicity. African-Americans and people of Asian descent have the lowest rates (2), whereas Caucasians and people of Finnish, Scandinavian, Scottish, and Sardinian descent have the highest (2). Prevalence rates differ among ethnic groups living in the same geographic region: Caucasian children living in Allegheny, Pennsylvania or Colorado are 50 to 70% more likely to develop type I diabetes than nonwhites living in the same area (2). Genetic factors associated with susceptibility are believed to explain these differences.

Type II diabetes occurs at an incidence of 300/100,000 per year and accounts for 80% of all diabetic cases (3). Among Caucasians it is more prevalent in females than males (3). Its prevalence is 10 to 15% among people older than age 50 (3). Type II diabetes is most prevalent among African-Americans (1.6 times as likely as the general population), Hispanics (twice as likely), and Native Americans (2.7 times as likely) (5). The Pima Indian tribe of Arizona has the highest rate of diabetes in the world: about 50% of Pimas age 35 years or older have diabetes (5).

SIGNS AND SYMPTOMS

The signs and symptoms of type I diabetes are (3):

Polyuria (increased frequency of urination)
Polydipsia (excessive thirst)
Polyphagia (extreme hunger), which is classic but not common
Anorexia that results in a 10 to 30% weight loss
Increased fatigue
Decreased energy
Chest pain and occasional difficulty breathing
Nausea
Muscle cramps
Irritability
Emotional lability
Blurred vision
Altered school and work behaviors
Headaches
Anxiety attacks
Abdominal pain and discomfort
Diarrhea or constipation

Some signs and symptoms of type II diabetes are the same as type I. These are polyuria, polydipsia, polyphagia, unusual weight loss, extreme weakness and fatigue, and irritability. Additional symptoms include frequent skin, gum, or bladder infections, cuts or bruises that are slow to heal, and numbness or tingling in the hands or feet (5). Finally, symptoms related to hyperglycemia and complications can occur (nephropathy, neuropathy, and retinopathy) (5).

COURSE AND PROGNOSIS

After initial diagnosis of type I diabetes, a temporary remission period usually occurs for 3 to 6 months. During this time, overall control of the disease is easier and insulin needs are less. Insulin production gradually regresses until levels are insignificant and a state of total diabetes is reached (3). Longevity and quality of life are currently better than in the past owing to improvements in insulin delivery regimens. Life expectancy is lower overall than for persons who do not have diabetes; however, in the past 20 years, the life expectancy of those with diabetes has increased dramatically (3). Quality of life depends on development of potential complications common to people who have type I diabetes. Whether the vascular and neuropathic complications of diabetes can be prevented or delayed by improved glycemic control has been debated for more than half a century (2). The National Institutes of Health (NIH) recently completed a 9-year study called the "Diabetes Control and Complications Trial" (DCCT). Its purpose was to learn if intensive insulin therapy could prevent diabetic complications or retard progression of mild retinopathy (2). Subjects were divided into intensive insulin and conventional care groups. The conclusion drawn from the results was that glucose control matters (2). The intensive insulin group showed significantly less development of retinopathies and neuropathies. However, it was noted that participants were highly motivated and more compliant than the average person with diabetes, which also may explain the results.

COMPLICATIONS

Following is a description of common complications that may occur during both types I and II diabetes disease processes.

Hypoglycemia or insulin shock is a condition of too much insulin and not enough glucose in the bloodstream (5). This is the most frequent complication of type I diabetes, affecting 10 to 25% of individuals per year (2). Symptoms are vague: fatigue, headache, drowsiness, lassitude, tremulousness, shallow breathing, and nausea (5). It may produce seizures, accidental injury, catecholamine response, or arrhythmia or cardiac ischemia in patients with underlying cardiac disease (2). The patient needs to ingest some form of sugar, such as orange juice, cola, candy, or jelly, if able to swallow. On an emotional level, this could become a great fear of the patient's, leading to less-than-optimal blood sugar control (2).

Hyperglycemia is a condition of too-little insulin causing abnormally high blood glucose levels. Signs are thirst, heartburn, fast and deep breathing, excessive urination, headache, nausea, abdominal pain, blurred vision, and constipation (5). If untreated, the patient is at risk for entering into a diabetic coma. Mortality from hyperglycemia increases with age and is usually caused by the presence of a comorbid condition (myocardial infarction, cerebral vascular accident, sepsis). Treatment depends on insulin to reverse metabolic abnormalities and on detection and successful treatment of the comorbid condition.

Diabetic ketoacidosis (DKA) is an emergency state of metabolic imbalance that usually signals onset of type I diabetes (2). It occurs in patients with established disease because of illness (infection), inappropriate reduction in insulin intake, or missed injection (2). It commonly occurs in patients who are sick and who fail to increase insulin and consume extra fluids accordingly.

Diabetic retinopathy is caused by many physiological changes in the eye (microaneurysm, neurological changes, or vascular leakage). It typically occurs 15 years after onset of diabetes (2). Blindness occurs 20 times more frequently for those with diabetes than in the general population; 10 to 15% of patients with type I diabetes and 5 to 8% of those with type II become legally blind (2). At present, medical therapy is restricted to optimization of glycemic control, which delays and slows progression of nonproliferative retinopathy. Little evidence suggests that improving glycemic control benefits the more advanced stages of retinopathy (2).

Diabetic nephropathy affects 25 to 30% of persons with type I and 15 to 20% of those with type II diabetes. Diabetes is the leading cause of ESRD; one-third of individuals with ESRD have diabetes (2). Gross protein in the urine appears about 15 years after diagnosis of diabetes. Subsequent development of renal failure is highly variable, especially among type II diabetics. Most patients develop ESRD approximately 10 years after creatinine in blood levels begins to rise. Initially, tight control of blood sugar levels and aggressive treatment of hypertension (HTN) may slow progression of renal failure. Once clinical nephropathy is present, blood sugar control is less effective.

People with diabetes tolerate uremia (toxic effects of waste products built up in the blood owing to renal failure) more poorly than those who do not have diabetes. Retinopathy and neuropathies deteriorate more quickly, HTN is more difficult to control, and generalized atherosclerosis increases. Treatment options are dialysis or kidney transplant. Dialysis is either by hemodialysis or continuous ambulatory peritoneal dialysis (CAPD).

Hemodialysis removes waste products from the patient's blood as it circulates through an artificial kidney. This requires the patient to be at a dialysis center and hooked up to a machine two or three times per week for 2 to 4 hours each treatment. Side effects of hemodialysis include weakness, fatigue, nausea, headaches, or hypotension.

Continuous ambulatory peritoneal dialysis is accomplished by infusing dialysis fluid into the abdomen through a catheter where waste products are collected by osmosis. These fluids are drained out to remove waste products from the body and the cycle is repeated. To do this, the patient must have sufficient grip, pinch, and peripheral sensation. Continuous ambulatory peritoneal dialysis patients are at risk for developing peritonitis (abdominal infection) because of the body's direct communication with the external environment. Hemodialysis is the most common intervention for persons with ESRD. However, often it is not tolerated well. Among individuals receiving dialysis, mortality is substantially higher for those with diabetes than for those who do not. This is primarily because of the more-rapid development of vascular insufficiency among persons with diabetes (2).

Diabetic neuropathy at symptomatic, potentially disabling levels affects nearly 50% of those with diabetes (2). Current treatment, which involves control of blood glucose, is primarily effective before clinical symptoms are present. Distal sensorimotor neuropathy is the most common form. Damage is typically more sensory than motor in nature. Symptoms include numbness and tingling in hands and feet, variable loss of distal reflexes, and intrinsic muscle wasting in the hands and feet. Axonal loss encompasses both small (pain and temperature) and large (position and touch) fibers (2). The individual also could develop autonomic neuropathy, which carries a poor prognosis. This may result in abnormal cardiovascular, skin, gastrointestinal, bladder, and sexual functioning. There is no treatment intervention to reverse neuropathies once developed. Pain control, however, is an important part of management.

Diabetic foot is the cause of 50% of nontraumatic limb amputations (2). In this condition, foot ulcers result from insignificant trauma; they heal slowly and may lead to gangrene. Diabetic foot is characterized by:

Chronic sensorimotor neuropathy
Autonomic neuropathy
Poor peripheral circulation
Visual loss that compromises ability to care for feet
Loss of sensation (inability to detect mild trauma)

Treatment aimed at prevention and education can reduce the risk of amputation by 50% (2).

The onset of atherosclerosis is both earlier and more severe for those with diabetes. The major cause of death among diabetics is atherosclerosis of cerebral, cardiac, and peripheral blood vessels (2). Smoking cigarettes compounds this risk.

DIAGNOSIS

Diabetes is diagnosed based on laboratory results of blood tests. Type I diabetes has a sudden or rapid onset. Diagnosis is based on excessive amounts of glucose in the blood and excessive amounts of glucose and ketones in the urine. Often, the first indicator of type I diabetes is DKA. Pathological findings include inflammatory changes in pancreatic tissue (2).

Onset of type II diabetes is more gradual and the patient may have it without being aware. Fasting blood sugar (FBS) levels of less than 140 mg/dL on two separate occasions or random plasma glucose ≥ 200 mg/dL plus presence of classic symptoms (polydipsia, polyuria, polyphagia, weight loss) are indicators of the disease (3).

MEDICAL/SURGICAL MANAGEMENT

Type I Diabetes

There is no known cure for diabetes. The primary focus of treatment is to replace insulin in the body, which is typically accomplished through subcutaneous injection. An alternate method is continuous subcutaneous insulin infusion (CSII), which is an external pump that delivers continuous basal rates of insulin (2). Oral hypoglycemics (to simultaneously lower blood glucose levels) are usually not indicated (3). Immunosuppressants (such as cyclosporine) may be given to reduce the rate of autoimmune destruction of pancreatic cells and must be started in initial weeks after diagnosis is made. (See Appendix II.)

Insulin regimens must be carefully designed and monitored for effectiveness. Commercial preparations differ in amount of time before onset and length of effectiveness (2). Absorption depends on the site of injection. It occurs faster when a) injected into the abdomen than into an extremity and b) injected into an upper extremity than a lower extremity (2). Absorption is accelerated if injection is in an extremity that is either exercised or massaged or warmed. Finally, absorption is faster if injection is deep or intramuscular (2).

The secondary focus of treatment is to make lifestyle changes to facilitate insulin therapy and optimize health (2). Diet must consist of nutritionally sound meals. There must be a careful balance between caloric intake and energy expenditure, adjusting for periods of increased activity by consuming more food (2). Long delays between meals should be avoided, as not eating in a predictable pattern according to insulin regimen may cause hypoglycemia. Frequent small snacks at time of peak insulin action should also be taken to avoid hypoglycemia.

Regular exercise is recommended to enhance general well being and decrease the likelihood of vascular complications. There is little evidence that exercise improves glycemic control for persons with type I diabetes (2). Exercise can, however, enhance insulin sensitivity and decrease overall insulin requirements (2).

Type II Diabetes

Lifestyle changes and dietary control are the key management interventions. Often, metabolic states can be normalized by these alone. Dietary recommendations for management of diabetes are similar to those of the American Heart Association: increased complex carbohydrates, decreased saturated fat, and moderation in salt and alcohol intake.

Regular exercise is recommended as an adjunctive treatment. It can help weight reduction, improve insulin action, and decrease risk of cardiovascular complications. When diet and exercise are ineffective in controlling blood glucose level, oral glucose-lowering agents are indicated. These are used if hyperglycemia is mild, the patient is older, or obesity is pronounced (see Glossary). Individuals with type II diabetes may initially respond to oral hypoglycemics but then not respond well after years of this therapy. This could be the result of decreased compliance with diet and exercise, progression of pancreatic failure to produce insulin, complications from comorbid medical conditions or drugs, or development of tolerance to medication. Insulin therapy is indicated at this point. Insulin is also the first-line intervention for those who are younger, nonobese, severely hypoglycemic, pregnant, or require temporary treatment owing to increased stress (injury, infection, surgery) (2).

Self-monitoring of blood glucose (SMBG) levels is crucial for both type I and type II diabetes. Urine testing is unreliable and should be used when the only goal is prevention of symptomatic hyperglycemia (2). Self monitoring requires that individuals with diabetes take active control of their own health and well-being, allows for more rapid treatment adjustments, and reinforces dietary guidelines.

Portable glucose meters are available that take blood for sampling, give a digital readout of glucose levels, and have a computerized memory for record keeping. People with type I diabetes should monitor glucose levels before each meal and at bedtime (2). People with type II who are insulin dependent should monitor before breakfast, dinner, and bedtime, with the goal of monitoring being to avoid hypoglycemia. Persons with type II who are non-insulin dependent should learn to do SMBG for urgent situations.

Intensive insulin treatment rarely restores glucose homeostasis to levels achieved by those who do not have diabetes (2). In severe cases, and based on availability, a transplant of pancreas insulin-producing tissue is performed. Most patients remain stabilized for many years postoperatively. However, transplantation is an option for only a small group of individuals because of the need for long-term immunosuppression (2). Individuals with type I diabetes who have received a kidney transplant benefit most from pancreas tissue transplantation, as it may be effective in preventing neuropathy of the transplanted kidney.

IMPACT ON OCCUPATIONAL PERFORMANCE

Occupational Performance Areas (Table 17.1)

Function in all performance areas may be impaired. The degree of impairment depends on progression of the disease. Functioning in activities of daily living (ADL) is particularly important in the realm of medication routine, health maintenance, and emergency response. Ineffective performance in these areas can be life threatening to someone with diabetes. Sexual expression is also affected. For males, libido generally is not affected, but 50% are impotent (1) and frequency of activity is diminished. Sexual practices may change due to fatigue, comorbid medical conditions, decreased sensation, and emotional issues (anxiety, fear, guilt, anger, or shame) (1).

There has been little research regarding female sexuality and diabetes (1). Diabetes in childhood may delay development and affect self image. It is thought that libido in adulthood is probably about the same as for the general female population. Fertility is slightly subnormal (1). Careful blood sugar control is essential before and during pregnancy to reduce the risk of birth defects associated with diabetic complications (1). The chances of live birth are decreased (1).

Occupational Performance Components

Complications during the course of the disease have the potential to impair function in all three performance components areas. The degree of impairment may range from minimal impact (and having little influence on performance area abilities) to very severe and extremely debilitating. The course is variable for each individual and depends only in part on patient compliance and successful self-management. Often medical intervention can do little to slow or prevent these impairments.

The sensorimotor component is primarily influenced by development of peripheral neuropathies and retinopathy. Diabetic retinopathy can lead to varying degrees of visual processing deficits and, ultimately, blindness. Peripheral neuropathies may result in diminished to absent tactile processing. This, in turn, may result in impaired fine and gross motor coordination and muscle atrophy and diminished strength and range of motion (especially distally). Finally, distal soft tissue integrity is threatened by diminished vascularization.

Insulin and blood glucose levels influence both endurance and level of arousal. Fatigue is a symptom of diabetes and must be managed throughout the course of the disease. Hypoglycemia also leads to fatigue. Hyperglycemia can lead to coma if not treated.

Perhaps the biggest impact is made in psychosocial skills and psychological components.

TABLE 17.1 Occupational Performance Categories

I. PERFORMANCE AREAS

A. Activities of Daily Living
  1. Grooming
  2. Oral Hygiene
  3. Bathing/Showering
  4. Toilet Hygiene
  5. Personal Device Care
  6. Dressing
  7. Feeding and Eating
  8. Medication Routine
  9. Health Maintenance
  10. Socialization
  11. Functional Communication
  12. Functional Mobility
  13. Community Mobility
  14. Emergency Response
  15. Sexual Expression
B. Work and Productive Activities
  1. Home Management
    a. Clothing Care
    b. Cleaning
    c. Meal Preparation/Cleanup
    d. Shopping
    e. Money Management
    f. Household Maintenance
    g. Safety Procedures
  2. Care of Others
  3. Educational Activities
  4. Vocational Activities
    a. Vocational Exploration
    b. Job Acquisition
    c. Work or Job
       Performance
    d. Retirement Planning
    e. Volunteer Participation
C. Play or Leisure Activities
  1. Play or Leisure Exploration
  2. Play or Leisure
     Performance

II. PERFORMANCE COMPONENTS

A. Sensorimotor Component
  1. Sensory
    a. Sensory Awareness
    b. Sensory Processing
      (1) Tactile
      (2) Proprioceptive
      (3) Vestibular
      (4) Visual
      (5) Auditory
      (6) Gustatory
      (7) Olfactory
    c. Perceptual Processing
      (1) Stereognosis
      (2) Kinesthesia
      (3) Pain Response
      (4) Body Scheme
      (5) Right–Left Discrimination
      (6) Form Constancy
      (7) Position in Space
      (8) Visual–Closure
      (9) Figure Ground
      (10) Depth Perception
      (11) Spatial Relations
      (12) Topographical Orientation
  2. Neuromusculoskeletal
    a. Reflex
    b. Range of Motion
    c. Muscle Tone
    d. Strength
    e. Endurance
    f. Postural Control
    g. Postural Alignment
    h. Soft Tissue Integrity
  3. Motor
    a. Gross Coordination
    b. Crossing the Midline
    c. Laterality
    d. Bilateral Integration
    e. Motor Control
    f. Praxis
    g. Fine Coordination/Dexterity
    h. Visual–Motor Control
    i. Oral–Motor Control

III. PERFORMANCE CONTEXTS

A. Temporal Aspects
  1. Chronological
  2. Developmental
  3. Lifecycle
  4. Disability Status
B. Environment
  1. Physical
  2. Social
  3. Cultural

(continued)

TABLE 17.1   Occupational Performance Profile   (Continued)

I. PERFORMANCE AREAS	II. PERFORMANCE COMPONENTS	III. PERFORMANCE CONTEXTS
	B. Cognitive Integration and Cognitive Components 　1. Level of Arousal 　2. Orientation 　3. Recognition 　4. Attention Span 　5. Initiation of Activity 　6. Termination of Activity 　7. Memory 　8. Sequencing 　9. Categorization 　10. Concept Formation 　11. Spatial Operations 　12. Problem Solving 　13. Learning 　14. Generalization C. Psychosocial Skills and Psychological Components 　**1. Psychological** 　　a. Values 　　**b. Interests** 　　c. Self-Concept 　**2. Social** 　　**a. Role Performance** 　　**b. Social Conduct** 　　**c. Interpersonal Skills** 　　**d. Self-Expression** 　3. Self-Management 　　a. Coping Skills 　　b. Time Management 　　c. Self-Control	

Time management and self control are important for most people but for individuals with diabetes they can mean life or death. A person with diabetes also may need to cope with having an invisible disability. To others, their strict dietary and medication regimens may appear hypochondriacal in nature. Variations in blood glucose levels can cause mood swings (depression, irritability) (4). Often, there is anger and frustration over lifestyle and body image changes. Finally, they must adjust to progressive impairment and feelings of lack of control over one's health and well-being.

Occupational Performance Contexts

Temporal aspects are at high risk to be affected. The disease can strike from childhood through adulthood. It can interfere with successful completion of developmental or lifecycle phases. Finally, many people with diabetes experience the entire continuum of disability status. The physical environment can present barriers to access in cases of extreme debilitation caused by the disease. His or her social environment can significantly facilitate or impede quality of life for a person living with diabetes. Cultural influences or beliefs also may influence acceptance of the disease and compliance with strict lifestyle changes that are required for successful management of this condition.

CASE STUDIES

CASE 1

Mrs. D. is a 44-year-old Caucasian female with a diagnosis of type I diabetes mellitus. Onset of her disease was at the age of 12 years. Mrs. D's. medical history includes diagnoses for HTN 5 years ago and diabetic retinopathy 10 years ago. She has had peripheral neuropathies in four extremities for 7 years. She has ESRD and is receiving hemodialysis three times a week, as she has been for 2.5 years. She will be undergoing bilateral nephrectomies in 1 week because of her history of chronic pyelonephritis (infected kidneys). She has been on a list for a kidney–pancreas transplantation for 2 years.

Mrs. D's medication routine is extensive. She takes 20 units of Humulin N subcutaneously twice a day (insulin); Catapres TTS #3 change weekly (once per week blood pressure patch); one nephrocap by mouth each day (multivitamin); 325 mg of ferrous sulfate twice a day for anemia; three 667 mg Phoslo tablets by mouth three times a day with meals (calcium binds phosphorus with foods eaten to prevent phosphorus from going into the body; normal kidneys eliminate extra phosphorus in body; secondary hyperparathyroidism can occur); Kayexalate 1 T in diet 7 UP by mouth daily (binds potassium so it can be eliminated with bowel movement); and 100 mg of Colace orally each day for constipation.

Mrs. D. has been married to a veterinarian for 19 years. They have two daughters, ages 12 and 14. She has a bachelor of arts degree in education and worked as an elementary school teacher for 4 years before having children. She has been a full-time homemaker and mother since then. Her hobbies include travel, gardening, and listening to recorded books.

Mrs. D. is right-hand dominant and receives dialysis through her left upper extremity (LUE). She has pain and numbness in her LUE because of an ischemic neuropathy that is the result of decreased blood flow because blood is diverted to her dialysis access site. She is legally blind as

a result of diabetic retinopathy. She has full bilateral UE active range of motion but decreased peripheral sensation (tactile, pain, and temperature). Mrs. D. recently stepped on a tack, did not feel it, and subsequently developed an infection that has been slow to heal. A moderate decrease in bilateral grip and pinch strength has been noted, with her left side weaker than her right. Her physician notes chronic flat affect that may be an indication of mild depression. She communicates little information to the physician during hemodialysis visits.

Transportation services bring her to and from dialysis, as blindness prevents driving. She ambulates independently with guidance owing to her decreased vision. Mrs. D. is independent in all transfers, feeding, dressing, bathing, and hygiene. Her laboratory results show poor compliance with fluid restriction (1800 cc fluid/day) and noncompliance with dietary restrictions. Her husband contacted the physician with concerns about her lack of interest in caring for their daughters, in gardening, and in sexual activity. Her husband seems supportive but notes recent marital tensions.

Mrs. D. is moderately disabled by the physical and emotional ramifications of diabetes, retinopathy, neuropathies, and renal failure. This is affecting her role of wife and mother. Her physical environment must be adapted to accommodate her disabilities. Socially, she is becoming withdrawn. The context of her occupational performance further reflects the impact that diabetes has on decreasing the quality of her life.

CASE 2 (TABLE 17.2)

S. is a 9-year-old boy who attends third grade at the local public school. He is the middle child, having an older brother and younger sister, and lives with both parents. S. is an extremely bright and athletic child. He enjoys playing sports and is especially competitive with his older brother. He has several good friends and typically enjoys spending time with them and his siblings.

He was in good health until 8 months ago when his parents found him in bed, lethargic, confused, weak, complaining of being very thirsty and cold, and vomiting. They also noticed that his breath was "sweet-smelling." After ambulance transportation to the local emergency room, S. was diagnosed as being in a state of DKA and having type I diabetes. Initially, management of his disease was easy. His parents monitored blood glucose levels four times per day and little insulin was

TABLE 17.2 Occupational Performance Categories

I. PERFORMANCE AREAS	II. PERFORMANCE COMPONENTS	III. PERFORMANCE CONTEXTS

A. Activities of Daily Living
  1. Grooming
  2. Oral Hygiene
  3. Bathing/Showering
  4. Toilet Hygiene
  5. Personal Device Care
  6. Dressing
  7. Feeding and Eating
  8. Medication Routine
  9. Health Maintenance
  10. Socialization
  11. Functional Communication
  12. Functional Mobility
  13. Community Mobility
  14. Emergency Response
  15. Sexual Expression
B. Work and Productive Activities
  1. Home Management
    a. Clothing Care
    b. Cleaning
    c. Meal Preparation/
      Cleanup
    d. Shopping
    e. Money Management
    f. Household Maintenance
    g. Safety Procedures
  2. Care of Others
  3. Educational Activities
  4. Vocational Activities
    a. Vocational Exploration
    b. Job Acquisition
    c. Work or Job
      Performance
    d. Retirement Planning
    e. Volunteer Participation
C. Play or Leisure Activities
  1. Play or Leisure Exploration
  **2. Play or Leisure
    Performance**
	A. Sensorimotor Component
	  1. Sensory
	    a. Sensory Awareness
	    b. Sensory Processing
	      (1) Tactile
	      (2) Proprioceptive
	      (3) Vestibular
	      (4) Visual
	      (5) Auditory
	      (6) Gustatory
	      (7) Olfactory
	    c. Perceptual Processing
	      (1) Stereognosis
	      (2) Kinesthesia
	      (3) Pain Response
	      (4) Body Scheme
	      (5) Right–Left Discrimination
	      (6) Form Constancy
	      (7) Position in Space
	      (8) Visual–Closure
	      (9) Figure Ground
	      (10) Depth Perception
	      (11) Spatial Relations
	      (12) Topographical Orientation
	  2. Neuromusculoskeletal
	    a. Reflex
	    b. Range of Motion
	    c. Muscle Tone
	    d. Strength
	    e. Endurance
	    f. Postural Control
	    g. Postural Alignment
	    h. Soft Tissue Integrity
	  3. Motor
	    a. Gross Coordination
	    b. Crossing the Midline
	    c. Laterality
	    d. Bilateral Integration
	    e. Motor Control
	    f. Praxis
	    g. Fine Coordination/Dexterity
	    h. Visual–Motor Control
	    i. Oral–Motor Control
		A. Temporal Aspects
		  1. Chronological
		  2. Developmental
		  3. Lifecycle
		  4. Disability Status
		B. Environment
		  1. Physical
		  2. Social
		  3. Cultural

(continued)

TABLE 17.2 Occupational Performance Categories (Continued)		
I. PERFORMANCE AREAS	**II. PERFORMANCE COMPONENTS**	**III. PERFORMANCE CONTEXTS**
	B. Cognitive Integration and Cognitive Components	
	1. Level of Arousal	
	2. Orientation	
	3. Recognition	
	4. Attention Span	
	5. Initiation of Activity	
	6. Termination of Activity	
	7. Memory	
	8. Sequencing	
	9. Categorization	
	10. Concept Formation	
	11. Spatial Operations	
	12. Problem Solving	
	13. Learning	
	14. Generalization	
	C. Psychosocial Skills and Psychological Components	
	1. Psychological	
	a. Values	
	b. Interests	
	c. Self-Concept	
	2. Social	
	a. Role Performance	
	b. Social Conduct	
	c. Interpersonal Skills	
	d. Self-Expression	
	3. Self-Management	
	a. Coping Skills	
	b. Time Management	
	c. Self-Control	

needed for control. After this "honeymoon period" ended, S.'s blood glucose levels became more difficult to manage.

S. says he's embarrassed and does not want his friends to know that he has diabetes. Subsequently, he often does not follow dietary restrictions. He becomes irritable and combative with his parents regarding SMBG and insulin injections. He avoids socializing with friends and his teachers report a significant decline in his academic performance. S. refuses to do homework and spends most of his time alone in his bedroom. He often says that he doesn't care what could happen to him if he doesn't follow dietary and medication requirements.

Sensorimotor and cognitive components are currently intact except level of arousal. As his glucose levels fluctuate, S. becomes drowsy and fatigued. This often occurs during school, when he lays his head on his desk and sleeps. These fluctuations obviously impair his ability to learn.

At this point, psychosocial skills and psychological component functioning are challenged. S. is having difficulty adjusting to the fact that he is "different" from his friends and often refuses to follow dietary restrictions in their presence. Recently he refused to attend his best friend's birthday party because he could not have the cake, ice cream, and candy the other kids would be enjoying. S.'s mother notes increased arguing and fighting between S. and his siblings and friends.

S.'s mother also is having difficulty coping with her son's diagnosis because her father died of complications from diabetes when she was 14. She is distressed that S. is not enjoying his friends and school like a "typical" 9-year-old boy would. She is also concerned that his physical, social, emotional, and intellectual development will lag because of his diabetes. S.'s father is spending more time at work than he used to. There are many extended family members living in the area who have voiced concern and support.

POINTS FOR REVIEW

1. Give a brief definition of diabetes.

2. What are the differences between type I and type II diabetes?

3. What causes hypoglycemia and hyperglycemia?

4. What are the differences in symptoms between type I and type II diabetes?

REFERENCES

1. Tilton M. Diabetes and amputation. In: Sipski M, Alexander C, eds. Sexual Function in People with Disability and Chronic Illness: A Health Professional's Guide. Gaithersburg, MD: Aspen, Inc. 1997;279–302.

2. Sherwin R. Endocrine and reproductive diseases. In: Bennett J, Plumb F, eds. Cecil Textbook of Medicine, vol. 2. 20th ed. Philadelphia: WB Saunders, 1996:1258–1277.

3. Dambro M. Griffith's Five Minute Clinical Consult. Baltimore: Williams & Wilkins, 1995:306–311.

4. Daniel M, Strickland R. Occupational Therapy Management in Adult Physical Dysfunction. Gaithersburg, MD: ASPEN, Inc. 1992:253–261.

5. American Diabetes Association. Diabetes Facts and Figures, copyright 1995. http://www.diabetes.org/ada/c20f.asp

GLOSSARY

Affect: The external expression of emotional content.

Affective disorders: A term sometimes used in place of *mood disorders.*

Afferent: In the nervous system, a nerve that transmits impulses from the periphery toward the central nervous system (sensory).

Agnosia: Inability to recognize the import of sensory impressions despite being able to recognize the elemental sensation of a stimulus. Language deficits must be absent for this diagnosis; the varieties correspond to several senses and are distinguished as auditory (acoustic), gustatory, olfactory, tactile, and visual. Specific sensory agnosias can occur when the connections are interrupted between the primary cortical receptor region for a stimulus and the memory of that abstraction (parietal lobe damage). An example is the incapacity to identify a familiar face despite seeing the face.

> Visual agnosia: Inability to recognize familiar objects by sight.
>
> Tactile agnosia (astereognosis): Inability to recognize objects by touch.

Agranulocytosis: A majority of cases are caused by sensitization to drugs or chemicals that affect the bone marrow, leading to a marked decrease of granular leukocytes (e.g., leukopenia often leading to an increased susceptibility to bacterial and fungal infections). Manifestations are high fever, chills, prostration, and ulceration of mucous membranes.

Akathisia: A condition marked by motor restlessness and anxiety (considered an extrapyramidal symptom and a common side effect of neuroleptic drugs). Individuals with this disorder feel quivering of muscles, an urge to move about constantly, and an inability to sit still.

Akinesia: The absence of movement.

Allograft (homograft): A graft of tissue harvested from an individual other than the recipient. It is most often taken from a cadaver.

Alogia: A decrease in speech fluency caused by a mental deficiency or an episode of dementia.

Alzheimer's disease: A primary degenerative dementia (PDD) of the Alzheimer type characterized by a loss of cognitive and intellectual abilities severe enough to impair social or occupational performance. The full clinical picture consists of impaired memory, abstract thinking, and judgment, with some degree of personality change.

Amnesia: Pathological impairment of memory usually resulting from physical damage to areas of the brain caused by injury, disease, or alcoholism.

> Anterograde amnesia: Inability to learn new material in an individual demonstrating a normal state of consciousness; a short-term memory deficit.
>
> Posttraumatic amnesia: Amnesia resulting from concussion or other head trauma.

Retrograde amnesia: Inability to recall material that was well known in the past; a long-term memory deficit. Also refers to memory loss for events immediately prior to injury.

ANA: See Antinuclear antibodies

Analgesic: Medication or modality used to relieve pain.

Anastomosis: Surgical, traumatic, or pathological formation of a connection between two normally distinct structures.

Anemia: A reduction below normal in the number of erythrocytes or quantity of hemoglobin in the blood. Anemia is not a disease but a symptom of a number of different disorders that upset the balance between blood loss through bleeding or destruction of blood cells and blood production in the bone marrow.

Aneurysm: A sac formed by the localized dilation of the wall of an artery, vein, or the heart; an actual bulging or outpouching of the weakened wall of the artery is evident. The chief sign of an arterial aneurysm is the formation of a pulsating tumor and often a bruit heard over the swelling. A true aneurysm results from sac formation by the arterial wall with at least one unbroken layer; it is most often associated with atherosclerosis. A false aneurysm usually is caused by trauma when the wall of the blood vessel is ruptured and blood escapes into surrounding tissues and forms a clot. Aneurysms tend to increase in size, presenting a problem of increasing pressure against adjacent tissues and organs and a danger of rupture. Atherosclerosis is responsible for most arterial aneurysms, although any injury to the middle or muscular layer of the arterial wall (tunica media) can predispose the vessel to stretching of the inner and outer layers of the artery and the formation of a sac. Other diseases that can lead to aneurysm include syphilis, cystic medionecrosis, certain nonspecific inflammations, and congenital defects.

Angina pectoris: Acute pain in the chest resulting from decreased blood supply to the heart muscle (myocardial ischemia). The disorder is sometimes called cardiac pain of effort and emotion because the pain is brought on by physical activity or emotional stress that places an added burden on the heart and increases the need for additional blood supply to the myocardium.

Anhedonia: Inability to experience or find pleasure.

Ankylosis: Immobility and consolidation of a joint because of disease, injury, or a surgical procedure. In arthritis, there is destruction of articular cartilage, allowing bony surfaces to fuse.

Bony ankylosis: Union of the bones of a joint by proliferation of bone cells, resulting in complete immobility.

Fibrous ankylosis: Reduced joint mobility as a result of a proliferation of fibrous tissue. Also called false ankylosis.

Anomalous: Irregular; deviating from or contrary to normal.

Anomaly: Marked deviation from normal.

Anomia: Loss of the ability to name objects or recognize/recall names; may be both receptive and expressive.

Anoxia: Absence of oxygen to the body tissues, to be differentiated from hypoxia.

Antiadrenergic: In the sympathetic nervous system, nerve impulses from ganglia—usually transmitted to organs or tissues—are blocked, inhibiting smooth muscle contraction and glandular secretion. Some medications produce this effect.

Antibodies: Special proteins produced by the body (plasma cells) in response to infectious agents or other foreign matter (antigens). Antibodies are immunoglobulin molecules having a specific amino acid sequence that gives each antibody the ability to adhere to and interact only with the antigen that induced its synthesis, thereby neutralizing or facilitating the destruction of the antigen.

Anticholinergic: Blocking the passage of impulses through the parasympathetic nerves (parasympatholytic).

Antidepressant: A drug used for relief of symptoms of depression.

Antigen: A foreign protein or protein polysaccharide complex that stimulates a specific immune response.

Antinuclear antibodies (ANA): A group of abnormal antibodies found in most people with systemic lupus erythematosus, Sjögren's syndrome, and scleroderma. Also found in juvenile and rheumatoid arthritis cases. ANAs are autoantibodies directed against components of the cell nucleus (e.g., DNA, RNA, and histones).

Antipsychotic drugs: Drugs that exert an antianxiety effect by blocking the dopamine receptor (except for clozapine).

Apathy: Dulled emotional tone associated with detachment or indifference.

Aphasia: A defect or loss of the power of expression by speech, writing, or signs (e.g., gestures) or of comprehension of spoken or written languages as a result of disease or injury of the brain centers.

Broca's aphasia: Expressive aphasia in which an individual understands written and spoken words and knows what he or she wants to say, but speech production is limited or absent, usually as a result of damage to the left inferior frontal lobe. Also called apraxia of speech, motor aphasia, and nonfluent aphasia.

Conduction dysphasia: Impairment of speech consisting of a lack of coordination and the failure to arrange words in their proper order, possibly caused by a lesion of the pathway between the sensory and motor speech centers (arcuate fasciculus).

Wernicke's aphasia: Receptive aphasia in which an individual is unable to understand written, spoken, or tactile speech symbols, usually as a result of damage to the left superior temporal gyrus (also called sensory aphasia).

Global aphasia: Both expressive and receptive deficits, usually caused by an occlusion of the internal carotid or middle cerebral artery.

Apophyseal: Pertaining to any outgrowth or swelling, especially a bony outgrowth that has never been entirely separated from the bone of which it forms a part, such as a process, tubercle, or tuberosity.

Apoplexy: Copious extravasation of blood into an organ; often used alone to designate extravasations into the brain (cerebral apoplexy) after rupture of an intracranial blood vessel. Synonymous with stroke, the term is extended by some to include occlusive cerebrovascular lesions.

Apraxia: A disorder of skilled purposeful movement that is caused by neither deficits in primary motor skills nor comprehension problems. It can affect the praxis components of ideation and concept formation as well as programming and planning of movement. Disturbances of motor execution, on the contrary, are usually related to primary motor skills.

Motor apraxia: Loss of the ability to make proper use of an object, although its proper nature is recognized.

Sensory apraxia: Loss of ability as a result of a lack of perception of an object's purpose.

Arcuate fasciculus: The bundle of fibers in the brain that connect Wernicke's area to Broca's area. The pattern of normal speech starts with the selection of desired words and their sequence in Wernicke's area. This information is transferred through the arcuate fasciculus to Broca's area, where a detailed and coordinated program for expression of language is created. Finally, the information is passed on to the motor cortex, and language is either spoken or written.

Areflexia: Absence of reflexes.

Arrhythmia: Variation from the normal rhythm, especially of the heartbeat.

Arteriosclerosis: A group of diseases characterized by thickening and loss of elasticity of the arterial walls; popularly called "hardening of the arteries."

Arteriovenous: Pertaining to both artery and vein.

Arteriovenous malformation: A congenital malformation in which there is an abnormal collection of blood vessels near the surface of the brain that can cause a subarachnoid hemorrhage.

Arteritis: Inflammation of an artery.

Arthralgia: Pain in a joint.

Arthritis: Inflammation of a joint. Arthritis and rheumatic diseases in general constitute the major cause of chronic disability in the United States, with osteoarthritis and rheumatoid arthritis as the most common forms.

Arthrodesis: Surgical procedure designed to produce fusion to a joint.

Asphyxia: Condition caused by an insufficient intake of oxygen.

Aspiration: The act of inhaling or withdrawing fluid by a method of suction. Pathological inhalation of mucus into the respiratory tract can occur when an individual is unconscious or under the effects of general anesthesia.

Associated reactions: Involuntary movements or reflexive increases of tone of the affected side in individuals with hemiplegia; movements duplicate synergy patterns and are often seen during stressful or new activities. For example, resisted grasp by the noninvolved hand causes a grasp reaction in the involved hand.

Astereognosis: Inability to recognize objects by touch (also called tactile agnosia; see Agnosia).

Ataxia: Inability to coordinate muscle activity during voluntary movement. In posterior column damage of the spinal cord, incoordination and a loss of proprioception is caused by misjudgment of limb position with balance problems. Cerebellar ataxia produces a reeling, wide-based gait.

Atheroma: An abnormal mass of fatty or lipid material with a fibrous covering, existing as a discrete, raised plaque within the intima of an artery.

Atherosclerosis: An extremely common form of arteriosclerosis in which deposits of yellowing plaques (atheromas) containing cholesterol, other lipoid material, and lipophages are formed within the inner layer (intima) of large- and medium-sized arteries.

Athetoid: Resembling athetosis or repetitive involuntary, slow, sinuous, writhing movements. Classification of cerebral palsy in which involuntary purposeless movement occurs when an individual attempts purposeful motion. The abnormal movements may not only occur in the limb being moved but also involve an "overflow" of activity to all the other limbs with an exaggeration of reflexes.

Athetosis: A condition characterized by slow, writhing, involuntary movements; usually caused by an extrapyramidal lesion.

Atonia: The absence or lack of normal muscle tone.

Atrophy: A wasting away or diminution in the size of a cell, tissue organ, or part.

Auscultation: Listening for sounds produced within the body, chiefly to ascertain the condition of thoracic or abdominal viscera.

Autograft: A graft of tissue harvested from the same individual who is also the recipient. It is taken from a site other than the burn wound.

Autoimmune disease: A disease in which the immune system malfunctions and attacks tissues of the body, causing tissue injury and inflammation.

Autonomic dysreflexia (hyperreflexia): An uninhibited and exaggerated reflex of the autonomic nervous system to stimulation. The response occurs in about 85% of all patients who have spinal cord injury above the level of the 6th thoracic vertebra. It is potentially dangerous because of attendant vasoconstriction and immediate elevation of blood pressure, which in turn can bring about hemorrhagic retinal damage or cerebrovascular accident. Less serious effects include severe headache, changes in heart rate, sweating and flushing above the level of the spinal cord injury, and pallor and "goose bumps" below that level.

Autorelease: The spontaneous tearing of tissue. It is usually caused by an outside applied force.

Avoidant disorder: Characterized by an excessive fear of contact with unfamiliar people that leads to social isolation.

Avolition: Lack of will and purposeful activity.

B cells: Lymphocytes capable of becoming antibody-secreting plasma cells.

Baker's cyst: Cystic swelling behind the knee in the popliteal fossa.

Benign: Not malignant; not recurrent; favorable for recovery.

Binding cleft: A biochemical term describing the cleft area of the human leukocyte antigen molecule that appears to determine whether an antibody will react (bind) with an antigen.

Biologic dressing: Biologic tissue used to cover a burn wound.

Blunt affect: Lack of emotional expression, affective flattening.

Boutonnière deformity: A finger deformity in which flexion of the proximal interphalangeal joint and hyperextension of the distal interphalangeal joint occurs.

Bradycardia: Slowness of the heartbeat, as evidenced by slowing of the pulse rate to less than 60 beats per minute.

Bradykinesia: Abnormally slow and sluggish movement.

Bronchospasm: Bronchial spasm; spasmodic contraction of the muscular coat of the smaller divisions of the bronchi, such as occurs in asthma.

Bruit: An abnormal sound or murmur heard in auscultation. When a stethoscope is placed over an artery, a slushing noise indicative of turbulent blood flow may indicate a significant degree of stenosis.

Aneurysmal bruit: A blowing sound heard over an aneurysm.

Asymptomatic carotid bruit: A bruit heard over the carotid artery.

Bunion: Hallux valgus with a painful bursitis over the medial aspect of the first metatarsophalangeal joint.

Bursa: A small sac (like a water balloon) that is not part of the joint but is located around the joints where tendons, ligaments, and bone rub against each other. Bursae contain a fluid that lubricates the movement of muscles and are similar to synovial sacs. There are more than 140 bursae located throughout the body.

Bursitis: Inflammation of a bursa that can be the result of frictional forces, trauma, or rheumatoid diseases.

CABG: See Coronary artery bypass grafting.

Callositas (callosity):   Circumscribed thickening and hypertrophy of the horny layer of the skin. Usually appears on the flexor surfaces of hands and feet and is caused by friction, pressure, or other irritation.

CAPD: See Continuous ambulatory peritoneal dialysis.

Capsule: A band of cartilaginous, fatty, fibrous, membranous tissue enveloping a joint.

Articular capsule: A saclike envelope enclosing the cavity of a synovial joint.

Carpal tunnel syndrome: Compression of the median nerve in the carpal tunnel of the wrist, causing atrophy in the thenar area and paralysis as well as trophic changes of the fingertips and sensory deficits of the first three fingers.

Cartilage: A specialized, fibrous connective tissue that covers the ends of bones to help them glide smoothly and absorbs shock to a joint by acting as a "sponge" to release and reabsorb.

Catalepsy: Diminished responsiveness as in a trance; the limbs remain immobile.

Catheterization: Passage of a catheter into a body channel or cavity, especially introduction of a catheter via the urethra into the urinary bladder.

Cauda equina: The collection of dorsal and ventral nerve roots descending from the lower spinal cord and occupying the vertebral canal below the cord at the L1 region.

CBC: See Complete blood count.

Cellulitis: Inflammation of cells usually caused by an infection. It is characterized by redness, tenderness, and warmth of the tissue.

Cephalohematoma: A swelling or mass of blood on the head caused by a break in a blood vessel.

Cerebral vascular accident (stroke) (CVA): A disorder of the blood vessels serving the cerebrum, resulting from impaired blood supply to and ischemia in parts of the brain. Four neurologic events are associated with a cerebral vascular accident: (*a*) transient ischemic attack (TIA) caused by a temporary interference in blood supply and lasts only a few minutes and no longer than 24 hours; (*b*) small strokes that last a day or longer and completely resolve or leave only minor neurological deficits. Reversible ischemic neurologic deficits (RIND) are small strokes that resolve completely. Partially reversible ischemic neurologic deficits (PRIND) are small strokes lasting longer than 72 hours, with resultant minor neurological impairment; (*c*) stroke in evolution (SIE), in which an individual experiences gradual weakness on one side of the body; (*d*) completed stroke (CS), in which an individual exhibits symptoms associated with severe cerebral ischemia resulting from an interrupted blood supply to the brain.

Cholinergic: Stimulated, activated, or transmitted by choline (acetylcholine), a neurotransmitter; a term applied to those nerve fibers that liberate acetylcholine at the synapse when a nerve impulse passes, such as at the parasympathetic nerve endings.

Chorioamnionitis: Inflammation of the membranes covering the fetus.

Chronic obstructive pulmonary disease (COPD): Generalized airway obstruction, particularly of the small airways, associated with varying combinations of chronic bronchitis, asthma, and emphysema. The term COPD was introduced because these conditions often coexist and it may be difficult to decide which is the major one producing the obstruction.

Circle of Willis: The union of the anterior and posterior circulation at the base of the brain, often providing a back-up supply of blood in case of occlusion of one of the larger arteries.

Circumlocution: An indirect or lengthy way of expressing something; speaking in a roundabout way, never getting to the point during conversation.

Clonus: Alternate involuntary muscular contraction and relaxation in rapid succession.

CMV: See Cytomegalovirus.

Cock-up toe: Deformity with dorsiflexion of the metatarsophalangeal joint and flexion of the interphalangeal/distal interphalangeal joint.

Cognition: A conscious thought process that refers to awareness and knowledge of objects, perceptions, thoughts, and memories. In addition to knowledge, it includes the abilities to understand, reason, make decisions, and apply judgment.

Cogwheel rigidity: Tension in a muscle that gives way in little jerks when the muscle is passively stretched.

Collagen: A basic structural fibrous protein found in all tissues. It is the greatest fibrous component of skin and scar tissue.

Collateral circulation: Secondary or accessory circulation that continues to an area of the brain following obstruction of a primary vessel and which can prevent major ischemia.

Coma: A state of unconsciousness from which the patient cannot be aroused, even by powerful stimuli.

Complete blood count (CBC): Diagnostic test showing the number of different cellular components of the blood, such as white blood cells, red blood cells, and platelets.

Completed stroke (CS): When an individual exhibits symptoms associated with severe cerebral ischemia resulting from an interrupted blood supply to the brain (see Cerebral vascular accident).

Computerized or computed tomography (CT): Tomography in which transverse planes of tissue are swept by a pinpoint radiographic beam, and a computerized analysis of the variance in absorption then produces a precise reconstructed image of that area. This technique has a greater sensitivity in showing the relationship of structures than does conventional radiography and has been used most successfully in diagnostic studies of the brain.

Conduction: Conveyance of energy, as of heat, sound, or electricity.

Conductive: Defects in the auditory system that interfere with sound waves reaching the cochlea. The locus of the lesion is usually in the outer or middle ear (e.g., external auditory meatus, tympanic membrane, auditory [eustachian] tube, auditory ossicles).

Confabulation (fabrication or fabulation): Unconscious filling in of gaps in memory with fabricated facts and experiences, commonly seen in organic amnestic syndromes. It differs from lying in that the individual has no intention to deceive and believes the fabricated memories to be real.

Constructional apraxia: A failure to produce or replicate a specific design or object from parts in two or three dimensions, either drawings or block designs. The failure may manifest spontaneously, on command, or by copying.

Continuous ambulatory peritoneal dialysis (CAPD): An alternative to hemodialysis for removing waste products from the body; solution is intermittently introduced into and removed from the abdomen, where the transfer of diffusible solutes and water occurs.

Contracture: Abnormal shortening of muscle tissue that renders the muscle highly resistant to stretching, which can lead to permanent disability. In many cases, contractures can be prevented by range-of-motion exercises (active or passive) and by adequate support of the joints to eliminate constant shortening or stretching of the muscles and surrounding tissue.

Contralateral: Pertaining to, situated on, or affecting the opposite side.

Convergence: The coordinated inclination of the two lines of sight toward their common point of fixation, or the point itself.

COPD: See Chronic obstructive pulmonary disease.

Coronary artery bypass grafting: A surgical procedure in which a section of vein from another part of the body is excised and grafted in the heart to replace an occluded artery.

Corpus striatum: A subcortical mass of gray and white substance in front of and lateral to the thalamus in each cerebral hemisphere.

Corticospinal pathways: The group of nerve cells connecting the cerebral cortex and the spinal cord.

Craniostenosis: Premature closure of cranial sutures resulting in malformation of the skull.

Creatinine: The waste product of the metabolism of phosphocreatine (a source of energy for muscle contraction); unusually large amounts appear in blood in advanced renal disease.

Crede's method: Use of manual pressure on the bladder to express urine, particularly in bladder training for individuals with paralysis. The hands are held flat against the abdomen, just below the umbilicus. A firm downward stroke toward the bladder is repeated six or seven times, followed by pressure from both hands placed directly over the bladder to manually remove all urine.

Crepitation: A dry, crackling sound or sensation, such as that produced by the grating of the ends of a fractured bone.

Cricoarytenoid: Pertaining to the cricoid and arytenoid cartilages.

> Cricoid cartilage: A ringlike cartilage forming the lower and back part of the larynx.

> Arytenoid cartilage: Shaped like a jug or pitcher, as in the cartilage of the larynx.

Cryogenic: Producing low temperatures.

CS: Completed stroke (see Cerebral vascular accident).

CT: See Computerized or computed tomography.

CVA: See Cerebral vascular accident.

Cytokines: Chemicals that are involved in growth regulation. They influence both bone resorption and bone formation.

Cytomegalovirus (CMV): One of a group of species-specific herpes viruses. The human CMV inhabits the salivary glands and causes cytomegalic inclusion disease.

DCA: See Diffuse axonal injury.

Debridement: The removal of damaged or necrotic tissue until healthy tissue is exposed.

Decerebrate: Bilateral or unilateral abnormal extensor responses in upper and lower extremities; in response to painful stimuli, the extremities extend rigidly and the palms turn outward. Decerebrate rigidity indicates damage to the brainstem and as a rule is a sign of greater cortical impairment than is decorticate rigidity.

Decorticate: Abnormal flexor responses in the upper extremity and extensor responses in the lower extremities. Decorticate rigidity usually indicates a lesion in the cerebral hemispheres or a disruption of the corticospinal tracts.

Decubitus ulcers: An ulcer caused by local interference with the circulation, usually occurring over a bony prominence at the sacrum, hip (trochanter), heel, shoulder, or elbow. It begins as a reddened area and can quickly involve deeper structures and become an ulcer; also called bedsore and pressure sore. Individuals most at risk for the development of decubitus ulcers are those who are emaciated, obese, or immobilized by traction or some other form of enforced immobility, and those who have diabetes mellitus or some type of circulatory disorder. Because urine and feces contribute to skin breakdown, incontinent patients are at high risk for pressure sores. Two major factors in their development are prolonged pressure on a part caused by the weight of the body or an extremity, and a shearing force that exerts downward and forward pressure on tissues beneath the skin. The shearing action can occur when a patient slides downward while sitting in a bed or chair, or when bedclothes are forcibly pulled from under a patient.

Decussation: A crossing over; decussation of pyramids: the anterior part of the lower medulla oblongata in which most of the fibers of each pyramid intersect as they cross the midline and descend as the lateral corticospinal tract.

Deep tendon reflexes: A reflected action or movement (reflex) elicited by a sharp tap on the appropriate tendon to induce brief stretch of the muscle.

Deep vein thrombosis (DVT): A thrombosis, most often in the legs or pelvis, that results from phlebitis, vein injury, or prolonged bed rest.

Deformity: Distortion of any part or general disfigurement of the body.

Degenerative joint disease: See Osteoarthritis.

Delirium: A mental disturbance of relatively short duration usually reflecting a toxic state and marked by illusions, hallucinations, delusions, excitement, restlessness, and incoherence. Almost any acute illness accompanied by extremely high fever can bring on delirium. Other causes are metabolic, neurological trauma, congestive heart failure, thyrotoxicosis, physical and mental exhaustion, and drug and alcohol intoxication and withdrawal.

Delusion: A false belief, based on incorrect inference about external reality, not consistent with an individual's intelligence and cultural background, which cannot be corrected by reasoning.

Dementia: An organic mental disorder characterized by a general loss of intellectual abilities involving impairment of memory, judgment, and abstract thinking, as well as changes in personality. It does not include a loss of intellectual functioning caused by clouding of consciousness (as occurs in delirium) nor that caused by depression or other functional mental disorders. Common causes are Alzheimer's disease, cerebrovascular disease (multi-infarct), central nervous infection, brain trauma or tumors, pernicious anemia, folic acid deficiency, Wernicke–Korsakoff syndrome, hydrocephalus, and neurological diseases such as Huntington's chorea, multiple sclerosis, and Parkinson's disease.

Demyelination: Destruction, removal, or loss of the myelin sheath of a nerve or nerves.

Depolarization: The process that takes place when neurotransmitter molecules diffuse across a synaptic cleft of a nerve cell and bind with specific receptors on the postsynaptic membrane, thereby transmitting nerve impulses.

de Quervain's disease: Stenosing (constricting) tenosynovitis of the dorsal compartment of the wrist involving the abductor pollicis longus and extensor pollicis brevis.

Dermis: The layer of skin under the epidermis.

Diabetes mellitus: A disorder of carbohydrate metabolism characterized by glucose in the urine, a high glucose level in the blood, and resulting from inadequate production or use of insulin.

Diabetic foot: A person who has diabetes is at increased risk for slow-healing injuries to distal extremities. It is caused by decreased vascularization; the risk of an infection that does not heal is higher. One possible intervention is limb amputation.

Diabetic ketoacidosis: State of medical emergency; life-threatening condition caused by a state of relative insulin deficiency characterized by hyperglycemia, ketonemia, metabolic acidosis, and electrolyte depletion. Often the first presenting sign of type I diabetes.

Diaphoresis: Perspiration, especially profuse perspiration.

Diastole: The phase of the cardiac cycle in which the heart relaxes between contractions; specifically, the period when the two ventricles are dilated by the blood flowing into them.

Diffuse: Not definitely limited or localized; usually involving several areas of the brain.

Diffuse axonal injury (DAI):   Shearing of white brain matter at time of impact during a traumatic brain injury so that transmission of normal neural impulses is disrupted. A rotational component during impact injuries to the head is believed essential for diffuse brain injury.

Diplegia: Paralysis of like parts on either side of the body. In cerebral palsy, diplegia describes involvement of the lower extremities predominantly, with only mildly affected upper extremities.

Dislocation: The temporary displacement of a bone from its normal position in a joint.

DJD: Degenerative joint disease (see Osteoarthritis).

Disorder: A derangement or abnormality of function; a morbid physical or mental state.

Donor site: The area from which skin has been harvested to use as an autograft to cover an open wound.

Dopamine: A neurotransmitter in the brain.

Dysarthria: Imperfect articulation of speech caused by disturbances of muscular control resulting from central or peripheral nervous system damage.

Dysesthesia: Impairment of any sense, especially of the sense of touch; a painful, persistent sensation induced by a gentle touch of the skin.

DVT: See Deep vein thrombosis.

Dyskinesia: Impairment of the power of voluntary movement.

Dysmetria: Difficulty judging distances when trying to coordinate limb movements; inability to properly direct or limit motions.

Dysphagia: Difficulty in swallowing. The condition can range from mild discomfort, such as a feeling that there is a lump in the throat, to a severe inability to control the muscles needed for chewing and swallowing. Dysphagia can seriously compromise the nutritional status of a patient. In general, placing the patient in an upright position, providing a pleasant and calm environment, being sure the lips are closed as the patient begins to swallow, and preparing and serving foods of the proper consistency are helpful. Stroke victims who have difficulty swallowing should be turned, or should turn their heads, to the unaffected side to facilitate swallowing.

Dyspnea: Labored or difficult breathing. A symptom of a variety of disorders and primarily an indication of inadequate ventilation or of insufficient amounts of oxygen in the circulating blood.

Dyspraxia: A partial loss of ability to perform coordinated movements.

Dystonia: Impairment of muscular tonus manifested as an abnormal persistence of limb and trunk postures; body is bent or twisted in abnormal, relatively fixed positions with possible accompanying muscular facial spasms or torticollis (considered an extrapyramidal symptom).

EBV: See Epstein–Barr virus.

Echolalia: Automatic repetition by an individual of what is said to him/her.

Echopraxia: The spasmodic and involuntary imitation of the movements of others.

Ectopic: Arising or produced at an abnormal site or in a tissue where it is not normally found.

Ectopic bone: Bone that is situated elsewhere than in the normal place.

Edema: An abnormal accumulation of fluid in the intercellular spaces (tissues) of the body.

EEG: See Electroencephalogram.

Efferent: In the nervous system, a nerve that conducts impulses away from the central nervous system toward the periphery (motor).

Effusion: Excess fluid in the joint indicating irritation or inflammation of the synovium; excess of fluid in a body cavity.

Elastin: A fibrous and stretchy protein found in tissue. It gives skin its elasticity.

Electroencephalogram (EEG): The record obtained during the amplification, recording, and subsequent analysis of the electrical activity of the brain using an instrument called an electroencephalograph.

Electrolyte depletion: Insufficient amounts of vital chemical constituents of the body, including sodium, potassium, and chlorine.

Electromyogram (EMG): A record of the intrinsic electrical properties of skeletal muscle.

Embolism: The sudden blocking of an artery by a moving clot of foreign material (embolus) that has been brought to its site of lodgment by the blood current. Obstructing material is often a blood clot but may be a fat globule, air bubble, piece of tissue, or clump of bacteria. Emboli usually lodge at divisions of an artery, where the vessel narrows.

EMG: See Electromyogram.

Emphysema: Enlargement of the airspaces distal to the terminal nonrespiratory bronchioles, accompanied by destructive changes of the alveolar walls.

Encephalitis: Inflammation of the brain.

Endarterectomy: Excision of thickened atheromatous areas of the innermost coat of an artery (intima).

Carotid endarterectomy: A surgical procedure in which the diseased carotid artery is opened, a clot removed, and an artificial graft is put in its place.

Endocardium: The endothelial lining membrane of the cavities of the heart and the connective tissue bed on which it lies.

Endomysium: The sheath of delicate reticular (resembling a net) fibrils that surround each muscle fiber.

Endotracheal: Within the trachea.

Endotracheal tube: An airway catheter inserted in the trachea during intubation to assure clearance in the upper airway by allowing for removal of secretions and maintenance of an adequate air passage.

Epicardium: The inner layer of the serous pericardium, which is in contact with the heart.

Episcleritis: Inflammation of the loose connective tissue forming the sclera and the conjunctiva of the eye.

Epidemiology: The science concerned with the study of the factors influencing and determining the frequency and distribution of disease, injury, and other health related events and their causes in a defined human population for the purpose of establishing programs to prevent and control their development and spread.

Epidermis: The outermost layer of skin.

Epilepsy: A recurrent paroxysmal disorder of cerebral function characterized by sudden, brief attacks of altered consciousness, motor activity, sensory phenomena, or inappropriate behavior caused by abnormal excessive discharge of cerebral neurons.

Episode: A noteworthy happening occurring in the course of a continuous series of events.

Epithelialization: The healing of a wound by growth from the epithelium.

Epstein–Barr virus (EBV): A herpesvirus that is the etiologic agent of infectious mononucleosis. It has been isolated from cells cultured from Burkitt's lymphoma (an undifferentiated malignant form usually found in central Africa) and has been found in certain cases of nasopharyngeal cancer. Epstein–Barr virus has been implicated in cases of chronic fatigue, and a high proportion of individuals with rheumatic arthritis have circulating antibodies in response to the antigen present in the EBV.

Equilibrium reactions: Balance in developmental positions is achieved by these reactions in which the postural muscles contract to maintain or regain an upright position during walking, standing, or sitting.

Equinovalgus (talipes equinovalgus): A foot deformity in which the heel is abducted (turned outward) and everted and the foot is plantar flexed.

Equinovarus (talipes equinovarus): A foot deformity in which the heel is adducted (turned inward) and inverted and the foot is plantar flexed.

Erythema: Redness of the skin caused by capillary dilation.

Erythrocyte sedimentation rate (ESR): A diagnostic test that measures how fast red blood cells fall to the bottom of a tube; it indicates the presence and degree of inflammation.

Eschar: Necrotic tissue produced by the original burn injury.

Escharotomy: An incision made through the eschar.

ESR: See Erythrocyte sedimentation rate.

Euphoria: A pervasive and sustained emotion of intense elation with feelings of grandeur.

Evoked potentials: Through repeated stimulation of specific receptors the subsequent response (evoked potential) of a particular area of the brain is measured. For example, the retina is repeatedly stimulated with light flashes and then the evoked electrical reponse is measured. Computers are used to average the response and to dampen the normal electroencephalographic activity.

Exacerbation: An increase in severity of a disease or any of its symptoms.

Executive functioning: The ability to think abstractly; the ability to plan, initiate, organize, sequence, pace, monitor, and terminate complex activity.

Existentialism: A philosophical movement of the 20th century that emphasized immediate individual existence as the focus of reality and meaning.

Extrapyramidal: Any of a group of clinical disorders marked by abnormal involuntary movements, alterations in muscle tone, and postural disturbances (including Parkinsonism, chorea, athetosis).

Extravasation: A discharge or escape, as of blood, from a vessel into the tissues.

Fasciculus: A tract or pathway in the nervous system.

Fasciotomy: An incision made through the fascia.

Fasting blood sugar (glucose) test: Blood glucose level after a 12-hour fast. Abnormally high levels may suggest problems with glucose metabolism.

Felty's syndrome: A disease consisting of rheumatoid arthritis, splenomegaly, anemia, and leukopenia.

Fibrillation: A small, local, involuntary muscular contraction caused by spontaneous activation of single muscle cells or muscle fibers.

> Atrial fibrillation: A cardiac arrhythmia marked by rapid randomized contractions of the atrial myocardium, causing a totally irregular, often rapid, ventricular rate.

> Ventricular fibrillation: A cardiac arrhythmia marked by fibrillary contractions of the ventricular muscle caused by rapid repetitive excitation of myocardial fibers without coordinated ventricular contraction.

Fibrosis: Formation of fibrous tissue; fibroid degeneration.

Figure ground: The ability to determine the shape or outline of an object against a background environment; differentiate between foreground and background forms and objects.

Fistula: Any abnormal, tubelike passage within body tissue, usually between two internal organs, or leading from an internal organ to the body surface.

Flaccid (hypotonicity): Paralysis of muscles in which there is an absence of reflexes (in lower motor neuron disorders such as poliomyelitis).

Flaccidity: Abnormal muscle tone felt as too little resistance to movement; also called hypotonus.

Focal: The chief center of a morbid process; usually involving one area of the brain. Linear movement of the head leads to focal lesions at the site of impact (coup) or the opposite side of the brain (countercoup).

Form constancy: The ability to recognize forms and objects as the same in various environments, positions, and sizes.

Fragile X syndrome: May account for a large number of persons who have been described as having mild familial mental retardation. Family studies often reveal affected male siblings and maternal uncles, leaving no doubt that a group of X-linked mutant genes causes mental retardation without major congenital anomalies. This at least in part accounts for the excess of retarded males. Some of these males have an X chromosome with a constriction near the end of the long arm, resulting in what looks like a small knob separated from the main portion of the chromosome by a thin stalk. The stalk, often broken in preparing the karyotype, is referred to as a fragile site, and its presence can be detected by using special cell culture techniques. The clinical features include large testes, especially after puberty, large protuberant ears, and prominent chin and forehead.

Friedreich's ataxia: A hereditary sclerosis of the dorsal and lateral columns of the spinal cord, usually beginning in childhood or youth, with resultant progressive ataxia, speech impairments, scoliosis, and peculiar swaying and irregular movements, with paralysis of the muscles, especially of the lower extremities.

Full thickness burn: Necrosis of the tissue through the dermal layer.

Functional unit: Nuclei and fibers (excluding the pyramidal tract) of the brain involved in motor activities that control and coordinate, especially the postural, static, supporting, and locomotor mechanisms. Structures include the corpus striatum, subthalamic nucleus, substantia nigra, and red nucleus, with their interconnections with the reticular formation, cerebellum, and cerebrum; some authorities include the cerebellum and vestibular nuclei.

Fusiform: Tapering at both ends; spindle-shaped.

Gangrene: Necrosis or death of tissue as a result of obstruction, loss, or decreased blood supply.

Genetic marker: A gene having alleles that are all expressed in the phenotype, that is, they are codominant. Markers are used to determine consistent and stable irregularities in the sequential order of bases in DNA to pinpoint disorders of heredity.

Gestational diabetes: Diabetic state that begins during pregnancy and usually resolves after delivery. Patient may be at higher risk for developing type II diabetes later.

Glycemia: Presence of glucose in blood.

Grand mal seizures: A type of epilepsy (recurrent paroxysmal disorder of cerebral function characterized by sudden, brief attack of altered consciousness, motor activity, or sensory phenomena) that is generalized and affects the entire brain. The seizure proceeds with loss of consciousness; falling; and tonic then clonic contractions of the muscles. The attack usually lasts 2 to 5 minutes.

Granulation tissue: Small islands of tissue that grow up through a wound.

Granulocytopenia: An acute or chronic reduction in peripheral blood granulocytes resulting in increased susceptibility to bacterial infection and mucous membrane ulcerations.

Granulomatous: Composed of granulomas or nodules representing a chronic inflammatory response associated with infectious (disease) or noninfectious (foreign body) agents.

Granulomatous aortitis: Inflammatory nodule in the aorta.

Graphesthesia: The ability by which outlines, numbers, words, or symbols traced or written on the skin are recognized.

Graphomotor: Pertaining to movements involved in writing.

***Haemophilus* influenzae:** A genus of aerobic to facultatively anaerobic, parasitic bacteria containing minute, Gram–negative rod-shaped cells.

Hallucination: False sensory perceptions not associated with real external stimuli; there may or may not be a delusional interpretation of the hallucinatory experience. Hallucinations indicate a psychotic disturbance only when associated with impairment in reality testing.

Hallux valgus: Lateral deviation at the first metatarsophalangeal joint.

Hammer toe: Deformity with hyperextension of the metatarsophalangeal joint, flexion of the proximal interphalangeal and hyperextension of the distal interphalangeal joints.

Hematoma: A localized collection of extravasated blood, usually clotted, in an organ, space, or tissue. Contusions (bruises) and black eyes are familiar forms of hematoma that are seldom serious. Hematomas can occur almost anywhere on the body; they are almost always present with a fracture and are especially serious when they occur inside the skull, where they may produce local pressure on the brain. The most common kinds are epidural (above the dura mater, between it and the skull) and subdural (beneath the dura mater, between the tough casing and the more delicate membranes covering the tissue of the brain, the pia–arachnoid).

Hemianesthesia: Anesthesia or absence of sensation on one side of the body.

Hemianopsia (hemianopia): Defective vision or blindness in one-half the visual field, usually applied to bilateral defects caused by a single lesion, often as a result of CVA. The individual is unable to perceive objects to the side of the visual midline. The visual loss is contralateral (i.e., it is on the side opposite of the brain lesion).

Hemiparesis: Paresis or weakness affecting one side of the body.

Hemiplegia: Paralysis of one side of the body; usually caused by a brain lesion, such as a tumor, or by a cerebral vascular accident. The paralysis occurs on the side opposite the brain disorder, as most of the fibers in the motor tracts of the brain cross to the opposite side in the medulla oblon-gata; therefore damage to the right hemisphere of the brain affects motor control of the left half of the body.

Hemodialysis: Removal of toxic waste products from the blood with an artificial kidney. Vascular access is achieved by insertion of a needle into an artery. Removal of wastes is accomplished by osmosis using dialysis fluid.

Hemoglobin: A substance in red blood cells that transports oxygen through the body.

Hemorrhage: Abnormal internal or external discharge of blood.

Hemorrhagic stroke: A type of stroke that occurs when blood escapes the normal vessels and enters the brain tissue or the subarachnoid space. Intracerebral hemorrhage: A type of hemorrhagic stroke that occurs when blood escapes a cerebral vessel and directly enters the brain tissue.

Herpes simplex virus II (HSV-II): A recurrent viral infection characterized by the appearance on the skin or mucous membranes of single or multiple clusters of small vesicles, filled with clear fluid, on slightly raised inflammatory bases. Herpes simplex virus II is usually genital, is transmitted primarily by direct contact with lesions, most often venereally, and produces skin lesions.

Heterotopic ossification: The formation of bone in soft tissue and periarticular locations. Early clinical signs include warmth, swelling, pain, and decreased joint motion. Common joints for heterotopic ossification are the shoulder, elbow, hip, and knee.

HLA: See Human leukocyte antigen.

HLA-DR4: A genetic marker associated with increased risk of development of rheumatoid arthritis.

Homograft: See Allograft.

Homonymous hemianopsia: Both visual fields, either the right halves or left halves, are defective on the same side.

Horner's syndrome: Sinking in of the eyeball, ptosis of the upper eyelid, slight elevation of the lower lid, constriction of the pupil, narrowing of the palpebral fissure, anhidrosis, and cooling on the affected side of the face caused by paralysis of the cervical sympathetic nerve supply at the T1 spinal level.

HSV-II: See Herpes simplex virus II.

Human leukocyte antigens (HLA): Specific genetic markers on the white blood cells (leukocytes), several of which are related to an increased tendency to develop certain rheumatic diseases.

Hunter's syndrome: An X-linked genetic condition characterized by increased urinary mucopolysaccharide excretion and variable systemic manifestations. In the severe form, death usually occurs before age 15, whereas in the mild form, persons survive to age 30 to 50.

Hydrocephalus: A condition characterized by enlargement of the cranium caused by abnormal accumulation of cerebrospinal fluid within the cerebral ventricular system; also called "water on the brain."

Hyperemia: An excess of blood in a part; after a stroke, an area of the brain in which blood vessels are congested and swollen.

Hyperglycemia: An abnormally high concentration of glucose (115–139 mg/dL) in the circulating blood, especially with reference to a fasting level.

Hyperlipidemia: Increased levels of fat in the blood that can develop secondary to diabetes.

Hypernatremia: An abnormally high concentration of sodium ions in blood. Normal range is 136 to 145 mEq/L.

Hyperphenylalaninemia: Abnormally high phenylalanine levels. Normal concentration is less than 8 mg/dL.

Hypermobility: Excess joint relaxation that permits increased mobility.

Hyperreflexia: see Autonomic dysreflexia.

Hypertension: Abnormally high blood pressure of ≥ 140 mm Hg systolic and/or ≥ 90 mm Hg diastolic.

Hyperthermia: Greatly increased body temperature of 104° to 106° F.

Hypertonicity (spasticity): Abnormal muscle tone felt as too much resistance to movement as a result of hyperactive reflexes and loss of inhibiting influences from higher brain centers.

Hypertrophic scar: Increased scar formation that grows above the level of the skin plane but does not exceed the boundaries of the original wound area.

Hypertrophy: Increase in volume of a tissue or organ produced entirely by enlargement of existing cells.

Hypoglycemia: An abnormally small concentration of glucose in circulating blood; i.e., < 50 mg/dL in men and < 45 mg/dL in women.

Hypotension: Abnormally low blood pressure. Normal blood pressure is 120 mm Hg systolic and 80 mm Hg diastolic.

Hypothyroidism: A condition resulting from deficiency of thyroid secretion, resulting in a lowered basal metabolism.

Hypotonicity: See Flaccid.

Hypotonus: See Flaccidity.

Hypoxia: Diminished availability of oxygen to the body tissues.

Iatrogenic diabetes: Diabetes caused by administration of certain drugs, such as corticosteroids, certain diuretics, and birth control pills.

Immune response: The reaction of the body to substances that are foreign or are treated as foreign. A cell-mediated immune response involves the production of lymphocytes by the thymus (T cells) in response to an antigen. A humeral immune response involves the production of plasma lymphocytes (B cells) in response to an antigen and results in the formation of antibodies.

Immune system: The body's natural defense system against injury or infection.

Immunosuppressant: Medications used to block or suppress excessive immune responses; used to slow or prevent rejection of transplanted organs.

Immunosuppression: Inhibition of the formation of antibodies; used in transplant procedures to prevent rejection of the transplanted organ or tissue.

Impulsion: A blind obedience to internal drives, without regard for acceptance by others or pressure from the superego; seen in children and in adults with weak defensive organization.

Impulsive: A tendency to obey internal drives, without regard for acceptance by others or pressure from society.

Incontinence: Inability to control excretory functions.

Infarct: An area of tissue on an organ or part that undergoes necrosis after cessation of blood supply.

Infarction: A localized area of ischemic necrosis produced by occlusion of the arterial supply or the venous drainage of the heart.

Inflammation: A local response to injury characterized by swelling, pain, increased temperature, and redness in the region of injury as a result of increased local blood flow.

Insulin: A hormone secreted by the beta cells of the islets of Langerhans of the pancreas; high blood glucose levels stimulate its secretion; essential for use of glucose by cells to produce energy.

Intima: The innermost coat of a blood vessel; also called the tunic intima.

Intrauterine: Within the uterus.

Ipsilateral: Pertaining to, situated on, or affecting the same side.

Ischemia: Deficiency of blood in a part, caused by functional constriction or actual obstruction of a blood vessel, often leading to necrosis of surrounding tissue.

Ischemic stroke: A deficiency of blood to the brain caused by an occlusion of an artery from a thrombus or embolism.

Isoenzymes: Any of the several forms of an enzyme, all of which catalyze the same reaction, but which may differ in reaction rate, inhibition by various substances, electrophoretic mobility, or immunological properties. Several enzymes, particularly alkaline phosphatase, lactate dehydrogenase, and creatine kinase, have clinically important isoenzymes. Isoenzymes are separated by electrophoresis, and the pattern indicates which damaged organ has released the enzymes.

Jaundice: Condition characterized by yellowness of the skin, whites of the eyes, mucous membranes, and body fluids caused by deposition of bile pigment as a result of excess bilirubin in the blood.

Joint: A meeting of two bones for the purpose of allowing movement.

JRA: see Juvenile rheumatoid arthritis.

Juvenile rheumatoid arthritis (JRA): Polyarticular (more than four joints) is the most common form. Pauciarticular (four or fewer joints) is the second most common. Systemic JRA affects many parts of the body, including organs and joints, and is the least common form.

Juxta-articular: Situated near (adjoining) or in the region of a joint.

Keloid: Increased scar formation that grows above the level of the skin plane and exceeds the wound boundaries.

Keratoconjunctivitis: Inflammation of the cornea and conjunctiva (the delicate membrane lining the eyelids and covering the eyeball).

Kernicterus: A form of hemolytic jaundice of the newborn. The basal ganglia and other areas of the brain and spinal cord are infiltrated with bilirubin, a yellow-pigmented substance produced by the breakdown of hemoglobin. Develops during the second to eighth day of life.

Ketosis: Accumulation of ketones in the body resulting from incomplete metabolism of fatty acids; commonly observed in uncontrolled diabetes (among other conditions); large amounts of ketones may be eliminated in urine.

Kinesthesia: The ability and sense by which position, weight, and movement are perceived.

Kinesiology: Scientific study of movement of body parts.

Kyphosis: Abnormally increased convexity in the curvature of the thoracic spine viewed from the side, resulting from an acquired disease, an injury, or a congenital disorder or disease.

Lability: The quality of being labile (i.e., unstable, fluctuating, moving from point to point). In psychiatry, emotional instability; a tendency to show alternating states of gaiety and somberness.

Lacuna: A small pit or hollow cavity.

Lacunar strokes: Small infarcts usually in the deep noncortical parts of the cerebrum and brainstem resulting from an occlusion of small branches of larger cerebral arteries.

Lag phenomenon: Difference between active and passive range of motion.

Lemniscus: A band or bundle of nerve fibers in the central nervous system; also called a tract or pathway.

Lesch–Nyhan syndrome: Usually, affected males are severely mentally and physically retarded, have significant hyperuricemia, and exhibit a peculiar propensity to self-mutilation by chewing their lips and fingertips, which leads to tissue loss and scarring. The basic enzymatic defect is known, and cases and carriers are detectable with almost 100% accuracy through biochemical studies on cultured cells.

Leukocyte: White blood cell; a colorless blood corpuscle whose chief function is to protect the body against microorganisms causing disease.

Leukopenia: Reduction of the number of leukocytes in the blood.

Ligament: A band of short, fibrous, elasticlike tissue that helps hold tendons in proper alignment and stabilizes joints by attaching one bone to another. The joint capsule is considered a ligament.

Capsular ligament: Fibrous layer of a joint capsule.

Lipohyalinosis: A condition characterized by fat and hyaline degeneration.

Listeria: A soil saprophyte that becomes pathogenic for animals or man under favorable circumstances. The most common manifestation in the adult is meningitis. It may be transmitted transplacentally to the fetus, in which case it may cause abortion.

Lordosis: Forward curvature of the lumbar spine.

Lymph nodes: Small organs containing lymphocytes.

Lymphocyte: A type of leukocyte responsible for specific defenses of the body against foreign matter divided into two classes, B (humoral) and T (cellular) lymphocytes.

Magnetic resonance imaging (MRI): When certain atomic nuclei with an odd number of protons, neutrons, or both are subjected to a strong magnetic field, they absorb and re-emit electromagnetic energy. Analysis of the net magnetization vector's deflection by application of a radiofrequency pulse provides image information. This technique is valuable in providing images of the heart, large blood vessels, brain, and soft tissues. It is an expensive procedure and involves keeping the patient immobile for a lengthy period.

Mallet finger deformity: Deformity involving only flexion of the distal interphalangeal joint; secondary to disruption of the insertion of the extensor tendon into the base off the distal phalanx.

Meningitis: Inflammation of the meninges.

Mental retardation: Below-normal intellectual function that has its cause or onset during the developmental period and usually within the first years after birth.

Mesencephalon: The midbrain.

Mesh graft: A skin graft that has been expanded by placing holes (interstices) in it to provide wound coverage over a greater surface area. Grafts are meshed 1:2, 1:3, 1:4.

Metabolic acidosis: Increase in acid level of blood that can result from ketosis (among other causes).

Mononeuritis multiplex: Simultaneous inflammation of several nerves remote from one another with sensory, motor, reflex, or vasomotor symptoms, or a combination of these.

Monozygotic: Pertaining to or derived from a single zygote (fertilized ovum); identical twins.

Mood: A pervasive and sustained emotion, subjectively experienced and reported by an individual; examples include depression, elation, and anger.

Mood episodes: Mood syndromes that have no known cause other than the mood disorder.

Morning stiffness: The term describing the prolonged generalized stiffness that is associated with inflammatory arthritis upon awakening. The stiffness is indicative of systemic involvement. The duration of the stiffness correlates with the intensity of the disease. The generalized stiffness is in contrast to the localized stiffness seen in osteoarthritis.

MRI: See Magnetic resonance imaging.

Mucopolysaccharidosis: A group of inherited disorders characterized by a deficiency of enzymes that are essential for the degradation of the mucopolysaccharides heparin sulfate, dermatan sulfate, and keratan sulfate. Clinically these disorders include some or all of the following: coarse facies, corneal clouding, hepatosplenomegaly, joint stiffness, hernias, skeletal dysplasia, and mental retardation. They can be diagnosed before birth by culturing amniotic fluid cells for specific enzyme activity or after birth by testing cultured skin fibroblasts for specific enzymes.

Mural thrombus: One attached to the wall of the endocardium in a diseased area. Venous thrombus: One attached to the wall of a vein.

Muscle: Elastic tissue that moves the joints by helping them flex, extend, or rotate, depending on how the joints are designed.

Muscular dystrophy: A group of genetically determined, painless, degenerative myopathies that are progressively crippling as muscles gradually weaken and atrophy.

Myalgia: Muscle pain.

Myelin: The lipid substance forming a sheath around the axons of certain nerve fibers, occurring predominantly in the cranial and spinal nerves that compose the white matter of the brain and spinal cord. The myelin sheath is formed by a glial cell, either an oligodendrocyte (in the central nervous system) or Schwann cell (in the peripheral nervous system).

Myelogram: A graphic representation of the differential count of cells found in a stained representation of bone marrow.

Myelography: A procedure used to examine the spinal cord. A substance that is opaque to radiographs is injected into the subarachnoid space. The area(s) are then x-rayed and examined on film for structural abnormalities.

Myocardium: The middle and thickest layer of the heart wall, composed of cardiac muscle.

Myoclonus: Shocklike contraction of part of a muscle, an entire muscle, or a group of muscles.

Myositis: Inflammation of a voluntary muscle.

Necrosis: The morphological changes indicative of cell death caused by enzymatic degradation.

Neologism: A newly coined word; in psychiatry, a word whose meaning may be known only to the patient using it; also seen in aphasics.

Nephrectomy: Surgical removal of the kidney.

Nephropathy: Any disease of the kidney.

Neuroendocrine: Pertaining to neural and endocrine influence and, particularly, to the interaction between the nervous and endocrine systems.

Neurofibrillary tangles: Neurofibrils are the delicate threads running in every direction through the cytoplasm of a nerve cell, extending into the axon and dendrites. These bundles of fibrous proteins are not normally present in large quantities in the human brain. In Alzheimer's disease, these threads proliferate and become tangled and disorganized, generally with an accumulation in the hippocampus, amygdala, and pyramidal cells of the neocortex.

Neurogenic bowel/bladder: Dysfunction resulting from congenital abnormality, injury, or disease process of the brain, spinal cord, or local nerve supply to the urinary bladder or rectum and their respective outlets. The dysfunction may manifest as partial or complete retention, incontinence, or frequency of elimination.

Neuroleptic: A medication having antipsychotic action affecting sensorimotor, cognitive, and psychologic function.

Neurologist: A specialist in diseases of the nervous system.

Neuromyopathy: A disease of the nervous system and muscle.

Neuropathy (peripheral): A syndrome of sensory loss, muscle weakness and atrophy, decreased deep tendon reflexes, and vasomotor symptoms, singly or in any combination.

Neuropathy: Pathology of the nervous system.

Neurotransmitter: A substance (e.g., norepinephrine, acetylcholine, dopamine) that is released from the axon terminal of a presynaptic neuron on excitation and that travels across the synaptic cleft to either excite or inhibit the target cell.

Neutropenia: Diminished number of neutrophils in the blood.

Nitrosamines: Amines substituted by a nitroso (NO) group, usually on a nitrogen atom, to yield *N*-nitrosamines. These compounds can be formed by direct combination of an amine and nitrous acid.

Nonreflex neurogenic bladder or bowel: Also called autonomic bladder/bowel. A neurogenic bladder/bowel resulting from a lesion or injury in the sacral portion of the spinal cord that interrupts the reflex arc that controls the bladder/bowel. The lesion may be in the cauda equina, conus medullaris, sacral roots, or pelvic nerve. It is marked by loss of normal bladder/bowel sensations and reflex activity, inability to initiate urination/elimination normally, and stress incontinence.

Norepinephrine: A neurotransmitter.

Nystagmus (nystaxis): Involuntary, rapid, rhythmic movement (horizontal, vertical, rotatory, or mixed, i.e., two types) of the eyeball.

Obsessive–compulsive disorder: A disorder characterized by the presence of recurrent ideas and fantasies (obsessions) and repetitive impulses or actions (compulsions) that the patient recognizes as morbid and toward which he or she feels a strong inner resistance.

Ophthalmologist: A physician who specializes in the treatment of disorders of the eye.

Optic neuritis: Inflammation of the optic nerve, affecting the part of the nerve within the eyeball (neuropapillitis) or the part behind the eyeball (retrobulbar neuritis), usually causing pain and partial blindness in one eye.

Orthopaedist: A specialist in the study of the prevention of and correction of disorders involving locomotor structures of the body, especially the skeleton, joints, muscles, fascia, and other supporting structures, such as ligaments and cartilage.

Orthosis: An orthopaedic appliance or apparatus used to support, align, prevent, or correct deformities or to improve function of movable parts of the body.

Orthostatic intolerance: An inability to tolerate sitting upright or standing, related to a fall in blood pressure that causes dizziness, syncope, and blurred vision.

Orthotic: Pertaining to the use or application of an orthosis.

Osmotic agent: An agent (e.g., drug) that increases osmosis, which is the passage of pure solvent from a solution of lesser to one of greater solute concentration when the two solutions are separated by a membrane that selectively prevents the passage of solute molecules but is permeable to the solvent.

Osteoarthritis: A noninflammatory joint disease marked by degeneration of the articular cartilage, hypertrophy of bone at the margins, and changes in the synovial membrane; also called degenerative joint disease (DJD).

Overflow: See Athetosis.

Pancreas: Salivary gland of the abdomen; extends from duodenum to spleen; secretes insulin.

Pannus: An inflammatory exudate overlying synovial cells on the inside of a joint capsule, which can damage the cartilage, usually occurring in rheumatoid arthritis or related articular rheumatism.

Paradigm: An example or model; a means for organizing thinking.

Paraplegia: Paralysis of the legs and, in some cases, the lower part of the body as a result of central nervous system paralysis affecting all of the muscles of the parts involved.

Paraphasia: Partial aphasia in which wrong words are used or words are used in wrong and senseless combinations.

> Paraphasic errors: substitution of words or sounds, which reduces intelligibility or distorts meaning.

Paresthesia: Morbid or perverted sensation; an abnormal sensation as burning, prickling, formication caused by a disorder of the central nervous system.

Parkinsonism: A group of neurological disorders marked by slowed movement, tremors, and muscular rigidity.

Partial thickness burn: A burn injury that extends through the epidermis and into the dermis.

Partially reversible ischemic neurological deficits (PRIND): Small strokes lasting longer than 72 hours, with resultant minor neurological impairment. See Cerebral vascular accident.

PDD: Primary degenerative dementia (see Alzheimer's disease).

Pedal edema: Swelling of the feet and ankles.

Penumbra: During an infarct, this refers to the zone of injury in the brain that is downstream from the infarcted zone that may be served by collateral blood vessels.

Perception: The process of transferring physical stimulation into psychological information; mental process by which sensory stimuli are brought to awareness.

Percutaneous transluminal coronary angioplasty (PTCA): A procedure to enlarge the lumen of a sclerotic coronary artery by using a balloon-tipped catheter that is guided under fluoroscopy to the site of an atheromatous lesion. It provides an alternative to cardiac bypass surgery for selected patients with ischemic heart disease.

Peristalsis: The wormlike movement by which the alimentary canal or other tubular organs with both longitudinal and circular muscle fibers propel their contents, consisting of a wave of contraction passing along the tube.

Peritonitis: Inflammation or infection of the peritoneal cavity.

Periventricular leukomalacia: Nerve fiber track degeneration around the cavities in the center of the brain filled with cerebrospinal fluid. The degeneration can destroy neural communication pathways between several areas of the brain or between brain and spinal cord. Cerebral palsy is a major consequence of this destruction.

Perseveration: The persistence or repetition of a response after the causative stimulus has ceased or in response to different stimuli; for example, a patient answers a question correctly but gives the same answer to succeeding questions. Perseveration is most often associated with organic brain lesions such as traumatic brain injury but is also seen in schizophrenia.

Personality disorder: Disordered patterns of behavior characterized by relatively fixed, inflexible, and stylized reactions to stress, representing the individual's way of dealing with other people and external events regardless of existing realities.

PET: See Positron emission tomography.

Pica: A depraved or perverted appetite. A hunger for substances not fit for food.

Placenta previa: Low implantation of the placenta so that it partially or completely covers the cervical os (orifice). The condition is more frequent in women who have had multiple pregnancies or who are over 35. When the cervix begins to dilate at the onset of labor and the upper and lower uterine segments differentiate, the placenta is stretched and pulled from the uterine wall, producing bleeding. The life of the fetus is in jeopardy because of anoxia resulting from separation of the placenta from its blood supply. If the bleeding continues, the life of the mother is also at risk.

Plaque: Any patch of flat area. Atheromatous plaque: A deposit of predominantly fatty material in the lining of blood vessels occurring in atherosclerosis.

Plaques: Senile plaques are microscopic lesions in the brain, representing tissue deterioration, composed of fragmented axon terminals and dendrites surrounding a core of amyloid. Neuritic plaques: Glycoproteins that collect in scaly patches, replacing degenerating nerve terminals. These plaques are present in the cerebral cortex, hippocampus, amygdala, corpus striatum, and thalamus.

Pleuritis: Inflammation of the pleura that may be caused by infection, injury, or tumor.

Pneumonitis: Inflammation of lung tissue.

Poikilothermy: The state of having body temperature that varies with that of the environment (e.g., cold-blooded). The body tends to assume the temperature of the external environment for at least 1 year after injury in a spinal cord injury.

Polycythemia: An increase in the total red cell mass of the blood (viscosity) that results in thickening of the blood and an increased tendency toward clotting. This increased viscosity limits proper flow, diminishing the supply of blood to the brain and other vital tissues, which may cause mental sluggishness, irritability, headache, dizziness, fainting, and acute pain.

Polydipsia: Excessive thirst that is fairly chronic.

Polymyositis: A chronic, progressive inflammatory disease of skeletal muscle, occurring in both children and adults, and characterized by symmetric weakness of the limb girdles, neck, and pharynx, usually associated with pain and tenderness, and sometimes preceded or followed by manifestations typical of scleroderma, arthritis, systemic lupus erythematosus, or Sjögren's syndrome.

Polyphagia: Excessive eating.

Polyuria: Excessive excretion of urine.

Position in space: The ability to determine the spatial relationships of figures and objects to self or other forms and objects.

Positron emission tomography (PET): A method of imaging the physiological function of the brain, such as the uptake of deoxyglucose in a specific area.

Primitive reflexes: Innate primary reactions found in newborns and indicative of severe brain damage if present beyond their usual time of disappearance. Adult patients with closed head injury or stroke may manifest these signs; absence on reevaluation is a sign of progress in recovery. Examples include placing reactions, Moro reflex, grasp reflex, rooting reflex, and sucking reflex.

PRIND: Partially reversible ischemic neurologic deficits (see Cerebral vascular accident).

Proprioception: From the Latin word for "one's own." Interpretation of stimuli originating in muscles, joints, and other internal tissues that give information about the position of one body part in relation to another. Perception is mediated by sensory nerve endings, chiefly in muscles, tendons, and the labyrinth. Proprioceptive input tells the brain when and how muscles are contracting or stretching, and when and how joints are bending, extending, or being pulled or compressed.

Psychodynamic theories: The study of mental forces and motivations that influence human behavior and mental activity, including recognition of the role of unconscious motivation in human behavior.

Psychomotor agitation: Motor restlessness or excessive overactivity, usually nonproductive and in response to inner tension.

Psychosis: Inability to distinguish reality from fantasy; impaired reality testing, with creation of new reality. Presence of delusions and hallucinations.

Psychotic disorder: Characterized by prominent hallucinations or delusions. Diagnosis is also based on evidence from the history, physical examination, or laboratory findings that the disturbance is the direct physiological consequence of a general medical condition. The disturbance is not better accounted for by another mental disorder. The disturbance does not occur exclusively during the course of delirium. Disorders include schizophrenia, schizophreniform disorder, schizoaffective disorder, delusional disorder, and brief psychotic disorder.

Psychotropic: Exerting an effect on the mind; capable of modifying mental activity; a drug that affects the mental state. There are several classes of psychotropic drugs. Antidepressants are used for the relief of symptoms of major depression; lithium for the treatment of manic episodes of manic–depressive illness; neuroleptics (major tranquilizers) for management of the manifestations of psychotic disorders (schizophrenia); and antianxiety agents (minor tranquilizers) for relief of symptoms of anxiety and tension (phobias, anxiety neurosis).

PTCA: see Percutaneous transluminal coronary angioplasty.

Ptosis: Paralytic drooping of the upper eyelid.

Purkinje fibers: Modified cardiac muscle fibers in the subendothelial tissue, concerned with conducting impulses to the heart.

Pyelonephritis: Inflammation of kidney as a result of bacterial infection.

Quadriplegia: Paralysis of all four limbs (e.g., tetraplegia).

RA: See Rheumatoid arthritis.

Rapid eye movement (REM): A phase of sleep associated with dreaming, mild involuntary muscle jerks, and rapid movements of the eyes.

RDS: see Respiratory distress syndrome.

Reflex: The total of any particular stereotyped, automatic response mediated by the nervous system. A reflex is built into the nervous system and does not need conscious thought to take effect. Reflex responses to stimuli begin to develop in fetal life and continue to be clearly apparent in motor behavior in early infancy. In adults, they become apparent in motor behavior as a result of stress or fatigue. Reflex motor patterns continue to underlie the organized voluntary movements used in daily activities and sports.

Reflex arc: A reflex is the total of any particular automatic response mediated by the nervous system, which is built in and does not need conscious thought to take effect. A reflex arc is usually a simple reflex such as a knee jerk, which involves only two nerves and one synapse. Other arcs may involve an interneuron. When the sensory nerve ending is stimulated, a nerve impulse travels along a sensory (afferent) neuron to the spinal cord. An association neuron or interneuron then transfers the impulse to a motor (efferent) neuron, which carries the impulse to a muscle, which then contracts and moves a body part.

Reflex neurogenic bladder or bowel: Also called autonomic or spastic bladder/bowel. A neurogenic bladder/bowel as a result of complete resection of the spinal cord above the sacral segments, marked by complete loss of micturition reflexes, violent voiding or eliminating, and an abnormal amount of residual urine/feces.

Reflex sympathetic dystrophy (shoulder–hand syndrome): A neurovascular disorder characterized by severe shoulder pain, along with stiffness, swelling, and pain in the hand, trophic changes, vasomotor instability, and resulting limitation in range of motion of the involved side. Prevention is by early frequent mobilization. Prompt treatment with an aggressive exercise program that includes active muscle contraction, joint movement, and light weightbearing activities is required to prevent permanent disability.

REM: See Rapid eye movement.

Remission: Diminution or abatement of the symptoms of a disease; the period during which diminution occurs.

Respiratory distress syndrome (RDS): Severe impairment in the function of respiration in the premature infant.

Resting tremor: Involuntary trembling or quivering occurring in a relaxed and supported extremity.

Retinopathy: Noninflammatory degenerative disease of the retina.

Retro virus: A large group of RNA viruses that includes the leukoviruses and lentiviruses; so called because they carry reverse transcriptase.

Reversible ischemic neurologic deficits (RIND): All strokes that resolve completely (see Cerebral vascular accident).

Rh factor: Genetically determined antigens present on the surface of erythrocytes (red blood cells). Presence or absence of Rh factor is especially important in pregnancies. If the mother is Rh negative and the fetus is Rh positive, the Rh antigens in the fetal tissues diffuse through the placental membrane and enter the mother's blood. Her body reacts by forming anti–Rh agglutinins, which diffuse back through the placental membrane into the fetal circulation and cause clumping of the fetal erythrocytes. This is known as Rh incompatibility.

Rheumatism: General term for acute and chronic conditions characterized by inflammation, muscle stiffness, soreness, and joint pain.

Rheumatoid arthritis (RA): A chronic, inflammatory systemic disease that causes pain, inflammation, mobility limitations, and joint deformity, with problems also seen with the tendons, sheaths, nerves, and muscles.

Rheumatoid carditis: Inflammation of the heart as a result of a rheumatic disorder.

Rheumatoid factor (RH factor): An abnormal antibody often present in people with rheumatoid arthritis.

Righting reactions: Response to stimuli in which an active righting movement brings the head and body into a normal relationship with each other in space; ability to assume an optimal position when there has been a departure from it.

Rigidity: Difficulties initiating movement and slow performance of active movements as well as increased resistance to passive movements as a result of increased muscle tone. There are different types of rigidity, including cogwheel seen in Parkinson's disease and clasp-knife rigidity seen in upper motor neuron diseases.

RIND: Reversible ischemic neurological deficits (see Cerebral vascular accident).

Roentgenology: That branch of radiology dealing with the diagnostic and therapeutic use of roentgen rays (x-rays).

Rubella: Acute infectious disease resembling both scarlet fever and measles but differing from these in its short course, slight fever, and freedom from sequelae.

Scleritis: Inflammation of the sclera, the tough, white outer coat of the eyeball.

Scleroderma: Chronic hardening and shrinking of the connective tissues of any organs of the body, including the skin, heart, esophagus, kidney, and lung. It may be generalized (systemic) or localized. Milder forms are most often seen in individuals in the 30- to 50-year-old age group and affect twice as many women as men. However, the severest forms usually affect men, blacks, and older persons. It is difficult to diagnose as it mimics symptoms of other diseases such as osteoarthritis and rheumatoid arthritis and other collagen disorders.

Scoliosis: Lateral curvature of the vertebral column. This deviation of the normally straight vertical line of the spine may or may not include rotation or deformity of the vertebrae.

Scotoma: An area of lost or depressed vision within the visual field, surrounded by an area of less depressed or of normal vision.

Seborrhea: Excessive oily secretion of the sebaceous glands.

Seizure: Sudden brief attacks of altered consciousness, motor activity, or sensory phenomena.

Self-injurious behavior: Examples include head banging and self biting. More frequent and more intense with increasingly severe mental retardation.

Sensorineural hearing loss: Defects to the auditory pathways within the central nervous system, beginning with the cochlea and auditory nerve and including the brainstem and cerebral cortex.

Sensory gating deficit: The inability to screen out irrelevant stimuli believed to be related to abnormalities in the limbic system and family genetics.

Septicemia: Presence of pathogenic bacteria in the blood.

Sequela: A morbid condition following or occurring as a consequence of another condition or event.

Serotonin: A hormone and neurotransmitter.

Sheet graft: A skin graft that is taken from the donor site and placed directly over the burn wound. It provides 1:1 coverage.

SIE: Stroke in evolution (see Cerebral vascular accident).

Sjögren's syndrome: A chronic disease of unknown etiology, usually occurring in middle-aged or older women, marked by the triad of keratoconjunctivitis with or without lacrimal gland enlargement, xerostomia with or without salivary gland enlargement, and the presence of a connective tissue disease, usually rheumatoid arthritis but sometimes systemic lupus erythematosus, scleroderma, or polymyositis. An abnormal immune response has been implicated and symptoms include dry eyes and mouth.

Smooth-pursuit eye movements (SPEM): The ability to track an item with the eyes without excessive jerking.

Spastic: Clonus or rapid series of rhythmic contractions during quick stretch of a muscle as a result of abnormally increased tension.

Spasticity: See Hypertonicity.

Spatial relation dysfunction: Difficulties in relating objects to each other or to the self. When the result of visual–spatial impairment, this term becomes synonymous with spatial-relations dysfunction.

Spatial-relations syndrome: Defects common to apraxias and agnosias, with related difficulties in areas such as constructional apraxia, figure–ground differentiation, interpretation of concepts related to spatial positioning of objects, spatial relations, impaired spatial memory, perceptual deficits related to depth and distance, and topographic disorientation.

Spatial relations: Ability to determine the relationship of one object to another in space.

SPEM: See Smooth-pursuit eye movements.

Spina bifida: A defect of the vertebral column involving imperfect union of the paired vertebral arches at the midline; it may be so extensive as to allow herniation of the spinal cord and meninges, which may or may not be covered by intact skin.

Spinal fusion: Surgical immobilization of adjacent vertebrae.

Spinal shock: Result of an acute transverse lesion of the spinal cord that causes immediate flaccid paralysis and loss of all sensation and reflex activity (including autonomic functions) below the level of injury. On return of reflex activity, there is increased spasticity of muscles and exaggerated tendon reflexes.

Splenomegaly: Enlargement of the spleen.

Static encephalopathy: A generalized disorder of cerebral function that is nonprogressive.

Stent: A thin cylinder of crushed metal, inserted into the diseased artery, that has tiny, stainless steel scaffolds designed to reduce the chance that the artery will reclose after angioplasty.

Stereognosis: The sense by which the form of objects is perceived, such as the ability to judge the shape of an object pressed against the skin.

Steroid myopathy: A disease of the muscle caused by the ingestion of steroids, complex molecules important in body chemistry.

Strabismus: Deviation of the eye in which the visual axes assume a position relative to each other different from that required by the physiological conditions; also called squint.

Stretch reflex: Reflex contraction of a muscle in response to passive longitudinal stretching.

Stroke: A sudden and severe attack.

Stroke in evolution (SIE): When an individual experiences gradual weakness on one side of the body (see Cerebral vascular accident).

Stroke syndrome: A condition with sudden onset caused by acute vascular lesions of the brain (hemorrhage, embolism, thrombosis, rupturing aneurysm), which may be marked by hemiplegia or hemiparesis, vertigo, numbness, aphasia, and dysarthria and often followed by permanent neurological damage. See Cerebral vascular accident.

Subarachnoid: Between the arachnoid and pia mater, which are membrane layers of the brain.

Subarachnoid hemorrhage: A type of hemorrhagic stroke that occurs when blood escapes its normal vessel, usually from an aneurysm, and spreads to the cerebrospinal fluid surrounding the brain.

Subclavian steal syndrome: A rare condition in which there is a narrowing of the subclavian artery. When the arm is exercised, blood is "stolen" from the brain and delivered to the exercised arm, often resulting in lightheadedness, weakness, and numbness.

Subluxation: Incomplete or partial dislocation. Shoulder subluxation at the glenohumeral joint is commonly seen after a stroke, or it can be caused by a contracture.

Subchondral: Below the cartilage.

Substantia nigra: The layer of gray substance separating the tegmentum of the midbrain from the crus cerebri.

Sudeck's atrophy: Potential complication in fracture healing characterized by pain, swelling (overlaying skin is stretched and glossy), and marked joint stiffness; Colles' fracture is one of the most common causes, although overall incidence is small.

Superficial burn: A burn injury that extends only through the epidermis.

Swan neck deformity: A finger deformity involving hyperextension of the proximal interphalangeal joint and flexion of the distal interphalangeal joint.

Syndrome: A combination of symptoms resulting from a single cause or so commonly occurring together as to constitute a distinct clinical picture.

Synergy: A grouping of stereotypic movements; correlated action or cooperation by two or more structures. Limb synergies may be elicited as associated reactions or as voluntary movements in early stages of recovery from stroke. When movement of a joint is initiated, all muscles that are linked in a synergy with that movement automatically contract, causing a stereotypic movement pattern.

Synovial membrane: The inner of the two layers of the articular capsule of a synovial joint, composed of loose connective tissue with a free, smooth surface that lines the joint cavity. Each joint capsule is lined with synovium for protection of the joint. Synovial tissue also is found on muscle, tendons, bursae, and some organs of the body. The synovial lining produces "fluid" to fill the joint space and aids the cartilage in absorbing shock. It also provides nourishment and aids in removing excess fluids from the joint.

Synovitis: Inflammation of the synovium.

Syphilis: An infectious, chronic venereal disease characterized by lesions that may involve any organ or tissue. It usually exhibits cutaneous manifestations, relapses are frequent, and it may exist without symptoms for many years.

Systole: The contraction, or period of contraction, of the heart, especially of the ventricles, during which blood is forced into the aorta and pulmonary artery.

T cells: Specialized lymphocytes that help remove antigens from the body or interact with B cells.

Tachycardia: Abnormally rapid heart rate, usually more than 100 beats per minute.

Tardive: Applied to a disease in which the characteristic lesion is late-appearing.

Tardive dyskinesia: Disturbed coordination and motor activity in the voluntary motor nervous system characterized by choreiform movements of the buccal–facial muscles and, less commonly, the extremities. Rarely, focal or generalized dystonia also may be seen.

Tay Sachs disease: The hereditary infantile form of a progressive disorder marked by degeneration of brain tissue and the maculas (with the formation of a cherry red spot on both retinas) and by dementia, blindness, and death. This disease is a sphingolipidosis in which the inborn error of metabolism is an enzyme deficiency that results in accumulation of gangliosides in the brain.

Tendon: A cord or band of strong, white, fibrous tissue that attaches muscles to bone. When the muscle contracts or shortens, it pulls on the tendon, which moves the bone.

Tendonitis: Inflammation of a tendon.

Tenosynovitis: Inflammation of a tendon and its sheath, the lubricated layer of tissue in which the tendon is housed and through which it moves. It occurs most frequently in the hands and wrists or feet and ankles and is often the result of intense and continued use. Rheumatoid and other types of arthritis frequently involve tendon sheaths. Treatment is by immobilization of the limb or, in severe cases, by surgery for the purpose of draining an infected sheath or releasing a tendon from a constricting sheath.

Teratogenic agents: Includes drugs taken by the mother during pregnancy, maternal illness such as diabetes mellitus and hypothyroidism, various infectious agents, and irradiation.

Thrombocytopenia: A decrease in the number of platelets in circulating blood, which can be caused by bleeding during trauma or by infections.

Thrombus: An aggregation of blood factors, primarily platelets and fibrin, with entrapment of cellular elements, frequently causing vascular obstruction at the point of its formation and resultant medical problems, such as stroke.

Thrombosis: The process by which a blood clot forms.

Thyrotoxicosis: Toxic condition as a result of hyperactivity of the thyroid gland.

TIA: See Transient ischemic attack.

Tonic labyrinthine reflex: Primitive reflex manifesting in humans as increased flexor tone when in prone position and increased extensor tone when supine.

Topagnosia: Loss of ability to localize site of tactile sensations.

Topagraphic orientation: The ability to adjust or become adjusted to the surface features of the environment or any changes therein; to determine the location of objects and settings and the route to the location, usually as a result of amnestic or agnostic problems.

Toxemia: The clinical syndrome caused by toxic substances in the blood.

Toxoplasmosis: A disease caused by infection with the protozoa *Toxoplasma gondii*. The organism is found in mammals and birds. Symptoms may be so mild as to be barely noticeable or may be more severe, with lymphadenopathy, malaise, muscle pain, and little, if any, fever.

Transient ischemic attack (TIA):   A sudden episode of temporary or passing symptoms, typically as a result of diminished blood flow through the carotid blood vessels but sometimes related to impaired blood flow through the vertebrobasilar vessels. The symptoms warn of impending stroke; approximately one in three individuals experiencing a TIA will have a cerebral vascular accident (stroke) within 5 years. Symptoms can range from obvious loss of sensation or motor function to more subtle changes in speech or mental activity. The person may feel numbness or weakness on one or both sides of the body, slurring of speech or inability to talk, staggering or uncoordinated walking, or difficulty in thinking. Double vision or disturbance of vision in one eye is also common. See Cerebral vascular accident.

Transitional movements: Movements between positions, i.e., sit to kneel, kneel to stand, etc.

Tremor: An involuntary trembling of the body or limbs, occurring either at rest or during activity, depending on the origin of the lesion.

Trisomy 13 (Patau's syndrome):   Occurs in about 1/5000 births and is characterized by midline anomalies. Infants tend to be small at birth. Apneic spells in early infancy are frequent, and mental retardation is severe. Many infants appear to be deaf. Moderate microcephaly with sloping forehead, wide sagittal sutures, and widely patent fontanelles are present. Most patients (70%) are so severely affected that they die before the age of 6 months; less than 20% survive beyond the age of 1 year.

Trisomy 18 (Edwards' syndrome): Occurs in about 1/3000 births and at a ratio of 3 females:1 male. The newborn infant is premature or small for gestational age, with significant hypoplasia of skeletal muscle and subcutaneous fat and hypotonia. The cry is weak, and response to sound is decreased. There often is a history of feeble fetal activity, polyhydramnios, a small placenta, and a single umbilical artery. Survival for more than a few months is rare, and mental retardation is severe in those who do survive.

Trisomy 21 (Down syndrome): In about 95% of cases of Down syndrome, there is an extra chromosome 21. The overall incidence is about 1/700 births, but there is considerable variability depending on maternal age—in the early child-bearing years, the incidence is about 1/2000 births; for mothers older than age 40, it rises to about 1/40 births. Infants tend to be placid, rarely cry, and demonstrate muscular hypotonicity. Physical and mental development are retarded. Microcephaly, brachycephaly, and a flattened occiput are characteristic. The eyes are slanted, and epicanthal folds usually are present. Life expectancy is decreased by heart disease and by susceptibility to acute leukemia.

Tuberous sclerosis: Multisystem hamartomas producing a typical triad: seizures, mental retardation, and skin nodules of the face. Autosomal dominant inheritance with variable penetrance and expression. The disease affects many organ systems other than the skin and brain, including the heart, kidney, eyes, lung, and bone.

Two-point discrimination: Ability to detect that the skin is being touched by two pointed objects at once.

Ulnar drift: Abnormal ulnar deviation of the fingers at the metacarpophalangeal joints.

Unilateral body inattention (neglect): Failure to report, respond, or orient to a unilateral stimulus presented to the body side contralateral to a cerebral lesion. It can result from either defective sensory processing or an attention deficit, resulting in ignoring or impaired use of the extremities.

Unilateral spatial neglect: Inattention to or neglect of visual stimuli presented in the extra-personal space on the side contralateral to a cerebral lesion, as a result of visual perceptual deficits or impaired attention. It may occur independently of visual deficits or with hemianopsia.

Uremia: Complex of symptoms resulting from build-up of waste products in the blood caused by renal failure; reversed by dialysis. Symptoms include headache, nausea, vomiting, dizziness, dimness of vision, coma or convulsions, urinous odor to breath, dry skin, hard rapid pulse, and elevated blood pressure.

Valgus: Bent outward; twisted; denoting a deformity in which the angulation is away from the midline of the body, as in talipes valgus.

Vertigo: A sensation of rotation or movement of one's self (subjective) or of one's surroundings (objective) in any plane. The term is sometimes used erroneously as a synonym for dizziness. Vertigo may result from diseases of the inner ear or may be caused by disturbances of the vestibular centers or pathways in the central nervous system.

Volition: The act of power of willing.

Wallenberg's syndrome: The result of lateral damage at the brainstem level (e.g., lateral medullary syndrome). Damaged structures may include the spinothalamic tract, spinal trigeminal tract, nucleus ambiguus, and descending sympathetic fibers. Symptoms of such damage are loss of pain and temperature sensations over the contralateral body (with relative sparing of tactile sensation), loss of pain and temperature sensations over the ipsilateral face, hoarseness and difficulty in swallowing, and ipsilateral Horner's syndrome. If the inferior cerebellar peduncles in the midbrain and vestibular nuclei are damaged, vertigo and ipsilateral cerebellar deficits, such as ataxia, may result.

Waxy flexibility: The immobile limbs of an individual in a trance can be moved into different positions and the limbs will hold the positions as if they were shaped in wax.

Xerostomia: Dryness of the mouth from salivary gland infection such as is found in Sjögren's syndrome.

Zig-zag effect: Ulnar drift at the metacarpophalangeal joints associated with radial deviation of the wrist.

UNIFORM TERMINOLOGY FOR OCCUPATIONAL THERAPY: THIRD EDITION

Uniform Terminology for Occupational Therapy, Third Edition is an official document of The American Occupational Therapy Association (AOTA). It is intended to provide a generic outline of the domain of concern of occupational therapy. Its purpose is to create common terminology for the profession and to capture succinctly the essence of occupational therapy for others.

It is recognized that the phenomena that constitute the profession's domain of concern can be categorized and labeled in many ways. This document is not meant to limit those in the field who may wish to combine or refine particular constructs. It is also not meant to limit those who would like to conceptualize the profession's domain of concern in a different manner.

INTRODUCTION

The first edition of *Uniform Terminology for Occupational Therapy* was approved and published in 1979 (AOTA, 1979). In 1989, *Uniform Terminology for Occupational Therapy, Second Edition* (AOTA, 1989) was approved and published. The second document presented an organized structure for understanding the areas of practice for the profession of occupational therapy. The document outlined two areas. *Performance areas* (activities of daily living [ADL], work and productive activities, and play or leisure) include activities that the occupational therapy practitioner emphasizes when determining functional abilities (*occupational therapy practitioner* refers to both registered occupational therapists and certified occupational therapy assistants). *Performance components* (sensorimotor, cognitive, psychosocial, and psychological aspects) are the elements of performance that occupa-

tional therapists assess and, when needed, in which they intervene for improved performance.

This third edition has been further expanded to reflect current practice and to incorporate contextual aspects of performance. *Performance areas, performance components,* and *performance contexts* are the parameters of occupational therapy's domain of concern. *Performance areas* are broad categories of human activity that are typically part of daily life. They are ADL, work and productive activities, and play or leisure activities. *Performance components* are fundamental human abilities that, to varying degrees and in different combinations, are required for successful engagement in performance areas. These components are sensorimotor, cognitive, psychosocial, and psychological. *Performance contexts* are situations or factors that influence an individual's engagement in desired or required performance areas. Performance contexts consist of *temporal* aspects (chronological age, developmental age, place in the lifecycle, and health status) and *environmental* aspects (physical, social, and cultural considerations). There is an interactive relationship among performance areas, performance components, and performance contexts. Function in performance areas is the ultimate concern of occupational therapy, with performance components considered as they relate to participation in performance areas. Performance areas and performance components are always viewed within performance contexts. Performance contexts are taken into consideration when determining function and dysfunction relative to performance areas and performance components and in planning intervention. For example, the occupational therapist does not evaluate strength (a performance component) in isolation. Strength is considered as it affects necessary or desired tasks (performance areas). If the individual is interested in homemaking, the occupational therapist would consider the interaction of strength with homemaking tasks. Strengthening could be addressed through kitchen activities, such as cooking and putting groceries away. In some cases, the practitioner would use an adaptive approach and recommend that the family switch from heavy cast iron to lighter-weight pots on the stove to enable the individual to make dinner safely without becoming fatigued or compromising safety.

Occupational therapy assessment involves examining performance areas, performance components, and performance contexts. Intervention may be directed toward elements of performance areas (e.g., dressing, vocational exploration), performance components (e.g., endurance, problem solving), or the environmental aspects of performance contexts. In the latter case, the physical and social environment may be altered or augmented to improve or maintain function. After identifying the performance areas the individual wishes or needs to address, the occupational therapist assesses the features of the environments in which the tasks will be performed. If an individual's job requires cooking in a restaurant as opposed to leisure cooking at home, the occupational therapy practitioner faces several challenges to enable the individual's success in different environments. Therefore, the third critical aspect of performance is the performance context—the features of the environment that affect the person's ability to engage in functional activities.

This document categorizes specific activities in each of the performance areas (ADL, work and productive activities, productivity or leisure). This categorization is based on what is considered "typical" and is not meant to imply that a particular individual characterizes personal activities in the same manner as someone else. Occupational therapy practitioners embrace individual differences, and so would document the unique pattern of the individual being served, rather than forcing the "typical" pattern on that person and his or her family. For example, because of experience or culture, a particular individual might think of home management as an ADL task rather than "work and productive activities" (current listing). Socialization might be considered part of a play or leisure activity instead of its current listing as part of "activities of daily living," because of life experience or cultural heritage.

EXAMPLES OF USE IN PRACTICE

Uniform Terminology, Third Edition defines occupational therapy's domain of concern, which includes performance areas, performance components, and performance contexts. Although this document may be used by occupational therapy practitioners in a number of different areas (e.g., practice, documentation, charge systems, education, program development, marketing, research, disability classifications, and regulations), it focuses on the use of uniform terminology in practice. This document is not intended to define specific occupational therapy programs or specific occupational therapy interventions. Examples of how performance areas, performance components, and performance contexts translate into practice are provided below.

- An individual who is injured on the job may have the potential to return to work and productive activities, which is a performance area. To achieve the outcome of returning to work and productive activities, the individual may need to address specific performance components, such as strength, endurance, soft tissue integrity, time management, and the physical features of performance contexts, like structures and objects in his or her environment. The occupational therapy practitioner, in collaboration with the individual and other members of the vocational team, uses planned interventions to achieve the desired outcome. These interventions may include activities such as an exercise program, body mechanics instruction, and job site modifications, all of which may be provided in a work-hardening program.

- An elderly individual recovering from a cerebrovascular accident may wish to live in a community setting, which combines the performance areas of ADL with work and productive activities. To achieve the outcome of community living, the individual may need to address specific performance components, such as muscle tone, gross motor coordination, postural control, and self-management. It is also necessary to consider the sociocultural and physical features of performance contexts, such as support available from other persons and adaptations of structures and objects within the environment. The occupational therapy practitioner, in cooperation with the team, uses planned interventions to achieve the desired outcome. Interventions may include neuromuscular facilitation, practice of object manipulation, and instruction in the use of adaptive and home safety equipment. The practitioner and individual also pursue the selection and training of a personal assistant to ensure the completion of ADL tasks. These interventions may be provided in a comprehensive inpatient rehabilitation unit.

- A child with learning disabilities is required to perform educational activities within a public school setting. Engaging in educational activities is considered the performance area of work and productive activities for this child. To achieve the educational outcome of efficient and effective completion of written classroom work, the child may need to address specific performance components. These include sensory processing, perceptual skills, postural control, motor skills, and the physical features of performance contexts, such as objects (e.g., desk, chair) in the environment. In cooperation with the team, occupational therapy interventions may include activities like adapting the student's seating in the classroom to improve postural control and stability and practicing motor control and coordination. This program could be developed by an occupational therapist and supported by school district personnel.

- The parents of an infant with cerebral palsy may ask to facilitate the child's involvement in the performance areas of ADL and play. Subsequent to assessment, the therapist identifies specific performance components, such as sensory awareness and neuromuscular control. The practitioner also addresses the physical and cultural features of performance contexts in collaboration with the parents. Occupational therapy interventions may include activities such as seating and positioning for play, neuromuscular facilitation techniques to enable eating, facilitating parents' skills in caring for and playing with their infant, and modifying the play space for accessibility. These interventions may be provided in a home-based occupational therapy program.

- An adult with schizophrenia may need and want to live independently in the community, which represents the performance areas of ADL, work and productive activities, and leisure activities. The specific performance categories may be medication routine, functional mobility, home management, vocational exploration, play or leisure performance, and social interaction. To achieve the outcome of living independently, the individual may need to address specific performance components, such as topographical orientation, memory, categorization, problem solving, interests, social conduct, time management, and sociocultural features of performance contexts, such as social factors (e.g., influence of family and friends) and roles. The occupational therapy practitioner, in cooperation with the team, uses planned interventions to achieve the desired outcome. Interventions may include activities such as training in the use of public transportation, instruction in

budgeting skills, selection and participation in social activities, instruction in social conduct, and participation in community reintegration activities. These interventions may be provided in a community-based mental health program.

- An individual with a history of substance abuse may need to reestablish family roles and responsibilities, which represent the performance areas of ADL, work and productive activities, and leisure activities. To achieve the outcome of family participation, the individual may need to address the performance components of roles, values, social conduct, self-expression, coping skills, self-control, and the sociocultural features of performance contexts, such as custom, behavior, rules, and rituals. The occupational therapy practitioner, in cooperation with the team, uses planned interventions to achieve the desired outcomes. Interventions may include roles and values exercises, instruction in stress management techniques, identification of family roles and activities, and support to develop family leisure routines. These interventions may be provided in an inpatient acute care unit.

PERSON–ACTIVITY–ENVIRONMENT FIT

Person–activity–environment fit refers to the match among the skills and abilities of the individual, the demands of the activity; and the characteristics of the physical, social, and cultural environments. It is the interaction among the performance areas, performance components, and performance contexts that is important and determines the success of the performance. When occupational therapy practitioners provide services, they attend to all of these aspects of performance as well as the interaction among them. The practitioners also attend to each individual's unique personal history. The personal history includes one's skills and abilities (performance components), the past performance of specific life tasks (performance areas), and experience within particular environments (performance contexts). In addition to personal history, anticipated life tasks and role demands influence performance.

When considering the person–activity–environment fit, variables such as novelty, importance, motivation, activity tolerance, and quality are salient. Situations range from those that are completely familiar to those that are novel and have never been experienced. Both the novelty and familiarity within a situation contribute to the overall task performance. Each situation includes an optimal level of novelty that engages the individual sufficiently and provides enough information to perform the task. When too little novelty is present, the individual may miss cues and opportunities to perform. When too much novelty is present, the individual may become confused and distracted, inhibiting effective task performance.

Humans determine that some stimuli and situations are more meaningful than others. Individuals perform tasks they deem important. It is critical to identify what the individual wants or needs to do when planning interventions.

The level of motivation an individual uses to perform a particular task is determined by both internal and external factors. An individual's behavioral state (e.g., amount of rest, arousal, tension) contributes to the potential to be responsive. The features of the social and physical environments (e.g., persons in the room, noise level) provide information that is either adequate or inadequate to produce a motivated state.

Activity tolerance is the individual's ability to sustain a purposeful activity over time. Individuals must select, initiate, and terminate activities as well as attend to a task for the needed length of time to complete that task and accomplish goals. The quality of performance is measured by standards generated by both the individual and others in the social and cultural environments in which the performance occurs. Quality is a continuum of expectations set within particular activities and contexts.

UNIFORM TERMINOLOGY FOR OCCUPATIONAL THERAPY, THIRD EDITION

Occupational therapy is the use of purposeful activity or interventions to promote health and achieve functional *outcomes. Achieving functional outcomes* means to develop, improve, or restore the highest possible level of independence of any individual who is limited by a physical injury or illness, a dysfunctional condition, a cognitive impairment, a psychosocial dysfunction, a mental illness, a developmental or learning disability, or an adverse environmental condition. *Assessment* means the use of skilled observation or evaluation by the administration and interpretation of standardized or nonstandardized tests and measurements to identify areas for occupational therapy services.

Occupational therapy services include but are not limited to:

1. The assessment, treatment, and education of or consultation with the individual, family, or other persons; or

2. Interventions directed toward developing, improving, or restoring daily living skills, work readiness or work performance, play skills or leisure capacities, or enhancing educational performance skills; or

3. Providing for the development, improvement, or restoration of sensorimotor, oral–motor, perceptual, or neuromuscular functioning; or emotional, motivational, cognitive, or psychosocial components of performance.

These services may require assessment of the need for and use of interventions such as the design, development, adaptation, application, or training in the use of assistive technology devices; the design, fabrication, or application of rehabilitative technology such as selected orthotic or prosthetic devices; the application of physical agent modalities as an adjunct to, or in preparation for, purposeful activity; the use of ergonomic principles; the adaptation of environments and processes to enhance functional performance; or the promotion of health and wellness (AOTA, 1993, p 1117).

I. Performance Areas

Throughout this document, activities have been described as if individuals performed the tasks themselves. Occupational therapy also recognizes that individuals arrange for tasks to be done by others. The profession views independence as the ability to self-determine activity performance, regardless of who actually performs the activity.

A. *ADL*—Self-maintenance tasks
   1. *Grooming.* Obtaining and using supplies; removing body hair (use of razors, tweezers, lotions, etc.); applying and removing cosmetics; washing, drying, combing, styling, and brushing hair; caring for nails (hands and feet); caring for skin, ears, and eyes; and applying deodorant.
   2. *Oral hygiene.* Obtaining and using supplies; cleaning mouth; brushing and flossing teeth; or removing, cleaning, and reinserting dental orthotics and prosthetics.
   3. *Bathing/showering.* Obtaining and using supplies; soaping, rinsing, and drying body parts; maintaining bathing position; and transferring to and from bathing positions.
   4. *Toilet hygiene.* Obtaining and using supplies; clothing management; maintaining toileting position; transferring to and from toileting position; cleaning body; and caring for menstrual and continence needs (including

catheters, colostomies, and suppository management).

5. *Personal device care.* Cleaning and maintaining personal care items, such as hearing aids, contact lenses, glasses, orthotics, prosthetics, adaptive equipment, and contraceptive and sexual devices.

6. *Dressing.* Selecting clothing and accessories appropriate to time of day, weather, and occasion; obtaining clothing from storage area; dressing and undressing in a sequential fashion; fastening and adjusting clothing and shoes; and applying and removing personal devices, prostheses, or orthoses.

7. *Feeding and eating.* Setting up food; selecting and using appropriate utensils and bringing food or drink to mouth, hands, and clothing; sucking, masticating, coughing, and swallowing; and management of alternative methods of nourishment.

8. *Medication routine.* Obtaining medication, opening and closing containers, following prescribed schedules, taking correct quantities, reporting problems and adverse effects, and administering correct quantities by using prescribed methods.

9. *Health maintenance.* Developing and maintaining routines for illness prevention and wellness promotion, such as physical fitness, nutrition, and decreasing health risk behaviors.

10. *Socialization.* Accessing opportunities and interacting with other people in appropriate contextual and cultural ways to meet emotional and physical needs.

11. *Functional communication.* Using equipment or systems to send and receive information, such as writing equipment, telephones, typewriters, computers, communication boards, call lights, emergency systems, Braille writers, telecommunication devices for the deaf, and augmentative communication systems.

12. *Functional mobility.* Moving from one position or place to another such as in-bed mobility, wheelchair mobility, transfers (wheelchair, bed, car tub), toilet, tub/shower, chair, floor). Performing functional ambulation and transporting object

13. *Community mobility.* Moving self in the community and using public or private transportation, such as driving, or accessing buses, taxis, or other public transportation systems.

14. *Emergency routine.* Recognizing sudden, unexpected hazardous situations, and initiating action to reduce the threat to health and safety.

15. *Sexual expression.* Engaging in desired sexual and intimate activities.

B. *Work and productive activities*—Purposeful activities for self-development, social contribution, and livelihood

1. *Home management.* Obtaining and maintaining personal and household possessions and environment.

   a. Clothing care. Obtaining and using supplies; sorting, laundering (hand, machine, and dry clean); folding; ironing; storing; and mending.

   b. Cleaning. Obtaining and using supplies; picking up; putting away; vacuuming; sweeping and mopping floors; dusting; polishing; scrubbing; washing windows; cleaning mirrors; making beds; and removing trash and recyclables.

   c. Meal preparation and cleanup. Planning nutritious meals; preparing and serving food; opening and closing containers, cabinets, and drawers; using kitchen utensils and appliances; cleaning up and storing food safely.

   d. Shopping. Preparing shopping lists (grocery and other); selecting and purchasing items; selecting method of payment; and completing money transactions.

   e. Money management. Budgeting, paying bills, and using bank systems.

   f. Household maintenance. Maintaining home, yard, garden, appliances, vehicles, and household items.

   g. Safety procedures. Knowing and performing preventive and emergency procedures to maintain a safe environment and to prevent injuries.

2. *Care of others.* Providing for children, spouse, parents, pets, or others, such as giving physical care, nurturing, communicating, and using age-appropriate activities.

3. *Educational activities.* Participating in a learning environment through school, community, or work-sponsored activities, such as exploring educational interests, attending to instruction, managing assignments, and contributing to group experiences.

4. *Vocational activities.* Participating in work-related activities.

   a. Vocational exploration. Determining aptitudes, developing interests and skills, and selecting appropriate vocational pursuits.

b. Job acquisition. Identifying and selecting work opportunities and completing application and interview processes.

c. Work or job performance. Performing job tasks in a timely and effective manner; incorporating necessary work behaviors.

d. Retirement planning. Determining aptitudes; developing interests and skills; and selecting appropriate avocational pursuits.

e. Volunteer participation. Performing unpaid activities for the benefit of selected individuals, groups, or causes.

C. *Play or leisure activities*—Intrinsically motivating activities for amusement, relaxation, spontaneous enjoyment, or self-expression

1. *Play or leisure exploration.* Identifying interests, skills, opportunities, and appropriate play or leisure activities.

2. *Play or leisure performance.* Planning and participating in play or leisure activities. Maintaining a balance of play or leisure activities with work and productive activities and activities of daily living. Obtaining, using, and maintaining equipment and supplies.

II. Performance Components

A. *Sensorimotor component*—The ability to receive input, process information, and produce output.

1. *Sensory*

a. Sensory awareness. Receiving and differentiating sensory stimuli.

b. Sensory processing. Interpreting sensory stimuli.

2. *Tactile.* Interpreting light touch, pressure, temperature, pain, and vibration through skin contact/receptors.

3. *Proprioceptive.* Interpreting stimuli originating in muscles, joints, and other internal tissues that give information about the position of one body part in relation to another.

4. *Vestibular.* Interpreting stimuli from the inner ear receptors regarding head position and movement.

5. *Visual.* Interpreting stimuli through the eyes, including peripheral vision and acuity and awareness of color and pattern.

6. *Auditory.* Interpreting and localizing sounds and discriminating background sounds.

7. *Gustatory.* Interpreting tastes.

8. *Olfactory.* Interpreting odors.

a. Perceptual processing. Organizing sensory input into meaningful patterns.

1) Stereognosis. Identifying objects through proprioception, cognition, and the sense of touch.

2) Kinesthesia. Identifying the excursion and direction of joint movement.

3) Pain response. Interpreting noxious stimuli.

4) Body scheme. Acquiring an internal awareness of the body and the relationship of body parts to each other.

5) Right–left discrimination. Differentiating one side from the other.

6) Form constancy. Recognizing forms and objects as the same in various environments, positions, and sizes.

7) Position in space. Determining the spatial relationship of figures and objects to self or other forms and objects.

8) Visual–closure. Identifying forms or objects from incomplete presentations.

9) Figure ground. Differentiating between foreground and background forms and objects.

10) Depth perception. Determining the relative distance between objects, figures, or landmarks and the observer, and changes in planes of surfaces.

11) Spatial relations. Determining the position of objects relative to each other.

12) Topographical orientation. Determining the location of objects and settings and the route to the location.

B. *Neuromusculoskeletal*

1. Reflex. Eliciting an involuntary muscle response by sensory input.

2. Range of motion. Moving body parts through an arc.

3. Muscle tone. Demonstrating a degree of tension or resistance in a muscle at rest and in response to stretch.

4. Strength. Demonstrating a degree of muscle power when movement is resisted, as with objects or gravity.

5. Endurance. Sustaining cardiac, pulmonary, and musculoskeletal exertion over time.

6. Postural control. Using righting and equilibrium adjustments to maintain balance during functional movements.

7. Postural Alignment. Maintaining biomechanical integrity among body parts.

8. Soft tissue integrity. Maintaining anatomical and physiological condition of interstitial tissue and skin.

9. *Motor*
   a. Gross coordination. Using large muscle groups for controlled, goal-directed movements.
   b. Crossing the midline. Moving limbs and eyes across the midsagittal plane of the body.
   c. Laterality. Using a preferred unilateral body part for activities requiring a high level of skill.
   d. Bilateral integration. Coordinating both body sides during activity.
   e. Motor control. Using the body in functional and versatile movement patterns.
   f. Praxis. Conceiving and planning a new motor act in response to an environmental demand.
   g. Fine motor coordination/dexterity. Using small muscle groups for controlled movements, particularly in object manipulation.
   h. Visual–motor integration. Coordinating the interaction of information from the eyes with body movement during activity.
   i. Oral motor control. Coordinating oropharyngeal musculature for controlled movements.
C. *Cognitive integration and cognitive components*—The ability to use higher brain functions.
   1. *Level of arousal.* Demonstrating responsiveness to environmental stimuli.
   2. *Orientation.* Identifying person, place, time, and situation.
   3. *Recognition.* Identifying familiar faces, objects, and other previously presented materials.
   4. *Attention span.* Focusing on a task over time.
   5. *Initiation of activity.* Starting a physical or mental activity.
   6. *Termination of activity.* Stopping an activity after an appropriate time.
   7. *Memory.* Recalling information after brief or long periods.
   8. *Sequencing.* Placing information, concepts, and actions in order.
   9. *Categorization.* Identifying similarities of and differences among pieces of environmental information.
   10. *Concept formation.* Organizing a variety of information to form thoughts and ideas.
   11. *Spatial orientation.* Mentally manipulating the position of objects in various relationships.
   12. *Problem solving.* Recognizing a problem, defining a problem, identifying alternative plans, selecting a plan, organizing steps in a plan, implementing a plan, and evaluating the outcome.
   13. *Learning.* Acquiring new concepts and behaviors.
   14. *Generalization.* Applying previously learned concepts and behaviors to a variety of new situations.
D. *Psychological skills and psychological components*—The ability to interact in society and to process emotions.
   1. *Psychological*
      a. Values. Identifying ideas or beliefs that are important to self and others.
      b. Interests. Identifying mental or physical activities that create pleasure and maintain attention.
      c. Self-concept. Developing the value of the physical, emotional, and sexual self.
   2. *Social*
      a. Role performance. Identifying, maintaining, and balancing functions one assumes or acquires in society (e.g., worker, student, parent, friend, religious participants).
      b. Social conduct. Interacting by using manners, personal space, eye contact, gestures, active listening, and self-expression appropriate to one's environment.
      c. Interpersonal skills. Using verbal and nonverbal communication to interact in a variety of settings.
      d. Self expression. Using a variety of styles and skills to express thoughts, feelings, and needs.
   3. *Self-management*
      a. Coping skills. Identifying and managing stress and related factors.
      b. Time management. Planning and participating in a balance of self-care, work, leisure, and rest activities to promote satisfaction and health.
      c. Self-control. Modifying one's own behavior in response to environmental needs, demands, constraints, personal aspirations, and feedback from others.

III. Performance Contexts

Assessment of function in performance areas is greatly influenced by the contexts in which the individual must perform. Occupational therapy practitioners consider performance contexts when determining feasibility and appropriateness of interventions. They may choose interventions based on understanding of contexts or those directly aimed at altering the contexts to improve performance.

A. *Temporal aspects*
   1. *Chronological.* Individual's age.
   2. *Developmental.* Stage or phase of maturation.
   3. *Lifecycle.* Place in important life phases, such as career cycle, parenting cycle, or educational process.
   4. *Disability status.* Place in continuum of disability, such as acuteness of injury, chronicity of disability, or terminal nature of illness.
B. *Environment*
   1. *Physical.* Nonhuman aspects of contexts. Includes the accessibility to and performance within environments having natural terrain, plants, animals, buildings, furniture, objects, tools, or devices.
   2. *Social.* Availability and expectations of significant individuals, such as spouse, friends, and caregivers. Also includes larger social groups that are influential in establishing norms, role expectations, and social routines.
   3. *Cultural.* Customs, beliefs, activity patterns, behavior standards, and expectations accepted by the society of which the individual is a member. Includes political aspects, such as laws that affect access to resources and affirm personal rights. Also includes opportunities for education, employment, and economic support.

SUGGESTED READINGS

American Occupational Therapy Association. Occupational Therapy Product Output Reporting System and Uniform Terminology for Reporting Occupational Therapy Services. Rockville, MD, 1979.

American Occupational Therapy Association. Uniform terminology for occupational therapy, second edition. Am J Occup Ther 1989;43:808–815.

American Occupational Therapy Association. Association policies: definition of occupational therapy practice for state regulation (Policy 5.3.1). Am J Occup Ther 1993;47:1117–1121.

The Terminology Task Force. Winifred Dunn, Ph.D., OTR, FAOTA, Chairperson; Mary Foto, OTR, FAOTA; Jim Hinojosa, Ph.D., OTR, FAOTA; Barbara Schell, Ph.D., OTR., FAOTA; Linda Kohlman Thomson, MOT, OIR, FAOTA; Sarah Hertfelder, M.Ed., MOT, OTR/Staff Liaison, for The Commission on Practice (Jim Hinojosa, Chairperson). Adopted by the Representative Assembly, July 1994.

This document replaces the following documents, all of which were rescinded by the 1994 Representative Assembly: Occupational Therapy Product Output Reporting System (1979); Uniform Terminology for Reporting Occupational Therapy Services—First Edition (1979); Uniform occupational therapy evaluation checklist. Am J Occup Ther 1981;35:817–818; Uniform terminology for occupational therapy—second edition. Am J Occup Ther 1989;43:808–815. Reprinted with permission of the American Occupational Therapy Association.

Uniform terminology for occupational therapy, third edition. Am J Occup Therapy 1994; 48:1047–1054.

MEDICATIONS

Drugs are listed alphabetically to allow for quick location and reference. Many of the people with whom occupational therapists work take multiple medications for an array of medical problems.

DRUG	BRAND NAMES	ACTION	POSSIBLE SIDE EFFECTS
Acetaminophen	Tylenol	Analgesic	Minimal to none
Amantadine	Symmetrel	Antiviral	Swelling of feet, anxiety, compound rigidity and depression, bradykinesia, hallucinations, urinary retention, blotchy legs, insomnia
Amitriptyline	Elavil Emitrip Endep Enovil Etrafon Triavil Limbitrol	Antidepressant	Cardiac effects: high incidence of anticholinergic sedative side effects; sexual dysfunction
Amoxapine	Asendin	Antidepressant	Moderate anticholinergic effects, sexual dysfunction. Only tricyclic known to cause tardive dyskinesia
Aspirin	Anacin Bayer	Antiplatelet	Gastrointestinal disorders, gastrointestinalbleeding, ulcers, tinnitus, dizziness

(continued)

DRUG	BRAND NAMES	ACTION	POSSIBLE SIDE EFFECTS
Baclofen	Lioresal	Antispasticity agent	Sedation, dizziness, nausea, vomiting, constipation, decreased attention and memory, possible liver toxicity
Benztropine	Cogentin	Blocks action of acetylcholine	
Bethanechol	Urecholine	Cholinergic; increases bladder tone	Sweating, hypotension, headache, loose stool
Bisacodyl	Dulcolax	Laxative; stimulates sensory nerve endings in bowel to produce evacuation of stool	Bitter taste, throat irritation, nausea
Bupropion	Wellbutrin	Antidepressant	Blocks reuptake of dopamine
Carbamazepine	Tegretol Epitol Mazepine	Antimanic	Dry mouth and throat; constipation; impaired urination, dizziness, vertigo, sedation, nausea, blurred vision, rash
Carisoprodol	Soma	Muscle relaxant; prevents flexor and extensor spasms	Sedation, insomnia, dizziness weakness, ataxia, confusion, respiratory depression, seizure; sudden withdrawal from chronic use may cause anxiety, tachycardia, and hallucinations
Casanthranol and docusate sodium	Peri-Colace Colace	Mild stimulant laxative combined with stool softener	Nausea, abdominal cramps, diarrhea, rash among rare side effects noted
Choline magnesium trisalicylate	Trilisate	Analgesic Anti-inflammatory	Nausea, vomiting, tinnitus, decreased hearing
Clonazepam	Klonopin Rivotril	Petit mal, atypical petit mal, myoclonic, akinetic seizures; infantile spasm	Drowsiness, lethargy, unsteadiness, increased salivation, ataxia, behavioral disturbances
Clozapine	Clozaril	Reduces psychoses, disorganization, and negative symptoms	Lesions appear in the throat and other mucous membranes, gastrointestinal tract, and skin; weight gain, excessive salivation, especially when beginning the medication. Other side effects are tachycardia, hypotension, fever
Codeine	Empirin Aspirin with codeine	Analgesic	Constipation, diverticulitis, depression, sedation

(continued)

DRUG	BRAND NAMES	ACTION	POSSIBLE SIDE EFFECTS
Cyclobenzaprine	Flexeril	Muscle relaxant; prevents flexor and extensor spasms	Sedation, insomnia, dizziness weakness, ataxia, confusion, respiratory distress, depression, seizure; sudden withdrawal from chronic use may cause anxiety, tachycardia, and hallucination
Dantrolene sodium	Dantrium	Antispasticity agent	Drowsiness, muscle weakness, liver toxicity, gastrointestinal complaints
Desipramine	Norpramin	Antidepressant	Cardiac arrhythmias; less severe anticholinergic and sedative effects than other tricylics
Diazepam	Valium Diastat Zetran	Antispasticity agent	Drowsiness, lethargy, unsteadiness, "hangover effects" the day after bedtime use
Diflunisal	Dolobid	Analgesic Anti-inflammatory	Gastrointestinal distress, severe headache, vertigo, confusion, depression
Diltiazem	Cardizem	Calcium channel blocker Antihypertensive Antianginal	Hypotension, reflex tachycardia, peripheral edema, headache; CNS signs: tremors, mood changes fatigue
Disopyramide	Norpace	Antiarrhythmic	Cardiac decompensation
Docusate sodium	Colace	Laxative: stool softener	Bitter taste, throat irritation, nausea
Doxepin	Sinequan	Antidepressant	Anticholinergic, sedative, orthostatic hypotension effects
Ethosuximide	Zarontin	Petit mal seizures	Drowsiness, lethargy, fatigue, ataxia, irritability, depression, nausea, vomiting, weight loss, cramps
Ethotoin	Peganone	Tonic-clonic or complex partial seizures	Nausea, vomiting, diarrhea
Fenoprofen	Nalfon	Analgesic Anti-inflammatory	Irritation of stomach lining, nausea, heartburn, vomiting, fluid retention
Fluoxetine	Prozac	Antidepressant	Nausea, sexual dysfunction
Fluphenazine	Prolixin Permitil	Antipsychotic	Extrapyramidal side effects contractions, or spasms that involve the neck, jaw, tongue, eyes, and entire body; akathisia, agitation, pacing, restlessness; parkinsonism: motor rigidity, tremor, akinesia, bradykinesia

(continued)

DRUG	BRAND NAMES	ACTION	POSSIBLE SIDE EFFECTS
Fluvoxamine	Luvox	Antidepressant	Gastrointestinal side effects, sexual dysfunction
Gabapentin	Neurontin	Adjunctive treatment of partial seizures	Fatigue, somnolence, dizziness, ataxia, nystagmus, tremor, diplopia, rhinitis
Gold salts	Myochrysine Solganal	Anti-inflammatory (when not responsive to less hazardous medication or when rheumatoid arthritis is severe and rapidly progressing)	Rash, itchy skin, kidney damage, mouth ulcers, nausea, liver damage; usually occur after prolonged use
Haloperidol	Haldol	High potency antipsychotic	Exrapyramidal side effects: dystonia, slow muscle contractions or spasms that involve the neck, jaw, tongue, eyes, and entire body; akathisia, agitation, restlessness, pacing; parkinsonism: motor rigidity, tremor, akinesia, bradykinesia
Heparin sodium	Heparin	Anticoagulant	Thrombocytopenia, increased risk of hemorrhage
Hydralazine hydrochloride	Apresoline	Antihypertensive; appears to lower blood pressure by relaxation of vascular smooth tissue	Headache, anorexia, nausea, vomiting, diarrhea, palpitations, tachycardia angina
Hydromorphone	Dilaudid	Narcotic analgesic	Sedation, physical dependence, gastrointestinal distress, respiratory depression
Ibuprofen	Motrin Rufen Advil	Analgesic Anti-inflammatory	Gastrointestinal effects: irritation of stomach lining, nausea, heartburn, indigestion, fluid retention, aseptic meningitis syndrome; rash
Imipramine	Janimine Norfranil Tipramine Tofranil	Antidepressant	Moderate cardiac and anticholinergic effects; high orthostatic hypotension effects
Indomethacin	Indocin	Analgesic Anti-inflammatory	Irritation of stomach lining: nausea, indigestion, heartburn; headache, dizziness
Isocarboxazid	Marplan	Monoamine oxidase inhibitor	Severe orthostatic hypotension; follow dietary restrictions
Lamotrigine	Lamictal	Antidepressant	Dizziness, headache, ataxia, somnolence, diplopia blurred vision, nausea, vomiting, rhinitis, rash

(continued)

DRUG	BRAND NAMES	ACTION	POSSIBLE SIDE EFFECTS
Levodopa	Sinemet	Replaces/mimics actions of dopamine	Nausea, sleepiness, orthostatic hypotension, involuntary movements, reduced appetite, insomnia, cramping, amblyopia
Lidocaine	Xylocaine	Antiarrhythmic (ventricular)	Disorientation, seizures, hypotension
Lithium Lithium carbonate Lithium citrate	Cibalith-S Eskalith Lithane Lithonate Lithobid Lithotabs	Antimanic	Tremor, gastrointestinal and renal effects; memory loss, weight gain; requires monitoring blood levels
Magnesium hydroxide	Phillips' Milk of Magnesia	Laxative	Possible interaction with prescription drugs; should not be taken if abdominal pain, nausea, vomiting persist
Maprotiline	Ludiomil	Antidepressant	May potentiate seizures
Meclofenamate	Meclomen	Analgesic Anti-inflammatory	Gastrointestinal effects: nausea, diarrhea
Mephenytoin	Mesantoin	Tonic-clonic, simple partial, and complex partial seizures in patients refractory to less toxic anticonvulsants	Drowsiness, rash
Mephobarbital	Mebaral	Anticonvulsant Generalized tonic-clonic or absence seizures	Hangoverlike symptoms
Methsuximide	Celontin	Refractory absence seizures	Nausea, vomiting, anorexia, diarrhea, weight loss, abdominal or epigrastic pain, constipation
Methylpred-nisolone	Medrol	Corticosteroid: anti-inflammatory effect; modifies the body's immune responses to many stimuli	Fluid retention, muscle weakness, osteoporosis, peptic ulcers, convulsions, vertigo, headaches, congestive heart failure, hypertension
Nadolol	Corgard	Beta blocking agent Antihypertensive: angina, some arrhythmias	Bronchospasm, hypotension, drug fever, gastrointestinal disturbances, transient thrombocytopenia, fatigue, sleep disorders
Naproxen	Naprosyn	Analgesic Anti-inflammatory	Gastrointestinal side effects: nausea, indigestion, irritation of stomach lining, heartburn, fluid retention

(continued)

DRUG	BRAND NAMES	ACTION	POSSIBLE SIDE EFFECTS
Nifedipine	Procardia	Calcium channel blocker Antihypertensive	Hypotension, reflex tachy-cardia, peripheral edema, and headache; CNS signs: tremors, mood changes, fatigue
Nimodipine	Nimotop	Vasodilator	Edema, hypotension, angina, dizziness, depression, abdominal cramping, constipation
Nitroglycerin	Nitrostat Nitro-Bid Nitrol Nitro-Dur	Vasodilator	Tachycardia, hypotension, flushing, headache
Oxybutynin chloride	Ditropan	Relaxes spastic bladder	Dry mouth, drowsiness, constipation, blurred vision
Phenobarbital Hyoscyamine sulfate	Donnatol Levsin	Antispasmodic	
Imipramine hydrochloride	Tofranil		
Oxycodone	Percodan Percocet	Analgesic	Depression, sedation
Paroxetine	Paxil	Antidepressant	Gastrointestinal side effects, sexual dysfunction
Penicillamine	Cuprimine	Anti-inflammatory	Rash, protein leakage in urine, decreased production of blood cells, nausea, metal taste in mouth, decreased sense of taste, weakened connective tissue, slowed blood clotting process
Phenobarbital	Cafergot Solfoton Luminal sodium	Generalized motor and partial motor seizures	Mild fatigue, sluggishness, pink to red to brown coloration of urine, drowsiness, lethargy, hangover
Phenacemide	Phenurone	Severe epilepsy refractory to other drugs	Drowsiness, psychic changes, anorexia
Phenoxy-benzamine hydrochloride	Dibenzyline	Relaxes bladder, sphincter/urethra	Hypotension, nasal congestion, gastrointestinal irritation, loose stool
Phensuximide	Milontin	Absence seizures	Drowsiness, nausea, vomiting
Phenelzine	Nardil	Monoamine oxidase inhibitor	Severe orthostatic hypotension effects. Must follow dietary restrictions

(continued)

DRUG	BRAND NAMES	ACTION	POSSIBLE SIDE EFFECTS
Phenytoin	Dilantin	Generalized motor, partial motor, partial complex seizures	Drowsiness; impaired concentration; mental and physical sluggishness, ataxia, slurred speech, mental confusion, decreased coordination, nystagmus, diplopia, gingival hyperplasia, nausea, hirsutism, vomiting
Piroxicam	Feldene	Analgesic Anti-inflammatory	Gastrointestinal symptoms: nausea, stomach lining irritation, heartburn, peptic ulceration, headache, dizziness
Prazosin hydrochloride	Minipress	Antihypertensive; causes a decrease in total peripheral resistance	May cause syncope with lightheadedness, dizziness, tachycardia
Prednisolone Prednisone	Prelone Deltasone	Anti-inflammatory Immunosuppressive	Birth defects, mood changes, increased appetite, fluid retention, infection with bacteria, acne, increased facial and skin hair, easy bruising, stretch marks, calcium loss, cataracts, thinning of the skin, arteriosclerosis; side effects related to dose and duration
Primidone	Mysoline	Partial complex, generalized motor seizures	Drowsiness; impaired concentration; mental and physical sluggishness
Protriptyline	Vivactil	Antidepressant	Low incidence of sedative side effects and orthostatic hypotension; moderate anticholinergic effects
Propantheline bromide	Pro-BanthAne	Antispasmodic	Decreases gastrointestinal motility; headache, drowsiness, dry mouth
Propoxyphene	Darvon compound or Darvocet	Analgesic	Mentally dull feeling, dizziness, headache, sedation, somnolence, paradoxical excitement, rash, gastrointestinal disturbances
Propranolol	Inderal	Beta blocking agent Antihypertensive Angina Migraines	Bronchospasm, hypotension, drug fever, gastrointestinal disturbances, transient thrombocytopenia, fatigue, sleep disorders
Quinidine sulfate	Quinidex	Antiarrhythmic	Severe nausea, diarrhea
Quinidine gluconate	Quinaglute	Antiarrhythmic	Severe nausea, diarrhea
Sertraline	Zoloft	Antidepressant	Gastrointestinal side effects, sexual dysfunction

(continued)

DRUG	BRAND NAMES	ACTION	POSSIBLE SIDE EFFECTS
Sodium bicarbonate	Ceo-Two	Rectal suppository that melts to form CO_2, which builds pressure on the rectum and lower bowel, causing peristalsis or reflex evacuation	
Streptokinase	Kabikinase	Thrombolytic	Intracerebral hemorrhage
Temazepam	Restoril	Sedative	Drowsiness
Tissue plasminogen activator (TPA)	Actilyse Activase	Thrombolytic	Intracerebral hemorrhage
Tolmetin sodium	Tolectin	Analgesic Anti-inflammatory	Gastrointestinal effects: nausea, heartburn, upset stomach, fluid retention
Tranylcypromine	Parnate	Antidepressant	Severe orthostatic hypotension effects. Must follow dietary restrictions
Trazodone	Desyrel Trazon Trialodine	Antidepressant	Sedation
Trimethoprim	Bactrim	Antibacterial	Early signs of serious reactions may include rash, fever, cough, jaundice, arthralgia, shortness of breath, nausea, diarrhea, headaches
Trimipramine	Surmontil	Antidepressant	High incidence of anticholinergic and sedative effects; cardiac effects
Trihexyphenidyl	Artane	Anticholinergic; opposes action of acetylcholine	Tremor, nausea, drooling, vomiting, dry mouth, rigidity confusion, oral motor dysfunction, blurred vision, loss of appetite, depression, hallucinations, constipation, urinary retention
Valproic acid	Depakene Depakote	Antimanic	Gastrointestinal symptoms; remors, hair loss, weight gain
Venlafaxine	Effexor	Antidepressant	Gastrointestinal side effects

REFERENCES

Kaplan HI, Sadock BJ. *Synopsis of Psychiatry*. 8th ed. Baltimore: Williams & Wilkins, 1998.

Karb VB, Queener SF, Freeman JB. *Handbook of Drugs for Nursing Practice*. St Louis: Mosby, 1996.

Physicians' Desk Reference. 53rd ed. Oradell, NJ: Medical Economics, 1999.

INDEX

Page numbers in italics denote figures; those followed by "t" denote tables.

A

Acetaminophen, 349
Acetylated plasminogen-streptokinase complex
    (APSAC), 137
Acetylcholine, Alzheimer's disease and, 101
Activities of daily living, 6, 344–345. See also Occupational
    performance
  chronic pain and, 291
  myocardial infarction and, 155t–156t, 159
  progressive neurological disorders and, 226
  schizophrenia and, 68–69
  spinal cord injury and, 196–197
Adult occupations, 6
Affect, 311
  blunt, 58, 59t, 61, 315
Affective disorders, 311. See also Mood disorders
Afferent, defined, 311
Age
  coronary artery disease and, 151
  depression and, 84, 86
  stroke and, 132
  traumatic brain injury and, 166
Agnosia, 311
  dementia and, 103, 105, 114
  stroke and, 139
  tactile, 311
  visual, 311
Agranulocytosis, 65, 311
Akathisia, 64, 311
Akinesia, 64, 311
Alcoholism. See Substance use/abuse
Allografts, 212, 311
Alogia, 58, 59t, 311
ALS. See Amyotrophic lateral sclerosis
Altruism, 1

Alzheimer's disease, 99–101, 311. See also Dementia
  assessing functional decline in, 104
  case study of, 116–117
  course and prognosis for, 104–105
  diagnosis of, 100, 107
  etiology of, 101
    genetic factors, 101
    neurotransmitter abnormalities, 101
    other potential causes, 101
  impact on occupational performance, 109–114, 110t–113t,
    115t–116t
  neuropathology of, 100–101
    amyloid precursor protein, 100–101
    neurofibrillary tangles, 100
    senile plaques, 100
Amantadine, 349
American Association on Mental Retardation, 46
American Burn Association, 207–208
American College of Rheumatology, 251–252, 252t
American Occupational Therapy Association Uniform
    Terminology, 2–3, 341–348
American Spinal Injury Association Impairment Scale, 187
Amitriptyline, 349
Amnesia, 311–312
  anterograde, 311
  dementia and, 99–100, 103, 109
  electroconvulsive therapy and, 89
  posttraumatic, 168, 169, 311
  retrograde, 168, 312
  stroke and, 130–131
Amoxapine, 349
Amyloid precursor protein, 100–101
Amyotrophic lateral sclerosis (ALS)
  age at onset of, 223
  case study of, 228

course and prognosis for, 223
diagnosis of, 223
impact on occupational performance, 224t–225t, 225–227
incidence and prevalence of, 219
medications for, 225
signs and symptoms of, 219
Analgesics, 288, 312
Anastomosis, 312
Anemia, 312
Aneurysm, 312
  cardiac, 153
  cerebral, 126–127, 138
Aneurysmal bruit, 315
Angina pectoris, 152, 154, 312
Angiography, cerebral, 136
Angioplasty, percutaneous transluminal coronary, 157, *157*, 330
Anhedonia, 58, 59t, 312
Ankle
  ankle-foot orthoses for cerebral palsy, 15
  rheumatoid arthritis of, 245–246, *245–246*
Ankylosis, 312
  bony, 312
  fibrous, 233, 312
  in rheumatoid arthritis, 233, 238
Anomalous, defined, 312
Anomaly, 312
Anomia, 111, 114, 312
Anoxia, 312
Anterior communicating arteries, *123*, 124
Anterior cord syndrome, 185, *185*
Antiadrenergic effects, 64, 312
Antianxiety drugs, 109
Antibodies, 312
  antinuclear, 313
Anticholinergic effects, 64, 313
Anticholinesterase inhibitors, 107–108
Anticoagulants, 136
Antidepressants, 80, 87–88, 313
  classification of, 87
  heterocyclic, 87
  monoamine oxidase inhibitors, 87–88
  for pervasive developmental disorders, 33
  selective serotonin reuptake inhibitors, 88
  time required to experience effects of, 88
  toxicity of, 88
Antigens, 313
  human leukocyte, 232, 325
Antiplatelet therapy, 136–137
Antipsychotic drugs, 313
  clozapine, 64–65
  for dementia, 109
  efficacy of, 65
  newer drugs, 65
  for pervasive developmental disorders, 32–33

risperidone, 65
  for schizophrenia, 63–65
  side effects of, 33, 63–64
    anticholinergic and antiadrenergic effects, 64
    extrapyramidal effects, 64
    neuroleptic malignant syndrome, 64
    sedation, 63–64
Antirheumatic drugs, 253–254
Anxiety, post-myocardial infarction, 158
Aorta, *148*
Aortic valve, *148*
Apathy, 313
Aphasia, 313
  Broca's, 313
  dementia and, 103, 105, 111
  global, 313
  stroke and, 130
  Wernicke's, 313
Apophyseal, defined, 313
Apoplexy, 122, 313
Apraxia, 313
  constructional, 317
  dementia and, 103, 105
  motor, 313
  sensory, 313
  stroke and, 131, 139
  traumatic brain injury and, 168
APSAC. *See* Acetylated plasminogen-streptokinase complex
Arcuate fasciculus, 313
Areflexia, 11, 313
Arrhythmias, 150t, 153, 313
Arteriosclerosis, 151, 152, 314
Arteriovenous, defined, 314
Arteriovenous malformation, 127, 138, 314
Arteritis, 314
Arthralgia, 314
Arthritis, 230, 314
  rheumatoid, 230–259
Arthrodesis, 314
Asperger's disorder, 22, 29, 30. *See also* Pervasive developmental disorders
  communication skills in, 29
  diagnosis of, 29
  historical recognition of, 30
  intelligence in, 30
  signs and symptoms of, 30
Asphyxia, 314
  perinatal, 9
Aspiration, 314
Aspirin, 136–137, 349
Associated reactions, 134, 140–141, 314
Astereognosis, 139, 314
Ataxia, 314
  cerebral palsy and, 11
  Friedreich's, 323

multiple sclerosis and, 220
stroke and, 130
traumatic brain injury and, 168
Atheroma, 125, 126, 314
Atherosclerosis, 124, 125, 132, 301, 314
Athetoid, defined, 314
Athetosis, 11, 13, 314
Atonia, 314
Atria of heart, 148, *148*
Atrial fibrillation, 322
Atrioventricular node, 149
Atrioventricular valves, 148, *148*
Atrophy, 314
Attentional deficit, 3
  schizophrenia and, 58, 59t
  traumatic brain injury and, 168
Auscultation, 314
Autism Diagnostic Interview, 27
Autism Diagnostic Observation Schedule, 27
Autism Society of America, 24, 27, 31, 41
Autistic disorder, 22, 30–31. *See also* Pervasive
    developmental disorders
  age at diagnosis of, 29
  course and prognosis for, 29
  definition of, 29, 31
  derivation of eponym, 23
  diagnosis of, 27, 28, 30–31
  etiology of, 31
  gender distribution of, 31
  Grandin's description of, 22–23
  historical recognition of, 23
  incidence and prevalence of, 31
  macrocephaly and, 25
  mental retardation and, 28, 31, 36
  neuroimaging in, 25, 33
  parents of children with, 27
  range of severity of, 31
  serotonin dysregulation and, 32, 33
  signs and symptoms of, 27–29, 31
  tuberous sclerosis and, 25
Autografts, 211–212, 314
Autoimmune disease, 314
  rheumatoid arthritis, 232–233
Autonomic dysreflexia, 188, 314–315
Autonomic nervous system, 188
Autorelease, 315
Avoidant disorder, 315
Avolition, 58, 59t, 315

B

B cells, 315
Baclofen, 15, 171, 350
Baker's cyst, 244, *244*, 315
Basilar artery, 123, 124

Behavior
  bipolar disorder and, 94
  dementia and, 108–109, 114
  depression and, 83–84
  mental retardation and, 47, 49, 51
  pervasive developmental disorders and, 23, 27, 28
  schizophrenia and, 58
  stroke and, 132
  traumatic brain injury and, 168
Benign, defined, 315
Benztropine, 350
Bethanechol, 350
Binding cleft, 315
Biologic dressing, 315
Bipolar disorders, 76, 92–96. *See also* Mood disorders
  case study of, 95–96
  complications of, 94
  course and prognosis for, 93–94
  diagnosis of, 94
  etiology of, 92
  impact on occupational performance, 90t–91t, 95
  incidence and prevalence of, 92–93
  medical/surgical management of, 94–95
  mood episodes in, 77–78, 77t–79t
  signs and symptoms of, 93
  types of, 76, 78
Bisacodyl, 350
Bladder complications of spinal cord injury, 187, *190*,
    190–191
Blessed Information-Memory-Concentration test, 105
Blessed Orientation-Memory-Concentration test, 105
Bleuler, Eugene, 55, 58
Blood glucose monitoring, 302–303
Blunt affect, 58, 59t, 61, 315
Boutonnière deformity, 238, *238*, 315
Bowel complications of spinal cord injury, 187, *191*,
    191–192
Bradycardia, 154, 315
Bradykinesia, 64, 221, 315
Brain, 176–177, *177*
  blood supply of, 122–124, *123*
Brain disorders
  cerebral palsy, 8–20
  dementia and, 100, 104, 105
  injury, 165–174 (*See also* Traumatic brain injury)
  pervasive developmental disorders and, 24–25
  schizophrenia and, 55–56
  stroke, 121–145
Brainstem stroke, 131
Bronchospasm, 315
Brown-Séquard syndrome, 186, *186*
Bruit, 315
  aneurysmal, 315
  carotid, 133, 315
"Bulge" sign, 244

Bunion, 315
Bupropion, 350
Burns, 205–216
  case studies of, 215–216
  complications of, 212
  depth and severity of, 206–208
    diagnosis of, 208
    full thickness (third degree) burns, 207–208, 323
    minor, moderate, and major burns, 207–208, 208t
    partial thickness (second degree) burns, 206, 207, 330
    superficial (first degree) burns, 206, 336
  estimating size of, 209
    Lund and Browder method, 209, *210*
    rule of nines, 209, *209*
  etiology of, 205
  impact on occupational performance, 212–215, 213t–214t
  incidence and prevalence of, 208
  integumentary system and, 206
  medical/surgical management of, 209–212
    acute stage, 210–212
    emergent stage, 209–210
    rehabilitative stage, 212
    skin grafting, 211–212
    wound care, 211
  mortality from, 205, 210
Bursa, 315
Bursitis, 315
  of shoulder, 242
Buspirone, 109

C

CAD. *See* Coronary artery disease
Calcarine artery, 124
Calcium antagonists, 137
Callositas (callosity), 315
CAPD. *See* Continuous ambulatory peritoneal dialysis
Capillaries, 148
Capsule, 315
  articular, 315
Carbamazepine, 109, 171, 350
Cardiac anatomy, 147–148, *148*
Cardiac circulation, 148–149, *149*
Cardiac conduction system, 148–150, *149, 150*
Cardiac rehabilitation, 155, 155t–156t, 158
Cardiopulmonary resuscitation, 153
Carisoprodol, 350
Carotid arteries, 123, *123*
Carotid bruit, 133, 315
  stroke and, 133
Carotid endarterectomy, 138, 321
Carpal tunnel syndrome, 285, 295, 315
  in rheumatoid arthritis, 240, *241*
Carpometacarpal joints in rheumatoid arthritis, 239
Cartilage, 316
  cricoarytenoid, 318

Casanthranol and docusate sodium, 350
Case management for schizophrenia, 66
Case studies, 3
  bipolar disorder, 95–96
  burns, 215–216
  cerebral palsy, 18–20
  chronic pain, 279, 293–295
  coronary artery disease, 160–161
  fractures, 268, 276–278
  major depression, 91–92
  mental retardation, 42–43, 50–52
  pervasive developmental disorders, 36–39
  progressive neurological disorders, 218, 227–228
  rheumatoid arthritis, 257–258
  schizophrenia, 54, 71–73
  spinal cord injury, 202–203
  stroke, 121, 142–145
  traumatic brain injury, 173–174
Catabolites, 282
Catalepsy, 61, 316
Catastrophic reactions, post–stroke, 141
Catatonia, 61
Catheterization, 316
  urinary, 187, 190
Cauda equina, *177,* 316
  injuries to, 186–187, 193
Cellulitis, 316
Central cervical cord syndrome, 186, *186*
Central nervous system (CNS), 176–181
  dermatome map, *182*
  muscle innervations and functions, 180t–181t
  progressive neurological disorders, 218–229
  reflex arc, 179–181, *183*
  response to pain, 280–282
  in rheumatoid arthritis, 247–248
  sensory and motor tracts, *178,* 178–179, 179t
  spinal cord and spinal nerves, *177,* 177–179
  spinal cord injury, 176–203
  traumatic brain injury, 165–174
Cephalohematoma, 316
Cerebellar arteries, *123,* 123–124
Cerebral aneurysm, 126–127, 138
Cerebral angiography, 136
Cerebral arteries, *123,* 123–124
  anterior cerebral artery stroke, 130
  middle cerebral artery stroke, 129–130
Cerebral atrophy, 56
Cerebral circulation, 122–124, *123*
  communicating arteries, 124
  extracranial vessels, 123
  intracranial vessels, 123–124
Cerebral infarct, 122, 124–126. *See also* Cerebrovascular
    accident
Cerebral palsy, 8–20
  ataxia in, 11
  athetoid, 11, 13

case studies of, 18–20
characteristics of, 8–9
course and prognosis for, 14
definition of, 8
diagnosis of, 8–9, 14
disorders associated with, 13–14
    mental retardation, 13
    seizures, 13
    visual and hearing impairments, 13–14
etiology of, 9–10, 10t
historical recognition of, 8, 9
impact on occupational performance, 15–17, 16t–17t
incidence and prevalence of, 10
medical/surgical management of, 14–15
mixed type, 13
racial distribution of, 10
related to multiple births, 10
signs and symptoms of, 11
spastic, 12–13
    definition of, 11
    diplegia, 12
    hemiplegia, 12
    quadriplegia, 13, 18
types of, 11–12
Cerebral thrombosis, 125
Cerebrospinal fluid evaluation, 127, 136
Cerebrovascular accident (CVA), 121–145
case studies of, 121, 142–145
cerebral circulation and, 122–124, *123*
cerebral palsy and, 9
in children, 128
course and prognosis after, 134
definition of, 122, 316
diagnosis of, 134–136
    invasive procedures, 136
    neuroimaging, 135
    noninvasive procedures, 135–136
etiology of, 122–124, *123* (*See also* Cerebral circulation)
hemorrhagic, 122, 126–127, 324
    due to ruptured aneurysm, 126
    intracerebral hemorrhage, 127
    subarachnoid hemorrhage, 127
historical perspectives on, 122
impact on occupational performance, 138–141, 143t–144t
    cognitive integration, 141
    neuromusculoskeletal and motor components, 139–141
    psychosocial changes, 141
    sensory and perceptual processing, 138–139
incidence and prevalence of, 127–128
ischemic, 122, 124–126, 326
    due to embolism, 126
    due to thrombosis, 125
    lacunar strokes, 125–126, 327
    pathophysiology of, 124–125
medical/surgical management of, 136–138
    anticoagulants, 136

    antiplatelet therapy, 136–137
    cerebral hemorrhage, 137–138
    thrombolysis, 137
neurological effects of, 129–131
anterior cerebral artery stroke, 130
left-sided cerebral injuries: middle cerebral artery, 129–130
right-sided cerebral injuries: middle cerebral artery, 130
vertebrobasilar stroke, 130–131
Wallenberg's syndrome, 131, 338–339
risk factors for, 132–134
secondary complications of, 131–132, 134
    infection, 131
    seizures, 131
    thromboembolism, 131–132
warning signs for, 128–129
    small strokes, 129
    subclavian steal syndrome, 129, 335
    transient ischemic attacks, 126, 128–129, 131–133, 337
Cervical spine in rheumatoid arthritis, 242–243, *243*
Childhood disintegrative disorder, 22, 29, 31. *See also*
    Pervasive developmental disorders
diagnosis of, 31
gender distribution of, 31
prognosis for, 29
Childhood occupations, 6
Chlorpromazine, 64
Choline magnesium trisalicylate, 350
Cholinergic, defined, 316
Cholinergic hypothesis of Alzheimer's disease, 101
Chorioamnionitis, 316
Chronic obstructive pulmonary disease, 316
Circle of Willis, *123*, 124, 316
Circulation
    cardiac, 148–149, *149*
    cerebral, 122–124, *123*
    collateral, 317
Circumflex coronary arteries, 148, 149
Circumlocution, 114, 316
Claw toes, 245
Clinical reasoning procedure, 1
Clomipramine, 33
Clonus, 316
Clozapine, 33, 63–65, 350
CNS. *See* Central nervous system
Cock-up toes, 245, *245*, 316
Codeine, 350
Cognition, 316
    cerebral palsy and, 13
    chronic pain and, 289–290
    depression and, 82–83
    disturbances of, 99–100
        delirium, 99–100, 318–319
        dementia, 98–119
    mental retardation, 42–52
    multiple sclerosis and, 221
    myocardial infarction and, 158

pervasive developmental disorders and, 28, 31, 36
rheumatoid arthritis and, 257
schizophrenia and, 58, 68
stroke and, 141
traumatic brain injury and, 166–168, 167t
Collagen, 316
Colles' fracture, 271–273, *272, 276,* 276–277
Coma, 317
  diabetic, 300, 303
  posttraumatic, 166–168 (*See also* Traumatic brain injury)
Communication
  chronic pain and, 290
  dementia and, 109–114
  pervasive developmental disorders and, 22–23, 27–29, 31, 36
  progressive neurological disorders and, 220, 221, 226
  schizophrenia and, 54, 58
  spinal cord injury and, 197
Complete blood count, 317
Computed tomography (CT), 317
  in amyotrophic lateral sclerosis, 223
  in autism, 25
  in dementia, 56
  in Parkinson's disease, 223
  in schizophrenia, 56
  in stroke, 135
  in traumatic brain injury, 170
Conduction, defined, 317
Conduction system of heart, 148–150, *149, 150*
Conductive, defined, 317
Confabulation, 317
Continuous ambulatory peritoneal dialysis (CAPD), 301, 317
Contractures, 317
  of burn scars, 212
  in cerebral palsy, 12
  due to spinal cord injury, 189
  in rheumatoid arthritis, 238
Contralateral, defined, 317
Contrecoup injury, 165
Conus medullaris, 177
Convergence, 317
Core values of occupational therapy, 1–2
Coronary artery bypass grafting, 157, 317
Coronary artery disease (CAD), 147–164
  cardiac anatomy, circulation, and conduction system and, 147–150, *148–150*
  course and prognosis for, 154
  diagnosis of, 154–155
  etiology of, 151
  impact on occupational performance, 158–160, 162t–163t
  incidence and prevalence of, 151
  medical/surgical management of, 157–158
  mortality from, 151
  pathophysiology of, 152

safe levels of activity for persons with, 155, 155t–156t
signs and symptoms of, 152–154
  angina pectoris, 152
  heart failure, 153
  myocardial infarction, 152–153
  sudden cardiac death, 153
Corpus striatum, 317
Cortical atrophy, 44
Corticospinal pathways, *178,* 179t, 317
Corticosteroids, 137, 193
Corticotropin, 101
Coup injury, 165
Craniostenosis, 44, 317
Creatine phosphokinase, 154
Creatinine, 317
Credé's method, 191, 317–318
Crepitation, 318
Creutzfeldt-Jakob disease, 100, 104, 105
Cricoarytenoid cartilage, 318
Cricoarytenoid joints in rheumatoid arthritis, 242–243
Cryogenic, defined, 318
CT. *See* Computed tomography
Cumulative trauma disorder, 285, 295. See also Pain, chronic
CVA. *See* Cerebrovascular accident
Cyclobenzaprine, 351
Cyclothymic disorder, 76
Cytokines, 318
Cytomegalovirus, 44, 45, 318

D

DAI. *See* Diffuse axonal injury
Dantrolene sodium, 15, 171, 351
Day care for persons with dementia, 109
de Quervain's disease, 239, *239,* 319
Debridement, 211, 318
Decerebrate posturing, 168, 318
Decorticate posturing, 168, 318
Decubitus ulcers, 188, 192, 318
Decussation, 129, 318
Deep tendon reflexes, 318
Deep vein thrombosis (DVT), 318
  myocardial infarction and, 153
  spinal cord injury and, 189
  stroke and, 131–132
Deformity, 318
Delirium, 99–100, 318–319
Delusions, 55, 58, 59t, 60–62, 319
  of grandeur, 61
  of persecution, 61
  of reference, 61
Dementia, 98–119
  caregivers of persons with, 107
  case studies of, 98, 116–118
  causes of death in persons with, 109

compared with delirium, 99–100
course and prognosis for, 104–105
definition of, 99, 319
diagnosis of, 105–107, 106t
etiology of, 100–101, 102t
  Alzheimer's disease, 99–101, 116–117
  medical conditions, 99, 101, 102t
  substance abuse, 99
  vascular dementia, 99, 101, 118
impact on occupational performance, 109–114
  in confusional phase, 111–114, 112t–113t
  in dementia phase, 114, 115t–116t
  in early or forgetful phase, 109–111, 110t–111t
incidence and prevalence of, 101–102
Lewy body, 107
medical/surgical management of, 107–109
  behavior management, 108–109
  environmental management, 109
  long-term care facilities, 109
  medications, 107–109
multi-infarct, 99
neuroimaging in, 105
praecox, 55 (*See also* Schizophrenia)
pugilistic, 104
screening elderly persons for, 107
senile, 99
signs and symptoms of, 103–104
Demyelination, 319
Depolarization, 149–150, 319
Depressive disorders, 76, 79–92. *See also* Mood disorders
case study of, 91–92
course and prognosis for, 86–87
dementia and, 111
depressive pseudodementia, 86, 107
diagnosis of, 87
economic costs of, 76
etiology of, 79–84
  behavioral theories, 83–84
  biological theories, 80–81
  cognitive theory, 82–83
  genetic factors, 81
  problems in research on, 80
  psychosocial theories, 81–82
  seasonal disorders, 81
impact on occupational performance, 89, 90t–91t
incidence and prevalence of, 84
major depressive episode, 77–78, 77t
medical/surgical management of, 87–89
  electroconvulsive therapy, 88–89
  medications, 80, 87–88 (*See also* Antidepressants)
  psychotherapy, 89
post-myocardial infarction, 158
post-stroke, 141
rheumatoid arthritis and, 249
signs and symptoms of, 77t, 85–86

sleep disruptions and, 81
substance abuse and, 87
suicide and, 81, 85–87
types of, 76
Dermatome map, 182
Dermis, 206, 319
Desipramine, 351
Diabetes mellitus (DM), 298–309
case studies of, 306–309, 307t–308t
complications of, 300–301
  atherosclerosis, 151, 301
  diabetic foot, 301, 319
  diabetic ketoacidosis, 300, 319
  diabetic nephropathy, 300–301
  diabetic neuropathy, 301
  diabetic retinopathy, 300
  hyperglycemia, 300
  hypoglycemia or insulin shock, 300
course and prognosis for, 299–300
definition of, 298, 319
diagnosis of, 301
dialysis for, 301
etiology of, 298
gestational diabetes, 323
iatrogenic diabetes, 325
impact on occupational performance, 303–306, 304t–305t, 307t–308t
incidence and prevalence of, 299
insulin-dependent (type I), 298, 302, 306–309
medical/surgical management of, 302–303
non-insulin-dependent (type II), 298, 302–303
signs and symptoms of, 298
stroke and, 133
Diagnostic and Statistical Manual of Mental Disorders (DSM-IV)
dementia in, 99, 105
mood disorders in, 76–79, 77t–79t, 85, 94
pervasive developmental disorders in, 22, 29
schizophrenia in, 60–61
Dialysis, 301
Diaphoresis, 319
Diastole, 319
Diazepam, 171, 351
Diffuse, defined, 319
Diffuse axonal injury (DAI), 166, 319
Diflunisal, 351
Dignity, 1–2
Diltiazem, 351
Diplegia, 12, 319
Dislocation, 319
Disopyramide, 351
Disorder, 319
Distal interphalangeal joints in rheumatoid arthritis, 238
DM. *See* Diabetes mellitus
Docusate sodium, 351

Donepezil hydrochloride, 107–108
Donor site for skin grafting, 211, 319
Dopamine, 319
Doppler ultrasound, 135–136
Down syndrome, 27, 42–44, 46, 49–51, 338. *See also* Mental retardation
Doxepin, 351
Drop attacks, 131
Drug addiction. *See* Substance use/abuse
Duchenne muscular dystrophy, 45
Duplex scanning, 135
DVT. *See* Deep vein thrombosis
Dysarthria, 320
  dementia and, 114
  progressive neurological disorders and, 220, 221, 226
  spastic quadriplegia and, 13
  stroke and, 130, 141
Dysesthesia, 220, 320
Dyskinesia, 11, 13, 320
  tardive, 33, 64, 336
Dysmetria, 130, 320
Dysphagia, 320
  amyotrophic lateral sclerosis and, 221
  multiple sclerosis and, 220
  stroke and, 131, 141
Dysphasia, conduction, 313
Dyspnea, 153, 320
Dyspraxia, 320
Dysthymic disorders, 76
Dystonia, 64, 320

E

EBV. *See* Epstein–Barr virus
ECG. *See* Electrocardiogram
Echolalia, 28, 61, 320
Echopraxia, 61, 320
ECT. *See* Electroconvulsive therapy
Ectopic, defined, 320
Ectopic bone, 189–190, 320
Edema, 320
  cerebral, 137
  pedal, 330
Edward's syndrome, 338
EEG. *See* Electroencephalogram
Efferent, defined, 320
Effusion, 320
Elastin, 320
Elbow
  in rheumatoid arthritis, 241
  "tennis," 241, 288
Electrocardiogram (ECG), *149*, 149–150
  arrhythmias on, 150t, 153
Electroconvulsive therapy (ECT)
  for depression, 88–89

  memory loss and, 89
  procedure for, 89
  for schizophrenia, 65
Electroencephalogram (EEG), 136, 223, 320
Electrolyte depletion, 320
Electromyogram (EMG), 320
Embolism, 320
  cerebral, 126, 131–132
  pulmonary, 153
EMG. *See* Electromyogram
Emotions. *See also* Mood disorders
  post-myocardial infarction, 158
  post-stroke lability of, 141
Emphysema, 321
Encephalitis, 321
  cerebral palsy and, 9
  mental retardation and, 46
Encephalopathy, 8
  static, 335
Endarterectomy, 138, 321
Endocardium, 148, 321
Endomysium, 321
Endotracheal, defined, 321
Endotracheal tube, 321
Environmental factors
  falls related to, 270
  mental retardation and, 45–46
  progressive neurological disorders and, 219
Epicardium, 321
Epidemiology, 321
Epidermis, 206, 321
Epilepsy, 321. *See also* Seizures
Episcleritis, 321
Episode, 321
  mood, 77–78, 328
Epstein-Barr virus (EBV), 231, 232, 321
Equality, 2
Equilibrium reactions, 321
Equinovalgus, 321
Equinovarus, 321
Erythema, 321
Erythrocyte sedimentation rate, 321
Eschar, 211, 322
Escharotomy, 322
Ethosuximide, 351
Ethotoin, 351
Euphoria, 322
Evoked potentials, 322
Exacerbation, 322
Executive functioning, 322
  dementia and, 103, 105
  traumatic brain injury and, 168
Exercise
  diabetes mellitus and, 302
  post-myocardial infarction, 155t–156t
Existentialism, 82, 322

Extrapyramidal effects, 64, 322
Extravasation, 322
Eye involvement in rheumatoid arthritis, *248*, 248–249

F

Fabulation, 317
Falls, 268–271
  disorders associated with, 270
  environmental factors and, 270
  fractures due to, 268–271
  medication-related, 270
Fasciculus, 178, *178*, 322
Fasciotomy, 322
FAST. *See* Functional Assessment Staging Scale
Fasting blood sugar test, 301, 322
Felty's syndrome, 247, 322
Fenfluramine, 33
Fenoprofen, 351
FES. *See* Functional electrical stimulation
Fibrillation, 322
  atrial, 322
  ventricular, 322
Fibrosis, 322
"Fight-or-flight" response, 188
Figure ground, 322
Finkelstein's test, *239*
Fistula, 322
Flaccidity, 139, 322
Fluid management for burned patients, 210
Fluoxetine, 33, 88, 351
Fluphenazine, 63, 64, 351
Fluvoxamine, 352
Focal, defined, 322
Foot
  ankle-foot orthoses for cerebral palsy, 15
  diabetic, 301, 319
  foot drop, 221
  in rheumatoid arthritis, 245–246, *245–246*
Form constancy, 322
Fountain House, 66
4AP, 193
Fractures, 268–278
  among elderly persons, 268–270
  case studies of, 268, 276–278
  Colles', 271–273, *272*, 276, *276–277*
  complications of, 271–273
    delayed union, 271
    healing time, 271
    malunion, 271
    nonunion, 271
    osteodystrophy, 272–273
  course and prognosis for, 271–273
  definition of, 268
  diagnosis of, 273

  etiology of, 270–271
  hip, 268, 271, 273, 277–278
  impact on occupational performance, 274–276, *275t–276t*
  incidence and prevalence of, 271
  medical/surgical management of, 273–274
    medications, 274
    reduction and fixation, 273
    open versus closed, 271
    signs and symptoms of, 271
    spontaneous, 270
Fragile X syndrome, 44, 45, 322–323
Framingham Heart Study, 132, 151
Freedom, 2
Freud, Sigmund, 8, 9
Friedreich's ataxia, 323
Functional Activities Questionnaire, 105
Functional Assessment Staging Scale (FAST), 104
Functional electrical stimulation (FES), 193
Functional unit, 323
Fusiform, defined, 323

G

Gabapentin, 352
Gangrene, 323
GCS. *See* Glasgow coma scale
"Gel phenomenon," 237
Genetic factors
  in Alzheimer's disease, 101
  in bipolar disorder, 92
  in depression, 81
  in mental retardation, 44–45
    chromosomal aberrations, 45
    single gene disorders, 44–45, 45t
  in pervasive developmental disorders, 24, 26–27
  in progressive neurological disorders, 219
  in rheumatoid arthritis, 232, 233
  in schizophrenia, 56–57
Genetic markers, 323
Gestational diabetes, 323
Glasgow coma scale (GCS), 168–169, 169t
Glasgow outcome scale (GOS), 169
Glycerol, 137
GM-1 ganglioside, 193
Gold salts, 352
GOS. *See* Glasgow outcome scale
Grandin, Temple, 22–23
Granulation tissue, 323
Granulocytopenia, 323
Granulomatous, defined, 323
Granulomatous aortitis, 323
Graphesthesia, 323
Graphomotor, 323
Group therapy for schizophrenia, 66
Gunshot wounds, 166

H

Haemophilus influenzae, 46, 323
Hallucinations, 55, 58, 59t, 60–62, 323–324
Hallux valgus, 245, *245–246,* 324
Haloperidol, 33, 63, 64, 352
Hammer toe, 245, 324
Hand
   fractures of, 271
   in rheumatoid arthritis, 238–240, *238–240*
Handedness, pervasive developmental disorders and, 26
Head
   involvement in rheumatoid arthritis, 242–243
   traumatic brain injury, 165–174
Health maintenance, spinal cord injury and, 197
Hearing impairment, cerebral palsy and, 13–14
Heart. *See also* Coronary artery disease; Myocardial infarction
   anatomy of, 147–148, *148*
   arteries of, 148–149, *149*
   conduction system of, 148–150, *149, 150*
   "pacemaker" of, 149
   in rheumatoid arthritis, 247
   transplantation of, 157–158
Heart failure, 153
Heart rate, 154
Heller's syndrome. *See* Childhood disintegrative disorder
Hematoma, 324
   cerebral, 127, 138
   subdural, 104, 105
Hemianesthesia, 129, 324
Hemianopsia, 324
   homonymous, 130, 139, 324
Hemiparesis, 130, 324
Hemiplegia, 324
   cerebral palsy and, 12
   flaccid, 139
   spastic, 12, 139
   stroke and, 130, 139–141
Hemodialysis, 301, 324
Hemoglobin, 324
Hemorrhage, 324
   intracerebral, 127, 137–138
   subarachnoid, 122, 127, 136, 138, 335
Hemorrhagic stroke, 122, 126–127, 324
Heparin sodium, 136, 352
Herpes simplex virus II, 324
Heterotopic ossification, 189–190, 324
Hip
   fracture of, 268, 271, 273, 277–278
   in rheumatoid arthritis, 243–244, *244*
HLA. *See* Human leukocyte antigens
Homelessness, 59–60
Homografts, 212, 311, 324
Horner's syndrome, 131, 325
Human Genome Project, 25
Human immunodeficiency virus (HIV) infection, 100

Human leukocyte antigens (HLA), 232, 325
Hunter's syndrome, 45, 325
Huntington's disease, 100, 101, 104, 105
Hydralazine hydrochloride, 352
Hydrocephalus, 325
   dementia and, 100, 101, 105
   mental retardation and, 44
   traumatic brain injury and, 170
Hydromorphone, 352
Hypercalcemia, 104
Hypercholesterolemia, 151
Hyperemia, 125, 325
Hyperglycemia, 299, 300, 303, 325.
      See also Diabetes mellitus
Hyperlipidemia, 325
Hypermobility, 325
Hypernatremia, 325
Hyperphenylalaninemia, 44, 325
Hyperreflexia, 11, 188, 314–315
Hypertension, 126, 132, 325
Hyperthermia, 325
Hyperthyroidism, 100
Hypertonicity, 325
   amyotrophic lateral sclerosis and, 221
   cerebral palsy and, 11
   stroke and, 139–140
   traumatic brain injury and, 168
Hypertrophic scar, 212, 325
Hypertrophy, defined, 325
Hypoglycemia, 104, 300, 325
Hypomanic episode, 78, 79t, 94. *See also* Bipolar disorders;
      Mood disorders
Hypotension, 325
   postural, 188
Hypothyroidism, 104, 325
Hypotonicity, 322
   cerebral palsy and, 11, 19
   stroke and, 139
Hypovolemic shock, 210
Hypoxia, 325
   perinatal, 9, 46

I

Ibuprofen, 352
Imipramine, 352
Immigration, schizophrenia and, 57
Immune response, 325
Immune system, 325
Immunosuppressants, 326
Immunosuppression, 326
Impulsion, 326
Impulsive, defined, 326
Incontinence, 141, 326
Indomethacin, 352
Infant occupations, 6

Infarct, 326
Infarction, 326
    cerebral, 122, 124–126
    myocardial, 151
Infection
    burns and, 211
    cerebral palsy and, 9
    dementia and, 104
    mental retardation and, 44–46
    pervasive developmental disorders and, 26
    progressive neurological disorders and, 219
    schizophrenia and, 57
    stroke and, 131
Inflammation, 326
    of joints in rheumatoid arthritis, 233, 236–237, 237t (*See also* specific joints)
Injuries
    cerebral palsy and, 9
    cumulative trauma disorder, 285
    fractures, 268–278
    mental retardation and, 46
    spinal cord injury, 176–203
    traumatic brain injury, 165–174
Insulin, 298–299, 326
Insulin therapy, 302–303
Integumentary system, 206, 207
International Statistical Classification of Diseases and Related Health Problems (ICD-10)
    mood disorders in, 78
    pervasive developmental disorders in, 29
Intima, 152, 326
Intracerebral hemorrhage
    stroke and, 127
    treatment of, 137–138
Intracranial pressure elevation, 127
Intracranial radiation, 100
Intrauterine, defined, 326
Ipsilateral, defined, 326
Ischemia, 326
ischemic stroke, 122, 124–126, 326
    myocardial, 152
    partially reversible ischemic neurological deficit, 330
    reversible ischemic neurological deficit, 129, 333
    soft tissue pain due to, 282
    transient ischemic attacks, 126, 128–129, 131–133, 337
Isocarboxazid, 352
Isoenzymes, 154, 326

J
Jaundice, 326
Joints, 326
    anatomy of, 231, 231
    in rheumatoid arthritis, 230–259, 232
JRA. *See* Juvenile rheumatoid arthritis
Justice, 2

Juvenile rheumatoid arthritis (JRA), 233–235, 326. *See also* Rheumatoid arthritis
    course and prognosis for, 249
    diagnosis of, 233, 234t, 252
    eye involvement in, 248, 248–249, 249t
    pauciarticular, 235, 235t
    polyarticular, 235, 235t
    prevalence of, 236
    resources about, 262–267
    signs and symptoms of, 237
    systemic, 235, 235t
Juxta–articular, defined, 326

K
Keloid, 326
Keratoconjunctivitis, 326
Kernicterus, 326–327
Ketoacidosis, diabetic, 300, 319
Ketones, 298
Ketosis, 327
Kinesiology, 327
Kinesthesia, 327
Knee in rheumatoid arthritis, 244, 244–245
Kraepelin, Emil, 55, 58
Kyphosis, 327

L
Labeling people, 2
Lability, 327
    emotional, 141
Lactic dehydrogenase, 154
Lacuna, 327
Lacunar stroke, 122, 125–126, 327
Lag phenomenon, 327
Lamotrigine, 352
Language usage, 2–3
    person-first, 2
    Uniform Terminology for Occupational Therapy, 2–3, 341–348
Lateral epicondylitis, 241, 288
Lateral medullary syndrome, 131
Left anterior descending artery, 148, 149
Leisure activities, 6, 346. *See also* Occupational performance
    chronic pain and, 291
    myocardial infarction and, 160
    progressive neurological disorders and, 227
    schizophrenia and, 69
    spinal cord injury and, 202
Lemniscus, 178, 327
Lesch-Nyhan syndrome, 45, 327
Leukocyte, 327
Leukopenia, 327
Levodopa, 353
Lidocaine, 353

Ligament, 327
  capsular, 327
Limbic system in schizophrenia, 56–57
Lipohyalinosis, 126, 327
Listeria, 327
Lithium, 94–95, 353
Lordosis, 327
Low back pain, 279, 285, 293–295. *See also* Pain, chronic
Low birth weight, mental retardation and, 45–46
Lower extremity bones and joints, *269*
Lower motor neuron injury, 185, *185*
Loxapine, 64
Lumbar puncture, 127, 136
Lymph nodes, 327
Lymphocytes, 327
  B, 315
  T, 232–233, 336

M

Macrocephaly, 25
Magnesium hydroxide, 353
Magnetic resonance imaging (MRI), 327
  in amyotrophic lateral sclerosis, 223
  in autism, 25, 33
  in dementia, 105
  in multiple sclerosis, 223
  in Parkinson's disease, 223
  in stroke, 135
Malingering, 283
Mallet finger deformity, 328
Managed care, 258
Manic episode, 76, 77, 78t, 92–96. *See also* Bipolar disorders; Mood disorders
Mannitol, 137
MAOIs. *See* Monoamine oxidase inhibitors
Maprotiline, 353
Meclofenamate, 353
Medications, 349–356
for bipolar disorder, 94–95
  for cerebral palsy, 15
  for chronic pain, 287–288
  for coronary artery disease, 157
  for dementia, 107–109
  for depression, 80, 87–88
  for diabetes mellitus, 302–303
  falls related to, 270
  for fractures, 274
  for pervasive developmental disorders, 32–33
  for progressive neurological disorders, 223
  for rheumatoid arthritis, 253, 253–254
  for schizophrenia, 63–65
  for spinal cord injury, 193
  for stroke, 136–138
  for traumatic brain injury, 171

Memory impairment. *See* Amnesia
Meningitis, 9, 46, 328
Mental illness
  dementia, 98–119
  mental retardation and, 47
  mood disorders, 75–96
  pervasive developmental disorders, 22–39
  schizophrenia, 54–73
Mental retardation (MR), 42–52
  autism and, 28, 31, 36
  case studies of, 42–43, 50–52
  cerebral palsy and, 13
  classifications of, 47
  conditions associated with, 46
  course and prognosis for, 49
  definition of, 46, 328
  diagnosis of, 43, 46–47, 49
  Down syndrome, 42–44, 46, 49–51
  etiology of, 43–46
    environmental factors, 45–46
    genetic factors, 44–45, 45t
  impact on occupational performance, 50
  incidence and prevalence of, 46
  levels of, 47, 48t
  medical/surgical management of, 49
  mental illness and, 47
  misconceptions about people with, 47
  signs and symptoms of, 46–47
Mephenytoin, 353
Mephobarbital, 353
Mesencephalon, 328
Mesh graft, 211, 328
Metabolic acidosis, 328
Metabolic equivalent (MET) levels for activities, 155, 155t–156t
Metacarpophalangeal joints in rheumatoid arthritis, 239, 240
Metatarsophalangeal joints in rheumatoid arthritis, 245, *245*
Methsuximide, 353
Methylphenidate, 33
Methylprednisolone, 193, 353
MI. *See* Myocardial infarction
Mini-Mental State Exam (MMSE), 104, 105
Mitral valve, 148, *148*
MMSE. *See* Mini-Mental State Exam
Mobility, functional
  progressive neurological disorders and, 226
  spinal cord injury and, 200
Monoamine oxidase inhibitors (MAOIs), 87–88
Mononeuritis multiplex, 328
Monozygotic twin, 328
Mood, defined, 328
Mood disorders, 75–96
  bipolar disorders, 92–96
  case studies of, 75
  classification of, 76–79

compared with normal mood variations, 76
continuum of, 78
depressive disorders, 79–92
economic costs of, 76
misconceptions about, 76
mood episodes, 77–78, 328
    hypomanic episode, 78, 79t
    major depressive episode, 77–78, 77t
    manic episode, 77, 78t
    mixed episode, 77, 79t
multiple sclerosis and, 221
post-stroke, 141
terminology for, 78
Morning stiffness, 237, 328
Mortality
    coronary artery disease and, 151–153
    dementia and, 109
    schizophrenia and, 59
Motor vehicle accidents
    fractures due to, 270
    spinal cord injury due to, 183, *183,* 184
    traumatic brain injury due to, 165, 166
Movement abnormalities
    antipsychotic-induced, 64
    cerebral palsy and, 11
    Parkinson's disease and, 64, 221
    post-myocardial infarction, 158
    spinal cord injury and, 188, 189
    stroke and, 139–141
    traumatic brain injury and, 168
MR. *See* Mental retardation
MRI. *See* Magnetic resonance imaging
MS. *See* Multiple sclerosis
Mucopolysaccharidosis, 328
Multiple sclerosis (MS)
    age at diagnosis of, 222
    case studies of, 218, 227
    course and prognosis for, 222
    dementia and, 104, 105
    diagnosis of, 223
    etiology of, 219
    impact on occupational performance, 224t–225t, 225–227
    incidence and prevalence of, 219
    medications for, 225
    signs and symptoms of, 218, 220–221, 220t
Mural thrombus, 328
Muscle(s), 328
    innervation and functions of, 180t–181t
    in rheumatoid arthritis, 246
    tone abnormalities of, 322, 325
        in amyotrophic lateral sclerosis, 221
        in cerebral palsy, 11
        due to spinal cord injury, 188
        due to stroke, 139–140
        due to traumatic brain injury, 168

    trigger points in, 282
    weakness of, in progressive neurological disorders, 220, 221
Muscular dystrophy, 328
Mutilans deformity, 240, *240*
Myalgia, 328
Myelin, 328
Myelogram, 328
Myelography, 328
Myocardial contraction, 149
Myocardial infarction (MI), 147, 152–153. *See also* Coronary
    artery disease
    angina and, 153
    arrhythmias and, 153
    case studies of, 160–161
    diagnosis of, 154
    heart failure and, 153
    heart structural damage and, 153
    impact on occupational performance, 158–160, 162t–163t
        activities of daily living, 159
        cognitive function, 158
        leisure activities, 160
        neuromuscular and motor performance, 158
        psychosocial skills and psychological effects, 158–159
        work, 159–160
    medical/surgical management of, *157,* 157–158
    mortality from, 151
    risk factors for, 151
    safe levels of activity after, 155, 155t–156t
    serum enzyme levels and, 154
    silent, 153
    thromboembolic disorders and, 153
Myocardium, 148, 328
Myoclonus, 168, 328
Myofascial pain, 282
Myositis, 328

N

Nadolol, 353
Naproxen, 353
Neck in rheumatoid arthritis, 242–243, *243*
Necrosis, 329
Neologism, 329
Nephrectomy, 329
Nephropathy, 329
    diabetic, 300–301
Nerves. *See also* Central nervous system; Peripheral nervous
    system
    in rheumatoid arthritis, 247–248
    spinal, 177, 177–179
Neuroendocrine, defined, 329
Neurofibrillary tangles, 100, 329
Neurogenic bowel/bladder, 187, *190,* 190–192, *191*
    nonreflex, 329
    reflex, 333

Neuroimaging
in amyotrophic lateral sclerosis, 223
in autism, 25, 33
in dementia, 105
in multiple sclerosis, 223
in Parkinson's disease, 223
in schizophrenia, 55–56
in stroke, 135
in traumatic brain injury, 170
Neuroleptic malignant syndrome, 64
Neuroleptics, 329. *See also* Antipsychotic drugs
Neurologist, 329
Neuromyopathy, 329
Neuropathy, 329
diabetic, 301
peripheral, 329
Neurotransmitters, 329
in Alzheimer's disease, 101
in depression, 80–81
in pain response, 280–281
Neutropenia, 329
Nifedipine, 354
Nimodipine, 137, 354
Nitroglycerin, 354
Nitrosamines, 329
Nociception, 280
Norepinephrine, 329
Alzheimer's disease and, 101
depression and, 80
Nutrition and diet
dementia and, 114
diabetes mellitus and, 302
monoamine oxidase inhibitors and, 88
pervasive developmental disorders and, 25–26
Nystagmus, 329

O

Obesity
coronary artery disease and, 151
stroke and, 132
Obsessive-compulsive disorder, 329
Obstetric factors
cerebral palsy and, 9
mental retardation and, 46
schizophrenia and, 57
Occupational dysfunction, 6–7
Occupational performance
bipolar disorder and, 90t–91t, 95
burns and, 212–215, 213t–214t
cerebral palsy and, 16t–17t
chronic pain and, 288–291, 292t–293t
coronary artery disease and, 158–160, 162t–163t
dementia and, 109–114, 110t–113t, 115t–116t
depression and, 89, 90t–91t
diabetes mellitus and, 303–306, 304t–305t, 307t–308t

fractures and, 274–276, 275t–276t
mental retardation and, 50
pervasive developmental disorders and, 33–36, 34t–35t
rheumatoid arthritis and, 254–257, 255t–256t
schizophrenia and, 68–69, 70t–71t
spinal cord injury and, 194–202, 194t–195t
stroke and, 138–141, 143t–144t
traumatic brain injury and, 171, 171t–172t
Occupational performance profile, 3–5, 4t–5t
Occupational therapy
core values of, 1–2
definition of, 344
services included in, 344
uniform terminology for, 2–3, 341–348
Occupation(s), 5–6
definition of, 5
developmental aspects of, 6
functions of, 6
of infant, child, and adult, 6
Olanzapine, 65
Opera glass hand, 240, *240*
Ophthalmic artery, 123, *123*
Ophthalmic involvement in rheumatoid arthritis, *248*, 248–249
Ophthalmologist, 329
Optic neuritis, 329
Oral contraceptives, stroke and, 133
Organization of book, 3–5
Orthopaedics, 268–278. *See also* Fractures
lower extremity bones and joints, *269*
Orthopaedist, 330
Orthosis, 330
Orthostatic hypotension, 188
Orthostatic intolerance, 330
Orthotics, 15, 330
Osmotic agents, 137–138, 330
Ossification, heterotopic, 189–190, 324
Osteoarthritis, 330
Osteodystrophy, 272–273
Osteoporosis, 270, 271
"Overlap syndrome," 252
Oxybutynin chloride, 354
Oxycodone, 354

P

P wave, 149, *149*
Pain
acute, 280
anatomy and physiology of, 280–281
compared with chronic pain, 284t
anginal, 152, 154
chronic, 279–296
among elderly persons, 285
case studies of, 279, 293–295
compared with acute pain, 284t

cumulative trauma disorder, 285, 295
   definition of, 280
   diagnosis of, 287
   drug dependency due to, 287
   economic costs of, 284, 285
   etiology of, 280
   impact on occupational performance, 288–291, 292t–293t
   incidence and prevalence of, 284–285
   low back pain, 279, 285, 293–295
   malingering and, 283
   medical/surgical management of, 287–288
   pathology of, 281–282
   psychology of, 282–284, *283*
   secondary gains from, 284
   signs and symptoms of, 286–287, 286t
  components to, 280
  definition of, 280
  of fracture, 271
  "gate theory" of, 281
  myofascial, 282
  referred, 282
  reflex sympathetic dystrophy, 333
  of rheumatoid arthritis, 236
  soft tissue, 282
  types of, 280
Pancreas, 330
Pannus, 233, *233*, 330
Papillary muscles, *148*
Paradigm, 330
Paranoid schizophrenia, 61, 71, 72
Paraphasia, 114, 330
Paraplegia, 187, 330
Paresthesia, 220, 330
Parkinsonism, 64, 330
Parkinson's disease
  age at diagnosis of, 222
  case study of, 227–228
  course and prognosis for, 222–223
  dementia and, 100, 101, 104
  diagnosis of, 223
  etiology of, 219
  impact on occupational performance, 224t–225t, 225–227
  incidence and prevalence of, 219
  medications for, 225
  signs and symptoms of, 218–219, 221, 221t
Paroxetine, 354
Partially reversible ischemic neurological deficits (PRIND), 330
Patau's syndrome, 337
PDD. *See* Pervasive developmental disorders
Penicillamine, 354
Penumbra, 125, 330
Perception, 330
Percutaneous transluminal coronary angioplasty (PTCA), 157, *157,* 330
Performance areas, 2–3, 4t, 344–346
Performance components, 3, 4t–5t, 346–347

Performance contexts, 3, 4t, 347–348
Pericarditis, rheumatoid arthritis and, 247
Peripheral nervous system, 176, 178
Peripheral neuropathy, 329
  diabetic, 301
  in rheumatoid arthritis, 247–248
Peristalsis, 331
Peritonitis, 331
Periventricular leukomalacia, 9, 331
Perphenazine, 64
Perseveration, 168, 331
Person-activity-environment fit, 33, 343–344
Person-first language, 2
Personality disorders, 331
Pervasive developmental disorders (PDD), 22–39
  Asperger's disorder, 30
  autistic disorder, 30–31
  case studies of, 36–39
  childhood disintegrative disorder, 31
  classification of, 22, 29
  course and prognosis for, 29
  diagnosis of, 26, 27, 29–30
  etiology of, 23–26
    brain morphology, 24–25
    developmental factors, 24
    genetic factors, 24, 26–27
    multiple causes, 26
    nutrition, 25–26
  gender distribution of, 26
  Grandin's description of, 22–23
  historical recognition of, 23
  impact on occupational performance, 33–36, 34t–35t
  incidence and prevalence of, 26–27
  institutionalization of persons with, 26–27
  medical/surgical management of, 32–33
  not otherwise classified, 22, 29, 31–32
  parents of children with, 27
  resources about, 41
  Rett's disorder, 32
  schizophrenia and, 61
  screening for, 30
  signs and symptoms of, 27, 29
PET. *See* Positron emission tomography
Phenacemide, 354
Phenelzine, 354
Phenobarbital, 171, 354
Phenoxybenzamine hydrochloride, 354
Phensuximide, 354
Phenylbutazone, 354
Phenylketonuria, 45
Phenytoin, 171, 355
Phototherapy for seasonal depression, 81
Pica, 331
Pick's disease, 100, 101, 104
Piroxicam, 355
Placenta previa, 331

Plaques, 331
  atherosclerotic, 125, 152
  senile, 100, 331
Pleuritis, 331
PNDs. *See* Progressive neurological disorders
Pneumonitis, 331
Poikilothermy, 189, 331
Polycythemia, 133, 331
Polydipsia, 299, 331
Polymyositis, 331
Polyphagia, 299, 331
Polyuria, 299, 331
Position in space, 331
Positron emission tomography (PET), 332
  in autism, 33
  in Parkinson's disease, 223
  in schizophrenia, 55
  in stroke, 135
Posterior communicating arteries, *123*, 123–124
Postural abnormalities
  cerebral palsy and, 11
  chronic pain and, 289
  Parkinson's disease and, 221
  traumatic brain injury and, 168, 170
Postural hypotension, 188
PR interval, *149*, 150
Prazosin, 355
Prednisolone, 355
Prednisone, 355
Pressure sores, 188, 192, 318
Primidone, 355
PRIND. *See* Partially reversible ischemic neurological
    deficits
Problem identification, 1
Program for Assertive Community Treatment, 66
Progressive neurological disorders (PNDs), 218–229
  case studies of, 218, 227–228
  course and prognosis for, 222–223
  diagnosis of, 223
  etiology of, 219
  impact on occupational performance, 224t–225t,
    225–227
    activities of daily living, 226
    play and leisure, 227
    work, 226–227
  incidence and prevalence of, 219–220
  medical/surgical management of, 223–225
  signs and symptoms of, 220–221, 220t–222t
Propantheline bromide, 355
Propoxyphene, 355
Propranolol, 109, 355
Proprioception, 332
  chronic pain and, 289
  stroke and, 129, 138
Protriptyline, 355

Proximal interphalangeal joints in rheumatoid arthritis, 238,
    238, 240
Prudence, 2
Psychodynamic theories, 332
  of depression, 81–82
Psychology of chronic pain, 282–284, *283*
Psychomotor agitation, 332
Psychosis, 54–73, 332. *See also* Schizophrenia
Psychosocial effects, 347
  of burns, 214
  of chronic pain, 290
  of depression, 81–82
  of myocardial infarction, 158–159
  of pervasive developmental disorders, 22–23, 28, 36
  of progressive neurological disorders, 226
  of rheumatoid arthritis, 257
  of schizophrenia, 67
  of spinal cord injury, 197
  of stroke, 141
Psychotherapy
  for depression, 89
  for schizophrenia, 66
Psychotic disorder, 332
Psychotropic drugs, 332
PTCA. *See* Percutaneous transluminal coronary
    angioplasty
Ptosis, 332
Pulmonary artery, *148*
Pulmonary complications
  of rheumatoid arthritis, 247
  of spinal cord injury, 189
Pulmonary embolism, 132
Pulmonary valve, *148*
Pulmonary veins, *148*
Purkinje fibers, 149, 332
Purpose of book, 3
Pyelonephritis, 332

Q

QRS complex, *149*, 149–150
Quadriplegia, 187, 332
  spastic, 13, 18
Quetiapine, 65
Quinidine gluconate, 355
Quinidine sulfate, 355

R

RA. *See* Rheumatoid arthritis
Race
  depression and, 84
  diabetes mellitus and, 299
  progressive neurological disorders and, 219–220

rheumatoid arthritis and, 236
stroke and, 132
Radiocarpal deviation in rheumatoid arthritis, 240, *240*
Rancho Los Amigos cognitive scale, 166–167, 167t
Rapid eye movement sleep, 81, 332
Recovery, Inc., 68
Reflex arc, 179–181, *183, 185,* 333
spinal cord injury and, 184–185, *185,* 188
Reflex sympathetic dystrophy, 333
Reflexes, 332–333
amyotrophic lateral sclerosis and, 221
primitive, 332
in cerebral palsy, 11, 12, 18
spinal cord injury and, 181, 184–185, 188
stroke and, 140–141
Rehabilitation
cardiac, 155, 155t–156t, 158
vocational
for schizophrenia, 67–68
for spinal cord injury, 201–202
for traumatic brain injury, 170
Remission, 333
Renal disease
dementia and, 104
diabetes mellitus and, 300–301
Reproductive function, spinal cord injury and, 200
Respiratory distress syndrome, 333
Retinopathy, 333
diabetic, 300
Retro virus, 231, 333
Rett's disorder, 22, 29, 32. *See also* Pervasive developmental
disorders
course of, 32
hyperammonemia and, 32
incidence of, 32
prognosis for, 29
signs and symptoms of, 32
Reversible ischemic neurological deficit (RIND), 129, 333
Rh factor, 333
Rheumatism, 333
Rheumatoid arthritis (RA), 230–259, 333
case studies of, 257–258
course and prognosis for, 236, 249–251
classification of functional capacity, 250–251, 250t
criteria for clinical remission, 250, 250t
diagnosis of, 251–252, 252t
"overlap syndrome," 252
economic costs of, 230–231
etiology and pathophysiology of, 231–233, *232, 233*
extra-articular systemic manifestations of, 246–249
cardiac, 247
changes in body composition, 249
depression, 249
Felty's syndrome, 247
nervous system, 247–248, *248*

ophthalmological, *248, 248*–249, 249t
pulmonary, 247
rheumatoid or subcutaneous nodules, 247, *247*
impact on occupational performance, 254–257, 255t–256t
cognitive, 257
motor, 256–257
neuromuscular, 254–256
psychosocial and psychological, 257
sensory integration, 254
incidence and prevalence of, 236
joint anatomy and, *231,* 231
juvenile, 233–235, 234t, 235t, 326
medical/surgical management of, 253–254
future challenges, 258–259
goals of, 253
interdisciplinary approach to, 253
under managed care, 258
medications, *253,* 253–254
self-help groups, 253
surgery, 254
muscle involvement in, 246
registry of families with, 233
resources about, 262–267
signs and symptoms of, 236–238
articular and periarticular involvement, 236–238
contractures, 237
"gel phenomenon," 237
pain, 236
stages of inflammatory process, 236, 237t, 251t
specific joint manifestations of, 238–246
ankle and foot, 245–246, *245–246*
elbow, 241
hand, 238–240, *238–240*
head, neck, and cervical spine, 242–243, *243*
hip, 243–244, *244*
knee, 244, 244–245
shoulder, 241–242, *242*
wrist, 240, *240–241*
tendon involvement in, 246
Rheumatoid carditis, 333
Rheumatoid factor, 333
Rhizotomy, 15
Righting reactions, 333
Rigidity, 334
cogwheel, 64, 221, 316
traumatic brain injury and, 168, 170
RIND. *See* Reversible ischemic neurological deficit
Risperidone, 63–65
Roentgenology, 334
Role changes
due to chronic pain, 290
due to progressive neurological disorders, 226
Rotator cuff in rheumatoid arthritis, 242, *242*
Rubella, 44, 45, 334
Rule of nines, 209, *209*

S

Savants, 29
Scars from burns, 212
  contractures of, 212
  hypertrophic, 212, 325
Schizophrenia, 54–73
  autism compared with, 23
  case studies of, 54, 71–73
  in children, 58
  course and prognosis for, 55, 58–60
  diagnosis of, 60–62
    catatonic type, 61
    criteria for, 60–61
    disorganized type, 61
    paranoid type, 61
    residual type, 62
    symptom rating scales, 60
    undifferentiated type, 62
  economic costs of, 58
  etiology of, 55–57
    approaches to, 55
    genetic factors, 56–57
    neuroanatomy, 55–56
    other risk factors, 57
  historical descriptions of, 55
  homelessness and, 59–60
  impact on occupational performance, 68–69, 70t–71t
    activities of daily living, 68–69
    play and leisure, 69
    work, 69
  incidence and prevalence of, 58
  medical illness and, 58
  medical/surgical management of, 62–68
    case management, 66
    clubhouses and lodges, 66–67
    cognitive rehabilitation and therapy, 68
    electroconvulsive therapy, 65
    hospitalization, 59, 65
    medications, 63–65 (*See also* Antipsychotic drugs)
    phases of treatment, 62–63
    Program for Assertive Community Treatment, 66
    psychotherapy, 66
    self-help groups, 68
    social skills training, 67
    treatment planning, 62
    treatment settings, 65–66
    vocational rehabilitation, 67–68
  mortality and, 59
  prognosis for, 58
  signs and symptoms of, 55, 58, 59t
    delusions and hallucinations, 55, 58
    negative symptoms, 55, 58
  substance abuse and, 59–60

SCI. *See* Spinal cord injury
Scleritis, 334
Scleroderma, 334
Scoliosis, 334
Scotoma, 334
Screening
  for dementia, 107
  for pervasive developmental disorders, 30
Seasonality
  depression and, 81
  pervasive developmental disorders and, 26
  schizophrenia and, 57
Seborrhea, 334
Sedation, antipsychotic-induced, 63–64
Seizures, 334
  cerebral palsy and, 13
  grand mal, 323
  pervasive developmental disorders and, 31
  stroke and, 126, 131
Selective serotonin reuptake inhibitors (SSRIs), 33, 88
Self-help groups
  for rheumatoid arthritis, 253
  for schizophrenia, 68
Self-injurious behavior, 334
Self-monitoring of blood glucose, 302–303
Sensorimotor function, 346
  burns and, 212–214
  chronic pain and, 288–289
  diabetes mellitus and, 303
  in elderly persons, 270
  progressive neurological disorders and, 220, 226
  rheumatoid arthritis and, 254–257
  stroke and, 138–139
Sensorineural hearing loss, 334
Sensory gating deficit, 56–57, 334
Septicemia, 334
Sequela, 334
Serotonin, 334
  depression and, 80, 88
  pervasive developmental disorders and, 32, 33
Sertindole, 65
Sertraline, 33, 355
Sexual expression
  chronic pain and, 291
  diabetes mellitus and, 303
  myocardial infarction and, 159
  progressive neurological disorders and, 226
  spinal cord injury and, 200–201
  traumatic brain injury and, 168
Sheet graft, 334
Sheltered workshops, 67–68
Shock
  hypovolemic, 210

insulin, 300
spinal, 187, 335
Shoulder dysfunction
"frozen shoulder," 242
in rheumatoid arthritis, 241–242, *242*
shoulder–hand syndrome, 140, 333
stroke and, 140
Single photon emission tomography, 136
Sinoatrial node, 149
Sjögren's syndrome, 248, *248*, 334
Skin, 206, *207*
complications of spinal cord injury, 192–193
dermis, 206, 319
epidermis, 206, 321
grafting of, 211–212
Smoking
coronary artery disease and, 151
stroke and, 132
Smooth-pursuit eye movements, 56, 334
Social skills training, 67
Socioeconomic factors
depression and, 84
mental retardation and, 46
pervasive developmental disorders and, 26
schizophrenia and, 57
Sodium bicarbonate, 356
Soft tissue pain, 282
Somatognosia, 139
Somatostatin, Alzheimer's disease and, 101
Spastic, defined, 335
Spasticity, 325, 335
amyotrophic lateral sclerosis and, 221
cerebral palsy and, 11
multiple sclerosis and, 220
spinal cord injury and, 188, 189
stroke and, 139–140
traumatic brain injury and, 168
Spatial relation dysfunction, 335
Spatial relations, 335
Spatial-relations syndrome, 335
Spina bifida, 44, 335
Spinal cord injury (SCI), 176–203
case study of, 202–203
central nervous system structure and function, 176–181
(*See also* Central nervous system)
classification of, 184–187
anterior cord syndrome, 185, *185*
based on "ASIA Impairment Scale," 187
Brown-Séquard syndrome, 186, *186*
cauda equina injuries, 186–187
central cervical cord syndrome, 186, *186*
complete lower motor neuron injury, 185, *185*
complete upper motor neuron injury, 184–185, *185*

incomplete injuries, 185
tetraplegia and paraplegia, 187
complications of, 188–193
autonomic dysreflexia, 188
bowel, 187, *191*, 191–192
deep vein thromboses, 189
dermal, 192–193
heterotopic ossification, 189–190
postural hypotension, 188
respiratory, 189
spasticity, 188, 189
thermal regulation, 189
urinary system, 187, *190*, 190–191
course and prognosis for, 193–194
expected functional outcome related to level of injury, 198t–199t
etiology of, *183*, 183–184, 184t
impact on occupational performance, 194–202, 194t–195t
activities of daily living, 196–197
functional mobility, 200
health maintenance, 197
leisure activities, 202
personal device care, 197, 198t–199t
sexual expression, 200–201
socialization, functional communication, and emergency response, 197
work activities, 201–202
incidence and prevalence of, 184
posttraumatic progression, 187–188
spinal shock, 187, 335
prevention of, 184
Spinal fusion, 335
Splenomegaly, 335
SSRIs. *See* Selective serotonin reuptake inhibitors
Stent, 335
Stereognosis, 335
Steroid myopathy, 335
Stimulants, 33
Strabismus, 335
Streptokinase, 137, 356
Stretch reflex, 11, 335
Stroke, 335. *See also* Cerebrovascular accident
completed, 317
in evolution, 335
"Stroke belt," 133
Stroke syndrome, 335
Subarachnoid, defined, 335
Subarachnoid hemorrhage, 122, 127, 136, 335
treatment of, 138
Subchondral, defined, 336
Subclavian steal syndrome, 129, 335
Subdural hematoma, 104, 105
Subluxation, 336

Substance use/abuse
  alcoholism and stroke, 133
  dementia and, 100, 101
  depression and, 87
  homelessness and, 60
  schizophrenia and, 59–60
  traumatic brain injury and, 166
Substantia nigra, 336
Sudden cardiac death, 153
Sudeck's atrophy, 272–273, 336
Suicide, 81, 85–87
Superficial temporal artery bypass, 138
Supportive employment, 67–68
Supramalleolar orthoses (SMOs), 15
Surgery
  for cerebral palsy, 15
  for rheumatoid arthritis, 254
Swan-neck deformity, 238, *239,* 336
Syndrome, 336
Synergy, 336
Synovial membrane, 336
Synovitis, 336
Syphilis, 44, 45, 336
Systole, 336

T

T cells, 336
  rheumatoid arthritis and, 232–233
T wave, *149,* 149–150
Tachycardia, 154, 336
  antipsychotic–induced, 64, 65
Tacrine, 107–108
Talipes equinovalgus, 321
Talipes equinovarus, 321
Tardive, defined, 336
Tardive dyskinesia, 33, 64, 336
Tarsal joints in rheumatoid arthritis, 245–246
Tay-Sachs disease, 45, 336
TBI. *See* Traumatic brain injury
Temazepam, 356
Temporomandibular joints in rheumatoid
    arthritis, 242
Tendonitis, 337
Tendon(s), 336
  in rheumatoid arthritis, 246
"Tennis" elbow, 241, 288
Tenosynovitis, 239, *239,* 337

Teratogenic agents, 44, 46, 337
Terminology, 311–339
  Uniform Terminology for Occupational Therapy, 2–3,
      341–348
Tetraplegia, 187
Thermal regulation after spinal cord injury, 189
Thioridazine, 33, 64
Thrombocytopenia, 337
Thrombolysis, 137
Thrombosis, 337
  myocardial infarction and, 153
  spinal cord injury and, 189
  stroke and, 125–126, 131–132
Thrombus, 337
Thumb deformities in rheumatoid arthritis, 239, 240
Thyrotoxicosis, 337
TIAs. *See* Transient ischemic attacks
Ticlopidine, 136–137
Tissue plasminogen activator, 356
Tolmetin sodium, 356
Tonic labyrinthine reflex, 13, 337
Topagnosia, 337
Topagraphic orientation, 337
Toxemia, 44, 46, 337
Toxoplasmosis, 45, 337
Transient ischemic attacks (TIAs), 126, 128–129,
      131–133, 337
Transitional employment, 67–68
Transitional movements, 337
Tranylcypromine, 356
Traumatic brain injury (TBI), 165–174
  case studies of, 173–174
  course and prognosis for, 168–170
      factors affecting, 166, 169
      Glasgow coma scale, 168–169, 169t
      Glasgow outcome scale, 169
  dementia and, 100, 101
  economic costs of, 166
  etiology of, 165–166
      coup and contrecoup injuries, 165
      diffuse axonal injury, 166
  impact on occupational performance, 171, 171t–172t
  incidence and prevalence of, 166
  during infancy, 9–10
  medical/surgical management of, 170–171
  acute management, 170
  medications, 171
  rehabilitation, 170

mental retardation and, 46
signs and symptoms of, 166–168
  Rancho Los Amigos cognitive scale, 166–167, 167t
Trazodone, 109, 356
Tremor, 337
  in Parkinson's disease, 64, 221
  resting, 333
  traumatic brain injury and, 168
Tricuspid valve, 148, *148*
Trigger points, 282
Trihexyphenidyl, 356
Trimethoprim, 356
Trimipramine, 356
Trisomy 13, 337
Trisomy 18, 338
Trisomy 21, 338
Truth, 2
Tuberous sclerosis, 25, 44, 338
Two-point discrimination, 338

U

Ulnar drift, 338
Ultrasound, 135–136
Uniform Terminology for Occupational Therapy, 2–3, 341–348
  examples of use in practice, 342–343
  performance areas, 344–346
  performance components, 346–347
  performance contexts, 347–348
  person-activity-environment fit, 343–344
Unilateral body inattention (neglect), 338
  stroke and, 131, 139
  traumatic brain injury and, 168
Unilateral spatial neglect, 338
Upper motor neuron injury, 184–185, *185*
Uremia, 338
Urinary tract infection (UTI), 188, 190–191
Urokinase, 137
UTI. *See* Urinary tract infection

V

Valgus, 338
Valproic acid, 356
Vasculitis, in rheumatoid arthritis, 248, *248*
Vena cava, *148*
Venlafaxine, 356

Ventricles of heart, 148, *148*
  enlargement in schizophrenia, 55–56
Ventricular fibrillation, 322
Vertebrae, 177, *177, 178*
Vertebral arteries, 123, *123*
Vertebrobasilar stroke, 130–131
Vertigo, 338
Viruses. *See also* Infection
  progressive neurological disorders and, 219
  rheumatoid arthritis and, 231
Visual deficits
  cerebral palsy and, 13–14
  diabetes mellitus and, 298, 300
  homonymous hemianopsia, 130, 139, 324
  multiple sclerosis and, 220
  stroke and, 130, 131, 138–139
  traumatic brain injury and, 168
Vitamin deficiencies, 100, 104
Vocational rehabilitation
  for schizophrenia, 67–68
  for spinal cord injury, 201–202
  for traumatic brain injury, 170
Volition, 338

W

Wallenberg's syndrome, 131, 338–339
Waxy flexibility, 61, 339
Wheelchair use, 200
Work, 6, 345–346. *See also* Occupational performance
  chronic pain and, 291
  myocardial infarction and, 159–160
  progressive neurological disorders and, 226–227
  schizophrenia and, 67–69
  spinal cord injury and, 201–202
World Health Organization (WHO), 58
Wound care for burns, 211
Wrist
  fractures of, 271
  in rheumatoid arthritis, 240, *240–241*

X

Xerostomia, 339

Z

Zig-zag effect, 240, *240–241,* 339